Sociology: insights in health care

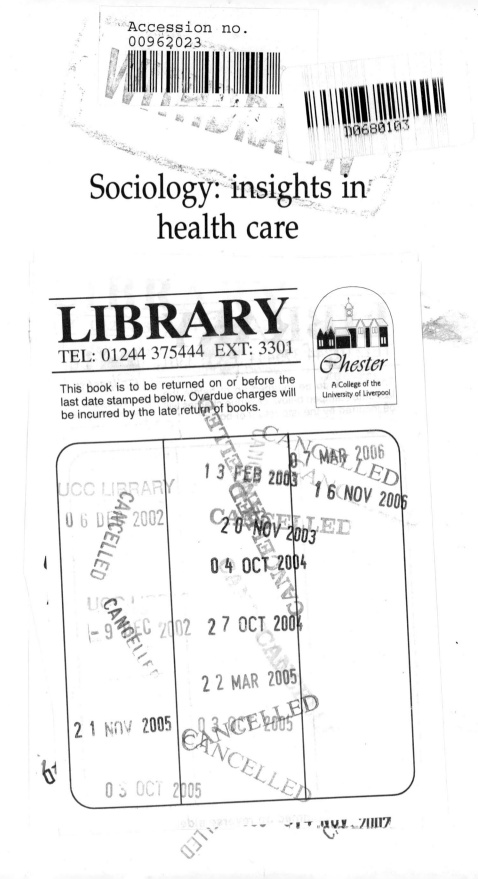

Sociology: insights in health care

Edited by

Abbie Perry

Medical Sociologist, Department of Human Science and Medical Ethics,
St Bartholomew's and Royal London Hospital School of Medicine, London, UK

ARNOLD

A member of the Hodder Headline Group
LONDON • SYDNEY • AUCKLAND

First published in Great Britain 1996 by
Arnold, a member of the Hodder Headline Group,
338 Euston Road, London NW1 3BH

British Library Cataloguing in Publication Data
A catalogue record for this book is available from the British Library

Library of Congress Cataloging-in-Publication Data
A catalog record for this book is available from the Library of Congress

ISBN 0 340 66200 X

Typeset in 10/12pt Palatino by J&L Composition Ltd, Filey, North Yorkshire

Printed and bound in Great Britain by J.W. Arrowsmith Ltd, Bristol

Contents

Preface

This book provides critiques of health care agencies; a high profile social issue. Such concern is reflected in the curricula of many courses apart from those directly involved in the education of health practitioners. For instance, health care is a subject studied by those undertaking qualifying courses in sociology, economics, political science, social policy, management and accountancy. Health knowledge, however, flows from people's lives and not just from a group of experts or an ideology. What happens in health is obviously a matter of concern to us all.

A whole industry of health workers descends upon the more or less integrated human body and the 'working gains' are divided among them. We hope to voice the concerns which have arisen from within the health service from both carers and clients, without supporting prescriptive accounts of practices which rely upon separations between groups. Using various analytical insights, the authors examine this system in terms of what it means for society. The main aim is to describe and explain how people think they should maintain or change those aspects of health care about which they feel most strongly.

An analysis is primarily objective and impartial, though not necessarily non-controversial. It outlines the structure of a body of knowledge and the institutions and population upon which it practises. But what is it like to be inside a body of knowledge and these structures as a student, a teacher, a researcher or as an object of research? The contributors to this book engage in current debates in health care from these differing positions. The sociological framework is mapped out in the introduction, along with details of specific chapter contents.

Abbie Perry, editor.
January 1996

Contributors

Paul Barber RN, RMN, RNMS, RNT, MSc, PhD
Director, Human Potential Resource Group, Department of Educational Studies, University of Surrey

Kate Beverley RN, RM, RCNT, MA, MSc
Senior Lecturer in Sociology, Thames Valley University

Joanne Coyle BSc, MSc
Lecturer in Social Policy, Queen Margaret College, Edinburgh

Patricia de Wolfe BA (Hons), BSc (Hons), MA
Doctoral student, Department of Sociology, Goldsmiths' College, University of London

Carolyn Featherstone BA, MPhil
Principal Lecturer in Sociology, Department of Social Science, Kingston University

Sally Glen RN, RSCN, Dip Ed(Lond), MA Ed
Acting Head of School, Education and Health Studies, South Bank University

June Greenwell RN, BA
Visiting Research Fellow, Department of Sociology, University of Bristol

Christopher Hibbert BA, Cert Ed, MA
Senior Lecturer in Law, Department of Professional Studies, Oxford College of Further Education

Moya Jolley RN, RNT, BSc Econ, Dip Nurs(Lond), Dip Ed(Lond), MA Ed
Formerly Lecturer in Sociology and Nursing Development, Royal College of Nursing Institute.

Abbie Perry RN, BSc(Hons), Cert FE, MSc
Medical Sociologist, St Bartholomew's and the Royal London School of Medicine, London, UK

Ann Pursey RN, HV Cert, BA Hons Nurs, PhD
Senior Research Fellow, Warwick Business School, University of Warwick

Nicki Thorogood BSc, PhD
Lecturer in Sociology, Unit of Dental Public Health, Guy's Hospital Medical School

Bridget Towers BA(Hons), Dip Soc Admin, PhD(Berkeley), PhD(Lond)
Senior Lecturer in Sociology, Faculty of Human Sciences, Kingston University

Introduction

What connection have chicken and cattle farming with medicine and contemporary health systems? At first glance, the organisation of fast-food chains such as Kentucky Fried Chicken or McDonald's Hamburgers and that of health care would appear to have nothing in common. Sociologist George Ritzer (1993), however, uses a concept of *'McDonaldization'* to analyse the process whereby all structures in American society are subject to the mechanisms of the market economy (consumerism) and the corporate mentality. Medicine is used throughout this text to illustrate that even this top profession is unprotected from the calculability and quantification of the market. In 'open-heart' and eye surgery in particular, standardisation procedures and control by scientific management assist in the inexorable drive to cost-cutting in the name of efficiency (profit). If professionals continue to use their own judgements, particularly in the case of doctors with their individualised technology, it is expensive, time consuming and unpredictable because healing practices necessitate involvement in messy human affairs. According to the analysis, McDonald's epitomises not only a successful restaurant business but also all manner of social institutions in America and other industrial societies developing along similar lines. The mass production of the 'perfect' predictable breakfast platter at McDonald's is equated with delivery of the 'perfect' cured patient, according to specified diseases, calculated procedures and predetermined levels of skill and costs, and within set time limits.

Such assembly-line techniques are not yet the norm in US medicine but 'one can imagine that they will grow increasingly common in coming years' (Ritzer 1993, p.53). High-speed, 'coldly' rational and purely physical production is nothing new in the food industry, dealing as it does with perishable food stuffs, livestock (dumb animals) and simplified tasks requiring manual workers or 'bodies' (pairs of hands). Henry Ford, who made a fortune from the mass production of automobiles (Model-T Fords) and lent his name to a whole industrial era (Fordism), was inspired by the precision and speed with which meatpackers in a Chicago abbatoir butchered the cattle (Ritzer 1993, p.58).

In Britain, the authors of *Medicine and nursing: professions in a changing health service* (Walby et al. 1994) argue that the National Health Service and the professionals who used to run it are at the forefront of the restructuring of the economy and work practices from which Ritzer's analysis stems. The NHS is the model for all developments in contemporary employment practices, not just in health. We know that people become ill and need hospital care, but this is by no means the whole story. The NHS is the largest employer in western Europe; half its workforce is female, in accordance with national trends, and it is a growth industry. It is of importance to the economy, and to the pay and conditions of the workforce and of women workers in particular.

Ritzer concentrates on major organisational change; our sociologists are concerned with its main outcome – the control of professional work or as it is commonly known, *'new wave management'*. Reorganisation precedes the introduction of a different management structure. The higher authority directing the changes is the government in power. We can no longer refer to the NHS as a purely medical, profession-led service. This does not mean that former hierarchies in health, with their set boundaries of authority and skill between occupations and work groups, have disappeared. Instead, a complex picture emerges of traditional practices coming up against new ways of working, centring on the changing relationships between bureaucrats, doctors, nurses and the patients. Professional roles are increasingly constituted within organisational agendas.

To those of us who are used to the old ways, it comes as a surprise to learn that administrators are now the most important people in health or other social institutions. Administrators make the policy to which everyone in the organisation must be loyal and which managers, acting as psychological 'healers', have to translate into unified working practices. This is the modern, middle-class version of the work ethic: employees belong, *emotionally* as well as physically, to those who pay and/or command them (Hochschild 1983). In the new structures, professionals become personalised 'instruments' with an expert technical function to diagnose problems in the front-line. As the 'brains' rather than the conscience or 'mind' of the organisation, they are measured by performance indicators. In straightforward language, this means that, in order to keep their jobs, they have an intense responsibility to make the system work. If this necessitates discharging the 'half-cured' to make room for new admissions, then this must be done. Patients are expected to have stable families and clean, comfortable homes to recover in, according to the rhetoric of community care. Management may make a mistake, but it is the professionals who have to rectify it – this is what quality assurance is all about. This is a confusing situation for nurses, due to their social location in the organisation. They are at the bottom of the professional line of responsibility, at the very organisation–patient interface. Whether or not they have been given the correct instructions or the appropriate equipment, their task is to keep the patient alive; theirs appears to be the ultimate responsibility, but the final accountability lies elsewhere. To locate this we must leave the nurse physically maintaining the patient and reverse up the hierarchy to a higher authority. Along with all the technological developments in hospital procedures (and in the wider society), it is small wonder that traditional nurse roles and nursing education have had to change.

Doctors have not been immune to developments in technologies, or to the changes in ways of working, given the increasing number of specialisms and the need, therefore, for greater co-operation between highly trained specialist teams. As well as acquiring skills in using the latest equipment, there are many related ethical and legal issues that demand attention, for example, organ transplants, technological definitions of death, patients' constitutional rights to treatments and the problem of informed consent, to name but a few. The doctor may be the professional charged with legal guardianship of the patient's body, but he or she is not the only authority concerned with the formulation of health concepts. In the current UK context, for instance, government policies are overt determinants of levels of health, expectations and definitions of health and levels of health provision (as several contributors to this book argue). Furthermore, if the poorest groups in society are the sickest (a combination of hardships and pressures), is the move from institutional care to an underfunded community and GP-administered service likely to improve the nation's statistics on ill health?

Occupational sociology is concerned with 'coalface' situations or the 'view from below'. The *Medicine and nursing* . . . research follows in this tradition and is, therefore, an attempt not to drown practitioners in social theory, but to rescue them. For direct practitioners may be too busy practising or too fearful of losing their practice to question publicly why they are doing it. In addition, professional ideology or ideal representations of work may not provide a true explanation of practice for those working at different levels in the organisation. We might reasonably object, along with many 'hard done by' nurses or junior hospital doctors, that their realities must be compared with those of the most successful members of their own profession or, indeed, with those pursuing careers in business or politics. However, when nurses or doctors are overwhelmed by the lack of beds, porters or trolleys to accommodate patients, they may need to think heroically in order to carry on acting as decent human beings; it may not be the explanation that has failed, but the 'social arrangements' surrounding their work.

Sociology, unlike the natural sciences, is not primarily concerned with presenting discoveries. Instead, it teaches new ways of looking at familiar things. In the discussion above, we see that changing structures can require new ways of thinking, perhaps a different language, as Ritzer's concept of 'McDonaldization' indicates. However, the power of the sociological imagination lies in its capacity to make connections between individuals and events which are usually taken to be totally unconnected and 'worlds apart'. It may not appear in any official manifesto, but the changes in nursing, medicine and professionalism generally may have more to do with a specific government response and an economy based on service industries, than with strategy on the part of nurses or doctors themselves. If professional caring philosophy continues to analyse nursing, for instance, in traditional ways of thinking, as a value largely independent of the institutional framework in which it 'happens', we shall never find out what prevents it from being. Professionalism may be a state of mind which involves intense socialisation throughout a long training, but it is also an objective social condition. Viewed through the sociological lens, nursing and other groups aspiring to a higher social status are first and foremost occupations. The purpose of sociology is not simply to pass on judgements of how professionals value themselves, but to assess their place in society.

The rise of the hospital medical establishment has been predicated on the cure–care divide. In their professionalising project, nurses have had little choice but to cling to a social model for maintenance and development (see Chapter 1). In contrast to the medical model, based upon the physical entity, namely the body, nurses have adopted a type of holistic approach which is almost anti-body: patients' needs stem not from biology alone but from a combination of individual temperament and social circumstances. The implication is that nursing care is the answer to all the patient's needs: care seems to take precedence over cure. While nursing theories and models continue to emphasise a personalised and privatised professional–client relationship, which only applies nowadays to the wealthy, the heavily insured or those with unusual diseases, we never reach the 'system', represented by the collective causes of much disease and illness and the collective nature of solutions such as social and welfare reforms. A truly social model takes us into the worlds of the needy, and thereby into political and economic affairs (see Chapters 2 and 9).

When there is not one doctor or one nurse for every person, needs must be rationalised. The way in which needs are defined, met or overlooked is a matter of social organisation and governance (see Chapter 6). The prioritising of patients' needs is not stable or fixed; like professionalism, it is a response to a restless and changing situation. Medicine and nursing analysed in a purely rational way as independent professions and mutually exclusive categories serve perhaps to reassure us that a healthy debate is going on. While we are thinking in terms of the normative order (dichotomies), we miss the underlying clarity, that professionals do not work alone but rely upon clients and other occupations, not just each other, to affect their practices (see Chapter 3). Methodology brings together critiques of what professionals do in terms of 'higher forms of work' and the immediacy of the 'worst mess of reality'. Academic research is a means by which professional accountability may be measured and tested, and thereby publicly scrutinised (see Chapters 4 and 8). It enables us to penetrate the surface mystique or the myth of open access (that professional help is available to everyone), to arrive at the reality – those who benefit have to be screened and seen to 'fit' into the framework of the prevailing system. For example, to be defined as sick implies a medical category, amenable to chemotherapy, surgery or psychiatric help (see Chapters 5 and 7). Meanwhile, health education writers frequently express optimism about the extent to which professionals have the power to influence the health status not only of individuals but also of whole communities (see Chapter 10).

Sociologists identify large-scale bureaucracy as a major institutional form in modern society, and the NHS is no exception. The story of medicine, nursing and the 'unfit classes' is intimately connected to the history of the hospital and the logic of industrialism. The social function of nurses is to assist in the provision of a system of help which has been under government sponsorship since the Medical (Registration) Act of 1858. At that time, British society was facing plagues and urban poverty on a massive scale, along with industrial unrest. While everyone else was questioning and living in fear of sickness or premature death, medical scientists were made responsible for the *control of illness as a social problem*.

While working-class patients and the poor loom small in conventional stories of medical progress, their contribution has not been overlooked. Richardson (1988), for example, argues that the 1832 Anatomy Act, which requisitioned for medical dissection unclaimed corpses from the poorhouses, contributed to the eventual public acceptability of medical specialism. Previously, under a law passed by Henry VIII in his endowment of medical education, the only legal source of corpses for dissection in England had been the gallows. Social histories of medicine reveal that the forging of the relationship between human misery, medical theory and technology was neither simple nor assured (Wear 1992).

In recent years, successive governments have found that plagues are no longer so prevalent, but the poor are still with us. They put pressure on the health and welfare services which governments are not so prepared to pay for. By 'the poor' and 'unfit classes' we now mean the unemployed, the incurable mentally ill, the disabled, low-income families, single mothers and the homeless; to these we may add the growing numbers of the chronically sick and the very elderly needing special treatment and care. Further cutbacks in welfare services and benefits are likely to increase the need for health care at the same time as changes in the NHS decrease its availability in the population generally, and the length of hospital stay is curtailed. While the suffering and misery appear to have increased, the formally defined objectives of profession-led public services, or those who authenticated them, such as the doctors, have been questioned.

Medicine has been used to inform the whole of contemporary health knowledge, yet in the process it has been reduced to a role of health control. As an elite profession and public service, it developed in an esoteric environment, relatively distanced and protected from market competition. In return for safeguarding the health of the nation's working population and their families (women's reproductivity and infant development), it was rewarded with teaching and research establishments, security of tenure, a guaranteed income and recruitment of patients, in other words, career progression. Medicine's knowledge base has developed because it has been under constant pressure to solve *all* of society's health problems. Doctors did not suddenly discover diseases of old age; they came up against problems, brought about by demographic changes, which existing knowledge could not explain. Similarly, advances in reproductive technology can be seen as medical responses to a combination of social factors, including changing patterns of fertility and reduced family size, the widespread use of contraceptives, greater opportunities for women in education and work and increased financial pressures on young couples, resulting in delay in starting a family. The development of a profession is a socially determined process and not only the outcome of scientific knowledge or the possession of technological expertise.

Although the demand for medical treatment continues to rise, its techniques have now outstripped capital funding, and politicians have imposed a cut-off point. The myth of professionals as independent practitioners has been revealed; public services are not autonomous practices with self-imposed tasks. Doctors have an immense responsibility but not absolute power. They are reliant upon a form of patronage, whether private client or public service, usually both, as in the American or Australian medical health systems. This should not mean that the old NHS order, medically prescribed as it was, has to be seen as decadent and its tools (knowledge and experience) pronounced obsolete. Interestingly, government policy may be directed at community care in *theory*, but in *practice* it is still heavily funding specific forms of highly technical and surgical medicine. As a consequence, hospitals have only recently been reduced to their professed specialist functions: it is labour-intensive care and the health service's informal capacity to house the old and lonely, the confused and the mad which have been seriously curtailed. While the money is there for the certain surgical cure or diagnostic performance, there are not enough nurses or beds to 'go round', wounds break down and dirty bandages pile up outside the ward lavatories.

The way in which health and social welfare is organised and government funded has been totally reshaped. Instead of rethinking our political choices, the debate appears to have been closed down. Many social scientists are asking, 'what happened to the crisis in health and health care?' Within a sociological framework we can raise some 'old' but pertinent questions. Despite all the technology and the money poured into the NHS, why are reported sickness rates increasing? Health expectations may have risen and more people may complain, but this is not an adequate explanation. It is more likely that changing patterns of work and family life across social classes have led to greater insecurity and pressures in people's lives. We should be asking the following questions. Who are the sick? What help is currently available to them? How are people managing to cope? What obstructions stand in the way of self-care? How can we move to a situation in which people can decide for themselves? These questions will be explored by the contributors to this book. The 'ensemble' of chapters covers the following areas: (1) knowledge claims of sociology, nursing and medicine; (2) moral and legal aspects of research methods; (3) dilemmas we face in illness, life-threatening disease and the hospital experience; and (4) our attempts to resolve these problems at personal and societal levels. Why have we chosen to analyse these structures?

The explosion of health knowledge and the commercial dissemination of information have not prevented people from falling ill or needing hospital medical treatment. The government's presumption that community care is the answer has not consolidated caring expertise – it has to cope with the 'hopeless cases', yet it is seriously under-resourced. Social inequality is still measured in terms of sickness and death rates, especially infant mortality. While health for many people may be an unobtainable ideal, research shows that illness is a common experience. Without a reasonable standard of health, people may not be able to earn a living, raise a family or fully participate as citizens in the life of society. In nursing, the majority of direct practitioners work in the clinical situation, and carry out basic physical care or tasks derived from traditional and innovative medical technology. The status of nursing, various paramedical occupations and patients continues to be dependent upon the hospital establishment. Finally, given the extent of the public ward and hospital closure movement and the new managerialism, it appears that there is no longer government support for a monopoly of the medical decision-making around which the hospital is organised. This has implications for medical education and research, as well as for the world of work in general, for medicine has been taken to be the model of development not only in health professionalism but also throughout society.

We rely upon professionals to tell the truth and to speak on behalf of others in the public domain. Like the medieval clergy, they are supposedly 'outside' the usual self-interested struggles for power and the need to benefit from people personally. The means by which this ancient virtue is upheld may only be possible in a state-protected system of 'protective' public services. In other words, professionals are not able to restructure solely from within; they require wider bureaucratic support. While employed individuals go to work, professionals 'practice'. The widespread use of the term 'practice', or more correctly 'modes of practice', can have misleading consequences: it may deny the factory logic of many a workplace which defines professional roles in terms of organisational function. For the majority of professionals in contemporary industrial societies are now part of the salariat, the employed and even the economically insecure. If we continue to reduce 'what is' to 'what ought to be', we shall never learn where the conflict comes in and how change takes place. Professionalism seeks to be as secure a 'property' on the market as land, but just as land tenure may be altered by political and economic changes, so may professionalism. In the current context of the health industry, it is impossible to keep the economics and politics out of professional care; what is government funded is, after all, government controlled.

The purpose of this book is to encourage readers, who are our clients, to be active and open to further studies on occupation and health care systems and on patterns of ill health and disease. The introductory chapter opens our eyes to the scope of the sociological imagination. This is a tool which reveals the shape of society which, in turn, we experience at the personal, local or institutional level. Some chapters are concerned primarily with theoretical problems, while others focus on research issues and the predicaments of both respondents and researchers. Overall, the chapters display a common methodological ideal, to lead the reader or practitioner out of their own experience into the comparative world, where this individual experience is analysed along with others in society. In this way, we enter the field of the social sciences.

The decision to invite authors from the spheres of teaching and research was taken by the editor at the outset of the project. The contributors share a concern to freshen their own thinking in the light of current changes in organisations and developments in theory. Professional accreditation is always conferred from above via the academy, but it is earned from below, in credentialising, organisational experience. An analysis of health structure and its main participants needs to take into account both 'worlds'. Furthermore, all students need the theory to be placed in context; this is especially the case when they are being introduced to a subject. The application of problems in the theory to problems in reality, and vice versa, usually reveals a high level of tension. This is an issue of which academics, including the authors of this book, are aware. They know from their own teaching or research that when the theoretical objectives confront a student's or a respondent's reality, with all the emotions and concerns involved, this may be far stronger than the internal integrity of their questions. Practitioners in any discipline have to deal with something which is stronger than them and not totally amenable to theoretical reasoning. Professionals may be ordering the theoretical sense of the universe, but that does not mean that they see themselves as set apart from the world as other people live it. This would be particularly difficult for sociologists and other social scientists; as members of society, they are an integral part of the subjects they study.

The chapters

In Chapter 1, co-authors Sally Glen, Kate Beverley and Joanne Coyle argue for the use of sociological perspectives to 'bridge' the gap between abstract nursing models and the diverse realities of direct practitioners. They show how professional judgements are influenced by the social characteristics of persons and the institutional framework in which nurses study and work. The devaluing of care in the current context is not just a nursing problem but a social one, which needs to be analysed sociologically.

In Chapter 2, Bridget Towers analyses the economics and politics of the market ideologues at government level in the UK, in terms of the financing and management of our system of health care. This national example is linked to strategic planning in health across the European community, and to the new methods of managing public services common to developed societies worldwide. Learning activities are provided in the discussion, with a case study at the end, as aids to the deconstruction of the language and administration of the new managerialism and the effects on the working lives of practitioners. Through sociological means this author demystifies a mass of public policy documents so that we, the readers, can make up our own minds.

Chapter 3 is a deeply personal study of subjective sociology. Paul Barber uses phenomenology and symbolic interactionism to explore his experiences as a patient, a nurse, a professional health educator, but most importantly of all, as a human being. His analysis focuses on the genuine loss of the 'sacred' and the 'soul' from modern scientific methods of care. Personal accounts are paralleled by academic analysis of the dynamics of professional–client relationships, especially in hospital. Phenomenology as a research approach is also considered by Ann Pursey in Chapter 4. She demonstrates that sociological methods, including that of feminists, contribute to health services and nursing research. The discussion is illustrated with examples to help us to distinguish between different approaches. Ann Pursey offers a substantial critique of the idea of the 'objective' or experimental method. It is precisely this method, used in numerous clinical trials, which forms the basis of analysis in Chapter 8.

In Chapter 5 Patricia de Wolfe takes us into the private worlds of the chronically sick and the problems that these people face in being accepted by their families, friends and other social networks on which we all depend. The discussion includes a critique of some of the qualitative methods used by social researchers investigating medicine and illness behaviour. The author refers to anecdotal, theoretical and research evidence from a wide spectrum of studies. Patricia de Wolfe leads the reader through a range of discourses about illness, all in current use, and many of which are in contradiction with each other.

June Greenwell (Chapter 6) puts the term 'community' under her sociologist's spotlight. We quickly realise that its use in health care tends to mean 'non-hospital' – it is defined negatively by what it is not. As a sociological concept, however, it has a history extending from shared occupation, geographical region and group identity to nationality. The author explores the policies and politics whereby a local community may or may not decide on patterns of health care provision. A clear finding emerges, that people everywhere are distressed by the extent of recent hospital closures. The interesting conclusion drawn is that this movement has been curtailed by, of all things, the Hospital Trusts, which cannot fully operate as entrepreneurs given the internalisation of the 'health market' and the government's budgetary constraints on local authorities generally. In terms of a definition of a consumer society, the 'health market' may really be no market at all.

In Chapter 7, Carolyn Featherstone offers her understanding of the cancer patient experience as a stigmatised condition. The patients' suffering is particularly poignant in consumer societies where youth, health and beauty have become individualised 'projects' or even products which can somehow be purchased, so the popularist theory runs, by everyone. Taking us through various notions of the body as an immutable part of nature or, by way of contrast, a social construct, the discussion centres on the debates concerning high- and low-level technological treatments in different types of cancer. A critique of the medical evaluation of these therapies, and others, follows in Chapter 8. Christopher Hibbert is particularly interested in ethical and legal issues arising from the use of randomised control trials. To test the efficacy of treatments, patients are not given full details about the research in which they are participants. The highly contentious issue of informed consent in randomisation trials is not confined to medical science; social researchers are confronted by this as they select their samples, and they, too, may withhold certain information from respondents, in an endeavour to eliminate 'human error' or bias. Professions are licentiate practices and must take into account legal as well as ethical concerns.

In Chapter 9, Moya Jolley and Abbie Perry examine a selection of social research in health inequalities. Social class location in British society strongly influences a person's predisposition to ill health, access to health care, and even premature death. Moya Jolley strongly believes that socio-economic factors in health need to be fully incorporated into nursing theories. Indeed, these material factors, along with gender, ethnicity and age, have been established areas in the medical curriculum for some time. For professionalism is the human face of an otherwise unacceptably harsh system based upon wealth divisions.

In the final chapter, Nicki Thorogood focuses on the study of power, a major subject in sociology and critical theory. Critical theory has direct links with grand philosophical debates which, over time, have devolved into analytical critiques across the sciences and not just sociology. An analysis of the distribution of power throughout society certainly deserves no less a treatment. In this framework, everything is scrutinised, including the very language used. For example, how do we recognise power and how does it operate in society? What type of behaviour is rational and appropriate and, by implication, who is 'self-excluded'? The example of HIV/AIDS is analysed in relation to the 'new' public health, in order to examine the proposition that all 'expert' knowledge is power and may be used to reproduce 'old' patterns of dependency rather than patient empowerment. We learn that those taken to be 'diseased' or 'deviant' are subject to social judgements, located in particular forms of conformity and society. Through critical theory we return to themes discussed in the opening chapter – the sociological imagination and its insights into many facets of human experience.

References

Hochschild, A.R. 1983: *The managed heart: commercialization of human feeling.* Berkeley: University of California Press.

Richardson, R. 1988: *Death, dissection and the destitute.* London: Penguin Books.

Ritzer, G. 1993: *The McDonaldization of society: an investigation into the changing character of contemporary social life.* California: Sage.

Walby, S., Greenwell, J., Mackay, L. and Soothill, K. 1994: *Medicine and nursing: professions in a changing health service.* London: Sage.

Wear, A. (ed.) 1992: *Medicine in society: historical essays.* Cambridge: Cambridge University Press.

What is the sociological imagination? The example of nursing education and work

Sally Glen, Kate Beverley and Joanne Coyle

Why use sociology?

The wisdom of sociology lies in its ability to help us to see that things are not what they seem and that social reality has many layers of meaning (Berger 1966). It encourages us to view the world around us, the things we take for granted, in a new light. This chapter will use a sociological approach and suggest frameworks so that nurses can analyse the situations that they face in their everyday practice.

Sociology is a way of conceptualising issues in nursing. It is a means by which nurses and other practitioners may critically reflect upon their education and occupation. We are making a break with the usual curricular approaches which have tended to present sociology as 'nuggets of theory' (Turnbull 1992) to be ingested and then regurgitated, without being used to evaluate what nurses think or do. Such approaches have done a disservice to both nursing and sociology. It is not the content of sociological theories which is at fault but the mode of presentation within curricula, which appears to be preoccupied with the need for approval by the academic establishment. We will, therefore, examine nursing's professionalising project (Witz 1992) in higher education and the tensions between abstract theories and the realities of many nurses. These issues, along with others, will be explored in detail later in the chapter.

What is nursing?

The absence of an agreed definition of nursing is a major problem for nurses. It is extremely difficult to develop and project a professional self-identity without a shared understanding of what constitutes a distinctive nurse role. Nursing theories and models have made some progress in attempting to define what nursing is, but there are problems. Direct practitioners feel that theoretical models fail to capture the complexity and diversity of their 'hands on' experiences. This is a valid criticism; nursing cannot be explained in isolation from 'what it is in action'. However, this is not the whole story; it is also necessary to take into account how it is constructed within contemporary and historical society. Nursing organisation in one society, such as the UK, for example, is not a universal model. Instead of viewing theoretical frameworks as blueprints in which to 'fit' every experience, these can be used to bring a variety of focuses, namely the means to interpret the realities of nurse-to-patient, nurse-to-nurse and nurse-to-health. Models and theoretical representations are, in this sense, the lenses offering a wider vision of the whole system.

Defining and using sociology

Nursing has been less theorised than medical practice in sociology. This may be related to the lower status of both nursing knowledge and nursing work within the worlds of academia and professionalism. Perhaps the perception of nurses' work as women's work, which is less valued in society, is reflected in mainstream sociology's preoccupation with medicine. Ann Oakley (1984), in her article exploring the role of nurses in health, begins with an apology:

In a 15-year career as a sociologist studying medical services, I confess that I have been particularly blind to the contribution made by nurses to health care.

(Oakley 1984, p.24)

It has mainly been left to an increasing number of nurses-who-are-sociologists to bring the sociological imagination to bear upon analyses of nursing education and practice during the past 15 years.

Perry (1987, p.139) describes sociology as the scientific and systematic study of people in relation to the social groups to which they belong. Anyone coming to sociological study for the first time arrives with an already established stock of ideas, beliefs and assumptions gained from their life experiences. This is also true of sociologists, and explains why sociology consists of a diverse range of theories about society. To move from *knowing about* life in society at an intuitive, *common-sense* level to developing *understanding which is sociological* requires that the person stand back from their experiences and reflect on these in the light of other, different versions. To participate in sociological thinking or research, a person needs to be prepared to allow important assumptions to be challenged or questioned.

Since *assumptions* are connected to *values and beliefs* which are *prized*, the *feelings and emotions* of students are necessarily involved. Nursing students encountering sociology for the first time may find that it is an uncomfortable experience. This may be one reason why some of them appear to lose interest after an introductory session. The subject may seem to threaten their self-identity if not handled sensitively. Reassurance that what is required is *exploration* of one's own assumptions and that of others, rather than abandonment of these, helps. Thus, the process of developing the *sociological imagination* is closely allied to the capacity for *empathetic understanding* as the basis for *critical reflective practice*. Without a practice of self-and-other reflexivity or self-criticism, which is an essential component of any *professional's accountability*, it is unlikely that improvements in practice will take place.

Sociology as a professional practice involves both theorising about, and researching, the *values* and *rules* which govern life in society, in accordance with the general principles of scientific enquiry (the rules of method).

This means that what the sociologist finds and says about the social phenomenon he (*sic*) studies occurs within a rather strictly defined frame of reference. One of the main characteristics of this scientific frame of reference is that operations are bound by certain rules . . . .

(Berger 1966, p.27)

Sociologists are identified as much by the rules or principles that they apply to research as by the areas of enquiry that they pursue. In asserting that sociology is a *scientific enterprise*, these theorists are claiming a widely acknowledged, academic rigour in the methods that they employ. There is, however, debate about the extent to which the elements of the social universe can be isolated and experimented with in quite the same way as, say, chemicals in a laboratory test-tube. Some sociologists argue that it is not possible to break society down in this way, proceeding on the basis that *social facts* exist independently of the people who make up a given society (see Chapter 4).

Instead, they suggest that what we know as *society* results from the actions and interactions of its members. Depending on where they stand in relation to this fundamental assumption about the nature of human society, sociologists frame particular kinds of questions within their *methods of enquiry.* These are referred to as *perspectives*, and it is usual to identify the four main ones which form the parameters within which most sociological work is done. In his introductory chapter, O'Donnell (1992) categorises these as follows:

- Structural functionalism
- Marxism
- Social action theory or interactionism
- Interpretive approaches: symbolic interactionism, ethnomethodology and phenomenology.

Feminism, a more recently developed framework, could be added to this list (see Chapter 4). In practice, the boundaries between one or other approach may be 'much less clear-cut and researchers may well draw on more than one tradition' (Robinson 1992, p.63).

Whatever the approach, the sociologist endeavours to conduct her or his research using systematic frameworks, so that a holistic picture may emerge. Thus the variety of sociological approaches has a potentially multi-dimensional effect, for the different fields of enquiry extend from the micro-level up to a macro-analysis of large-scale institutions. It is possible not only to look at and question social interaction on a small scale, such as the professional–client encounter, but also to query the purpose of the institution itself. We may therefore ask what mental hospitals have contributed to mental health. Is community or de-institutionalised care an improvement?

If we apply the sociologist's form of reasoning to the nursing context, questions can be raised concerning (1) the nature of taken-for-granted beliefs that form the normative stock of traditional nursing knowledge and (2) the consequences of such beliefs and value judgements in the course of the nurse's day-to-day experience. How are patients treated? Are they treated differently and, if so, why? Are the criteria which entitle young Mr Roberts to a bypass operation and not old Mr Edwards based purely on biological factors? How are patients categorised and labelled? Are these labels internalised by patients, and how does this affect their treatment and recovery? These questions require that theorising takes place on different levels which involves selecting the most appropriate method for further research. For instance, a structural approach, whether Marxist or functionalist, would provide us with a framework in which 'big' issues such as the fiscal crisis of the NHS, its relationship to the economy and the political system, can be analysed (see Chapter 2). Using the ideas of feminist theorists, issues of gender inequalities in health, including those of women in ethnic minority groups, can be raised as social (preventive) rather than natural (immutable) facts.

If we wished to focus more at the micro-level, for example, on analyses of illness experiences, we might use methods derived from interpretive or 'insider' sociology, with its focus on the perceptions of the individuals involved. This tradition looks at how meanings are constructed, the ways in which people are labelled, and the consequences of the process for the people labelled (see Chapters 3, 5 and 7).

Furthermore, the labelling process can also be linked to wider structures in society by using a Marxist class analysis. For instance, how could we explain the asymmetrical power relationship between a male doctor and a working-class female patient without reference to the lower status position of women and the working class in capitalist society? Without the concepts of *class* and *gender inequality*, how can we understand the subordinate place of nurses in medical health organisation?

The sociological imagination in nursing

Sociological perspectives and concepts may be thought of as the lenses through which we can clarify problems which all too often, particularly in nursing, are thought to be purely personal (it's your own fault), or peculiar to a particular occupational group, rather than organisational or social. To bring the sociological imagination to bear upon our experiences means making connections between the private/personal world and the public/impersonal world of institutions and social processes. The first lesson of social science:

> . . . is the idea that the individual can understand his (*sic*) own experi-
> ence and gauge his own fate only by locating himself within his period,
> that he can know his own chances in life only by becoming aware of
> those of all individuals in his circumstances (. . .)By the fact of his
> living he contributes, however minutely, to the shaping of this society
> and to the course of its history, even as he is made by society and by its
> historical push and shove. The sociological imagination enables us to
> grasp history and biography and the relations between the two within
> society. That is its task and promise . . . .
>
> (C.W. Mills 1959, p.12)

Nursing knowledge has benefited from the development of case studies or first-hand 'insider' accounts, which honestly portray what nursing is when it is happening (see Chapter 4). At the same time, what is needed is attention to analysis from the 'outside', so that nurses may locate their experiences and practices within the larger scheme of things. This is an oversight in nursing theories, guaranteeing an appeal only to the already initiated, that is, nursing theorists. Nursing is presented almost as if it had a separate existence in a parallel universe. The passionate quest for the definitive statement of nursing's unique contribution to health care has resulted in a one-track mindset (Hardy 1982, p.449) which, along with the biomedical model, fails to incorporate the complexity of nursing work.

Sociology, its tools and skills can be used to bring into focus the multi-dimensional aspects of nursing practices. To achieve this, however, means accepting that an analysis of nursing cannot be confined to narrow definitions of a professional interaction between nurse and patient or client. The structure of nursing and the changes which take place are often the results of policies and politics in the wider society. For instance, the expansion in nurse education probably has more to do with the pull from educational establishments seeking new markets in vocational fields, and a widening of educational opportunity for women generally, than with a specific push from within nursing itself (Perry 1991).

Sociology and reflective practice

The concept of *'the reflective practitioner'* (Schon 1983, 1987), adopted by nursing theorists, implies that theory is mediated by practice. A critical, that is, reflective practice, informed by sociology generates theory in a dialectical way; theory informs practice, and is in turn refined by practice, leading to the development of new theories/explanations of nursing. The development of sociological concepts in nursing theory can be regarded as contributing to new social theory.

In sociological analysis, nursing takes place within a set of institutional arrangements, through the active agencies of nurses-as-persons and patients-as-persons. Yet in nursing models and theories it is referred to as if it had an existence independent of nurses and patients themselves. Nurses as 'socially embedded persons' are rarely considered within such a theoretical world. The social context is viewed only in terms of patient needs, and nurses are taken to be passive instruments in the patient's right to health care. Furthermore, a nurse would find it difficult, no matter how stretched physically or emotionally, to raise the question of who cares for the carers (Mackay 1989). While nurses have a responsibility to help the patient, they may not have the necessary authority to act, given the constraints upon them in the organisational and professional setting. This may be one reason why nursing's status in the health hierarchy has remained relatively unchanged overall, despite a move towards higher education and more stratified grading systems.

Professionals are supposed to intervene and bring about real changes in people's lives, and to do this they need to be well placed in the organisational and social structure as well as vocationally inclined (Burrage and Torstendahl 1990). Insight into the social and occupational context in which nursing takes place is, therefore, an essential aspect of any theorising about the nature and extent of its caring practices. By way of illustration, two situations involving the contextual roles of nurses are presented below for discussion.

Situation one

This concerns a fairly ill patient who has been told that he has advanced cancer of the lung. The consultant visited to break the bad news, and afterwards informed the nursing staff that he had booked a course of radiotherapy for the patient, at a neighbouring hospital some miles away, to start 3 days later. Over the next 3 days, the nursing staff observed a marked deterioration in the patient's condition. He became very weak, breathless and withdrawn. On the morning of his first radiotherapy treatment, a student nurse was asked to prepare him for the journey and to accompany him. She was concerned about his poor condition, and reported this to the staff nurse in charge of the shift. The ward was very busy, and the staff nurse seemed rather stressed. He told the nurse that the patient should go for his treatment as planned, because the consultant had prescribed it.

The student accompanied the patient to the radiotherapy department, where treatment commenced. During the treatment the patient became ill. The doctor present curtailed the radiotherapy and told the student that the patient should not have been brought for the treatment in the first place, as he was obviously too ill. The student accompanied the patient back to the ward where, some hours later, he died. The student later related the account to her mentor. Analysing the events, she angrily attributed the responsibility and blame to the consultant. She defended the actions of the staff nurse, stating that he had been 'stressed and inexperienced'.

Reflection/analysis

In the above example, a number of questions could be asked relating to the *micro-level* of interactions between different health care staff and professional groups. This could involve the use of interactionist theories to help frame the questions. Here we can talk in terms of 'roles and actors'. What are the roles being played by the various actors? How do they see their roles? The story is told from the perspective of one of the actors, the student nurse. Her understanding of the situation, the *meanings* she attributes, are relative to her own *subordinate position* within the hierarchically structured 'team' of professionals concerned with the patient's care. Gender, class and age might also be factors which operate to reinforce her position within the organisation, compared with the medical professional. Witz (1992) emphasises the importance of gender in analysing the relative subordination of a predominantly female profession in the medical division of labour. Women, working-class people and the young have less power in society. We could also take into account concepts and issues relating to the *macro* and *political* dimensions of gender, class, race and age, known as *social stratification theories* (see Chapter 9).

The student attributes responsibility to the consultant; the staff nurse's action (or lack of action) is excused with reference to the busy workload and the stress which he, as a newly qualified nurse, is perceived by the student to be experiencing. Responsibility is thus mediated by these contextual circumstances. The staff nurse's subordinate position within the organisational structure of the hospital suggests that he has less power and status than the consultant. This results in the student having different expectations of the staff nurse's role and responsibility.

Salvage (1990) refers to an Australian hospital study which employed interactionist perspectives and in-depth interviewing methods to determine whether nurses viewed their primary allegiance in terms of patients or doctors. Using four hypothetical 'critical incidents', nurses were asked to choose between two sets of behaviours exemplifying the roles of handmaiden or patient advocate. The overwhelming majority of respondents 'failed to put the patient's needs first, even when it exposed the patient to serious risk'. The researchers concluded that the qualified nurse saw her main role as that of assistant to the doctor. Furthermore, student nurses arriving on the wards were:

> . . . presented with an image of themselves as subordinate members of a subordinate division of the health team. Internalisation of this image could then create a downward spiral of reduced self-esteem and acceptance of the handmaiden role.

> (Salvage 1990, p.44)

The patient, as well as the nurse, has a very *passive* role within these structures. How much is this accounted for by the specific circumstances relating to the individual and the context? If the patient had been unconscious, and thereby unable to take an active part in the decision to have the radiotherapy, then his passivity would have a particular meaning and explanation. In this case, the patient was very ill but fully conscious throughout the events described. This indicates that there may be a *general patient role*, where passivity is an *ascribed function*, an effect or consequence of the status and power which characterise professional roles. Patients and professionals alike 'learn' their parts and their place through socialisation. Functionalist, Marxist and feminist theories provide frameworks for understanding the structure of professional–patient relations within the organisation of health care and society.

Situation two

A 52-year-old woman was admitted to a ward having suffered her third heart attack. Two days after admission, the consultant physician responsible for her care visited her in the course of a formal ward round. Hence he was accompanied by his team, consisting of four doctors, a social worker and a physiotherapist. One of the staff nurses from the ward was also in attendance. Halting at the patient's bedside, which was located close to five others in a six-bed bay, the consultant asked how the patient was feeling, told her she'd had a severe heart attack, and enquired if she had given up smoking as advised. When the patient replied that she'd cut down but not stopped completely, the consultant told her in no uncertain terms that she had caused the heart attack. He then stated that, in view of the fact that his earlier advice had been ignored, he could see no point in wasting his time in continuing to care for the patient. He walked off, followed by his team. No-one stayed to speak to the patient, who had become very upset. Later, in the privacy of the ward office, the consultant stated that he had wanted to shock the patient into giving up smoking.

The staff nurse was deeply distressed by these events, and attempted to talk them through with peers. He was advised to do 'some health education' with the patient to persuade her to give up smoking.

Reflection/analysis

Questions can be framed which explore the micro-level of interactions between and among the various actors in this scenario, all playing their parts or roles according to the script (socialisation). Concepts drawn from interactionist sociological theories have a contribution to make, highlighting the *paternalistic* and *authoritarian* modes of interaction. The staff nurse might reflect, self-critically, on his reasons for non-intervention on behalf of the patient.

Social stratification theories which explore differences in *status* and *power* extend the analysis. The consultant is the powerful leader of the group, while the patient is rendered powerless, and thereby effectively silenced. Gender may contribute to an explanation; the patient is a woman, the consultant is a man. According to sociologists, biology alone does not account for the differences in social, political and economic status between men and women. They also question the dominance of medicine's knowledge claims in health. In accordance with biomedical definitions of disease causation, no attempt is made by the actors to acknowledge that factors other than smoking might have contributed to the patient's illness, nor is any attempt made to find out why the patient continued, against medical advice, her risky activity.

The comments made later to the staff nurse by his peers indicate that the consultant's actions are considered to be normative or taken-for-granted. The nurse's role is bound to an acceptance of the consultant's superiority and his view that the patient is the cause of her own illness.

According to interactionist, Marxist or feminist sociologists, health as a purely individual and personal responsibility can be criticised. This is because victim-blaming represents a particular political ideology which not only diverts attention away from the social factors which cause ill health but also negates the social reforms necessary for its improvement. Health problems are located in individual behaviour rather than environmental conditions such as poor housing, poverty or pollution. Consequently, it is the individual who must be changed and not society (Crawford 1977).

Who adheres to a political ideology which vaunts self-reliance and consumer sovereignty over state intervention and provision? In the British context, it is the Conservative government which, since 1979, has placed increasing emphasis on taking personal responsibility, while at the same time reducing the means or social welfare services which make it possible for many people to do so. Given that the government has shown a reluctance to continue fully funding the medical hospital establishment, to what extent is personal behaviour being used as a justification for the rationalisation of health care costs? If health behaviour increasingly becomes attached to notions of moral duty, the consequence is that illness as a moral failing will be emphasised (Crawford 1984). Moreover, if smoking is presented as a moral failure of individuals, it is unlikely that the power of the tobacco lobby will be seriously challenged at government level.

Sociological reflections on professional nursing

As previously mentioned, most nursing theorists are preoccupied with the search for the definitive nursing role, i.e. its absolute truth or scientific purity. Adopting an experimental method of one type or another, different models are tested against reality, and reality is found to be wanting. This is hardly surprising, given that these abstract notions are predicated upon a professional ideology which is seen to be the only acceptable explanation of practice. Similarly, prevailing social arrangements which develop or inhibit practice are rarely taken into account. We do not know what nursing is as an organisation or why its modes of practice continue to be defined by higher authorities in health, be they doctors, administrators or management consultants.

Nursing theories and models share a common belief that nursing is set in opposition to medicine. Whereas scientific or curative medicine engages with the disease, nursing is presented as an enterprise in which the nurse engages with the 'whole person'. Nursing becomes an activity centred on the personal experience of 'being ill', 'having treatment for a disease' or 'promoting health'. Different models express the basic premise in a variety of ways. It is, however, formally espoused in the ethical code of conduct put forward by nursing's foremost professional association, the United Kingdom Central Council for Nursing, Midwifery and Health Visiting (United Kingdom Central Council 1984). While the parallel universe of disease commands the attention of the medical scientist, nurses focus on the personal, human world. This distinction continues to be seen to arise out of individual choice alone (vocation), rather than as a consequence of nursing's place in the hospital structure (medical and management professionalism). Nurses are a continuous presence at the patient's bedside and, as such, they receive the full, emotional reactions of patients to illness, treatment and the organisation of care (Smith 1992).

Armstrong (1983) is critical of the claim that nursing has always espoused caring and person-centred approaches in its practices. He argues that this is a relatively recent orientation; until the 1970s, nursing was constructed within a medical paradigm which directed its interests to the doctor's rather than the patient's need. He cites as evidence the overwhelming biomedical content of nursing textbooks prior to the professionalising movement. This may be, however, only in reference to nursing's public face. 'Know-how' knowledge in nursing (Watkins 1991), passed on by the oral tradition from senior to junior staff, has certainly taken personalised caring into account. Perhaps this leads to the possibility that there are always dual agendas in operation: a private version that is well recognised by those at the nurse–patient interface, and a public account designed to 'woo' those with the power to grant legitimation of nursing's status.

Writers such as Hardy (1982, 1986) and Chapman (1990) believe that the caring orientation is an aspect of recent attempts to develop a distinct knowledge base for nursing. They argue that these developments represent the self-interested aspirations of the *'professionalisers'* rather than those of many nurses. Although nursing theorists borrow concepts from the sociology of the professions, the sharp, political edge of the meanings tends to be blunted or de-politicised. In other words, implicit sociological assumptions, critical of a preconceived harmony between professional practice and beneficial outcomes to clients (Perry 1991, p.187), are glossed over, if not totally ignored. It is almost as if nursing theory is the 'true' formula guaranteeing that the practitioner, in wielding the tool, will possess definitive solutions to every conceivable patient situation. Does this mean that only professional self-interest is being served by the development of a nursing knowledge base?

> The development of theoretical frameworks (. . .) have been created to bestow respectability and credibility upon our profession. They have provided a professionalising stance. This, in response to how other professions have evolved. Thus, it seemed important to follow the same path. This, in a way, is a knee-jerk response. Perhaps it is time to question the definitions of what a profession is, and indeed, whether or not professions utilizing models have served the public well.
>
> (Hardy 1986, p.106)

One assumption being made within critiques of this kind is that nursing as it is practised is different from and more authentic than the theorised versions. One problem may be that although nursing models are intended to act as guides to practice, most have never been tested empirically. Criticisms voiced by many nurses at the patient–nurse interface suggest a widespread dissonance between the 'authority' of the theory and the lack of authority experienced by direct practitioners. How are practising nurses supposed to implement and evaluate different approaches to care when they generally do not have the power needed in the health bureaucracy to express themselves? It appears, from the quote below, that the 'freedom' to question is not encouraged even within nursing itself:

> Academics trained in the much harsher but more realistic worlds of the natural sciences and perhaps sociology are shocked by the obvious back-slapping and 'hear, hear' attitude which prevails at nursing research conferences. Asking a searching question of a speaker at such an event is seen as terribly bad form – even worse form should the speaker be one of the eminent.
>
> (Johnson 1986, p.42, quoted in Chapman 1990, p.9)

Hardy (1986) suggests that instead of models and theories promoting 'pure' thinking about nursing, they should be used to aid critical thinking and improve practice. This is, after all, an important aspect of public account-ability and performance in the professional role.

Functionalist sociologists would analyse nursing's move towards profes-sionalism as a contribution to *system needs*. These theorists, commenting on recent developments, would demonstrate that this is part of society's rational response to recognised changing patterns of illness, from acute infectious diseases to chronic conditions and an increasingly elderly popula-tion. An important concept for these theorists is the *interdependence* of different parts or structures of society. If health care is viewed as one such structure contributing to the *'body of society'* as a whole, then nursing can be understood as a component of the health care system, in much the same kind of relationship as, say, between, the cardiovascular and respiratory systems in the *biological analogy* . To ensure overall functioning (or homeostasis) in either society or the human body, all systems and sub-systems need to work together.

Viewed from a Marxist perspective, the power of certain professionals in health, which emanates largely from a privileged position in the class structure, could be analysed. Nurses as a mainly female social group, with more working-class members than are found among physicians, are located in a subordinate position. However, first and foremost, health organisation is understood in terms of the ways in which it contributes to the maintenance of the capitalist system, that is, *social inequality* and the extraction of profit. For instance, the National Health Service helps to reproduce capitalism by providing a healthy, productive workforce. It also controls and disciplines certain aspects of social behaviour in the legitimation of illness. Doctors control entry to the sick role and access to all treatments; they also provide sick certificates to cover periods of absence from work. Marxists focus attention on the 'hidden' economic potential of health care. In the current British context, health is one of the largest industries.

Whereas functionalists and Marxists look at systems and structures, inter-actionists take into account how individuals and groups experience these at the interpersonal or micro-level. In particular, interpretive perspectives offer a critique of health services from the point of view of those on the receiving end, namely the users. When health users organise themselves into pressure groups they can provide, if consulted, insights into how professional practices might be improved to meet individual and local needs (see Chapter 6). These possibilities emerge from an analysis which at the outset recognises the importance of how 'ordinary' people view their lives and roles and what they may contribute to the professional's understanding of his or her own role. Applying this approach to the perspective of nurses who are actively engaged in working with patients, we suggest that alternatives to the professionalisation movement may be formulated.

What is the contribution of feminist sociology, given that nursing is a female-intensive occupation? Oakley (1984) and other feminist theorists tend to see this immersion in a female world as a potential strength; nurses and midwives are, in terms of gender and class, well placed to understand and promote women's health needs. Feminists are keen to show, using comparative research data, that women are not naturally best suited to be nurses, nor men to be doctors (Witz 1992). They do not, however, ignore nursing's relatively lower status in the health division of labour. The consequences for nurses are, and have been, a subservient role to doctors, who can claim status by virtue of expert (prescriptive) knowledge. According to Chandler (1991), Project 2000 courses on initial training situate the caring bases of nursing within the social and behavioural sciences because, if they did not, nursing on its own could be seen as devalued 'women's work'. Within these approaches, the role of sociology has been largely limited to explaining the world to the nurse so that, the logic runs, she can offer a 'better service'. The focus is on sociology for nurses rather than a sociological analysis of nursing.

While a sociological analysis of nursing would start from the premise that it is an occupation, albeit of a particular kind, this tends to be remarkable for its absence from the curriculum. Professionalism in nursing is assumed to be, in general, a 'good thing' and almost inevitable. However, Oakley's critique of professional dilemmas concludes that, for nurses, this may prove to be a counter-productive and counter-intuitive strategy:

> Alternatively, nurses might ask the truly radical question as to what is so wonderful about being a professional anyway? (. . .) the current crisis of confidence in medical care should tell us that professionalisation is not the only answer (. . .) indeed, it may be positively damaging to health.
>
> (Oakley 1984, p.27)

A consequence of professionalism is the creation of distance between nurses and patients. This would have implications for the nature of nursing work, such as the trend towards technical-instrumental extended roles at the cost of developing caring as a defining characteristic of nursing work (Melia 1987; Chapman 1990; Salvage 1990; Antrobus 1993). In other words, divisions in nursing organisation between higher status technical specialists and lower status 'routine' carers would widen.

Nursing's professionalising project

Theory in Project 2000 courses, and this includes sociology's contribution, is used as an instrument of policy and is therefore a political factor in education decision-making (Jarvis 1992). Project 2000 (United Kingdom Central Council 1986) justified the need to reform nurse education on the basis of two major demographic trends. First, a diminishing population of school leavers implied that nursing could no longer rely upon a steady stream of young recruits. Secondly, there is an increasing number of very elderly people in the population with specific social and health needs. The report advocated supernumerary status and a proper training environment. It emphasised the importance of attracting and retaining students of both sexes from a wider pool of school-leavers and mature recruits. Finally, recommendations were put forward to bring nurse training in line with higher education principles, in the provision of a broader curriculum, a more holistic consideration of health, and the introduction of research methodology for the purposes of academic validation for a diploma to accompany state registration. While none of this has been carried out with the courage and confidence of the original Project 2000 report, the parameters of nurse education have fundamentally shifted.

Academic knowledge determines professional status. Higher education in any form is intimately concerned with knowledge. The relationship is conceptual; a process is not entitled to be termed higher education unless the student experiences an encounter with knowledge. However, higher education is not about any kind of knowledge. Traditionally, it has been concerned with systematic, elaborated, conceptual frameworks, developed over time in the academic literature (see Chapter 10). For professions such as medicine and law, academic accreditation extends back as far as the medieval universities. In the case of nursing, the absence of such a research base, demonstrating a correlation between professional practice and the benefits to patients (Perry 1991, p.187), has prolonged its acceptance as a bona fide course in higher education. Not surprisingly, scientific knowledge derived from systematic enquiry is now of great significance in nursing education.

In contemporary British society, as in the past, the academy is vital to the interpretation of professionalism. In other words, public acceptance of a profession is based upon an occupation's assertion that its evaluation and training make it uniquely suitable to provide a specific service. For professionals:

> . . . must be adequately trained and socialised to provide recognisably distinct services. The process has been institutionalised in the modern university which gives professions the means to control their knowledge base as well as to award credentials certifying that practitioners possess this recognisably distinct type of knowledge.
>
> (Cevero 1988, p.5)

By way of contrast, nursing education/training has been carried out in small National Service-based schools, geographically and organisationally closely tied to service delivery. Qualifications were licences to practice, involving admittance to a professional register, specified by national nursing agencies/ boards, and not academically evaluated like diplomas or degrees. Students were a key part of the health work-force, and education was subordinate to this primary commitment. Schools of nursing achieved high standards of technical reliability and competence, but remained isolated from the broader values of higher education in terms of breadth of curriculum and access to a research base, university funding levels, library and other learning resources, and student lifestyle.

Until recently, nursing was constituted purely in terms of the manual labour content of hospital and medical tasks (Perry 1993). This applied both to qualified nursing staff and to those just entering the wards. It is not surprising that nurses, especially those who 'made it' through an ardu-ous training, developed a strong sense of injustice. These arrangements fostered a particular approach to education in which practical competence was paramount. Theoretical education was often taught in relatively short blocks prior to placement or work experience. A 'monotechnic' tradition grew up in which students were taught within the single-discipline group of nursing, and nurse tutors took responsibility for contributing subjects such as sociology.

Eventually, technological changes in the modern hospital affected not only medicine but also nursing roles. The traditional model of education was seen to be no longer appropriate to contemporary requirements (Cox 1992).

Since World War II, higher education has increasingly become a route for vocational groups seeking a higher social status. As a result, much has been heard about the tense relationship between theory and reality. In the struggle for professional status, it is one thing to adopt the strategy in theory, but another to have to live with it without the social conditions necessary for its maintenance, for example, increased public acceptability of the relevance of the work and government funding. It is, not surprising, therefore, to learn that some theorists do not feel that nurses can truly benefit from a univer-sity-based professional training. Indeed, some claim that practitioners 'have their heads filled with jargon and are no longer adequately prepared for the "real world"' (Squires 1990).

Sociologically speaking, this problem has more to do with the conditions under which nurses work and study, and their recruitment from the 'buffer zone' (just out of the working class), than with problems in the higher education environment *per se*. Decision-making in clinical nursing practice remains very particularistic or context-bound (Greenwood 1984), while judgement and scepticism are often systematically discouraged in the educa-tion setting. What tends to be overlooked is that the use of theory is to make morally defensible decisions and choices by developing the art of practical deliberation among practitioners and neophytes. The purpose of theory is to facilitate the improvement of practice. Chandler (1991) highlights a dichot-omy between the attainment of consensual knowledge, characteristic of nursing, and the more critical and enquiring stance implicit in academic learning, especially in the social sciences. In higher education, students are expected to go beyond the material they encompass and to form their own affinity with it. Learning this or that and being able to recall information is not sufficient. Insight, involvement and reflection are necessary, because the learning has to be *transcended*. Students have to show that they deeply understand what has been learnt, so that they are able to assess it critically for themselves and apply it for the benefit of others. One of the most important attributes of academic, professional education is to maintain a gap between what is learnt and what is practised, so that practitioners may respond imaginatively to people's needs and the distress in their lives. Even if students are not initially able to come up with alternative offerings of their own, they must be able, at the very least, to state honestly, 'I believe this to be the case, and this is why' (Barnett 1990). Discipline-based knowledge should be used by students, as previously discussed, reflectively.

Farley and Hendry (1992) suggest that the whole process of socialising nurses to a higher education level may be undermined in the clinical context, where they are expected to be non-critical and non-discerning. It appears that student nurses who move from an educational to a practice setting are subjected to 'a competing paradigm of occupational vocationalism' (Moore 1990). This paradigm seems to be consistent with Melia's (1984) description of student nurses' desire to get the work done with little reference to any explicit knowledge base.

In the meantime, some nurse educators continue to subscribe to a highly theoretical approach to diplomas or degrees in nursing. In the absence of a substantive knowledge base, it is necessary to 'borrow' from other disciplines. Professional knowledge in nursing is seen to consist of theoretical understandings or assumptions drawn from physiology, psychology, philosophy and sociology, and 'knowing how to apply them in particular situations'. In other words, what makes a person really professional is theoretical knowledge alone.

The establishment of links with higher education can be considered as a part of nursing's professionalising strategy. It has not, however, succeeded in bringing together accreditation and status in nursing. This is not the fault of nurses. It is perhaps more to do with the elevation of expert technical systems as solutions to all human problems. As a result, caring, taken to be natural, informal or vocational, is further devalued and carers demoralised. This affects not only nurses but also social workers and teachers (Seabrook 1985). Everyone knows that sick and vulnerable people need care. Caring is not just a nursing problem but a social one; hence it needs to be studied sociologically.

Conclusions

The theory–practice gap continues to be a contentious issue in nursing. In the absence of a substantive body of research, there is no 'bridge' or connection in nursing knowledge between what direct practioners do, the changes that they encounter as one NHS restructuring follows another, and the principles of care devised by theoreticians. Models and theories have been limited to promoting thinking about nursing as an abstract concept, rather than as an aid to reflecting critically upon practice.

In sociology, this problem is seen to stem from nursing's status location in the health hierarchy and an adherence to a professional ideology which obscures social function in health and society. Nursing is a vocation which has struggled to attain a semi-professional status, and change has not taken place in a uniform way. Nursing training is not wholly based within higher education, while alongside a rising number of nurse specialists, the majority continue to carry out basic physical care. The movement from traditional to more specialist roles is largely the effect of modern technology, in the hospital as well as other fields, and not solely the outcome of a nursing education policy.

In the past, nursing practices in health have been derived mainly from medical and bureaucratic imperatives. In the current context of the National Health Service, medical professionalism has been undermined by a government-led strategy of 'market forces'. This has taken medicine's professional associations by surprise. For the past 100 years or so they have been preoccupied with the market implications of an 'over-supply' of general practitioners. If this can happen to a powerful group such as doctors, where does it leave nurses? Caring work can too easily be seen to be something that many people, especially women, do naturally. It is little wonder that theories and tools such as the nursing process have attempted to formalise and elevate the status of caring work. Nursing's professionalising project may be more to do with survival tactics in modern society, where educational or 'paper' qualifications are essential credentials in the world of work generally, than with any notion of grandeur on the part of nurse 'professionalisers'. Many nurses may want simply to 'nurse', but in the current context they can no longer be just kind and concerned carers. They need 'new' theory to help them to understand the nature and extent of the competition they now face in the occupational and health structures in which they work.

Sociology is one of a number of disciplines which provide a wide range of insights into nursing activities. In this chapter we have tried to show that what happens in nursing is related to people, policies and politics in health organisation as a whole. Just as the personal experiences of an individual are inextricably linked to the institutions which characterise 'society', so the experiences of nurses and other health practitioners form part of a larger 'reality'. These structures and interconnections will be explored in the following chapters.

References

Antrobus, S. 1993: Nursing's nature and boundaries. *Senior Nurse* **13**(2), 46–50.

Armstrong, D. 1983: The fabrication of nurse–patient relationships. *Social Science and Medicine* **17**(8), 457–460.

Barnett, R. 1990: *The idea of higher education*. Buckingham: The Society for Research into Higher Education (SRHE) and Open University Press.

Berger, P. 1966: *Invitation to sociology*. Harmondsworth: Penguin.

Burrage, M. and Torstendahl, R. (eds) 1990: *Professions in theory and history: rethinking the study of the professions*. London: Sage.

Cevero, R. 1988: *Effective continuing education for professions*. San Francisco: Jossey-Bass.

Chandler, J. 1991: Reforming nurse education. 1. The reorganisation of nursing knowledge. *Nursing Education Today* **11**, 83–88.

Chapman, P. 1990: A critical perspective. In Kershaw, B. and Salvage, J. (eds), *Models for nursing*. 2. London: Scutari Press, 9–17.

Cox, D. 1992: *Working paper 10 – professional education in transition*. Paper presented to the International Sociological Association Conference, 'Professions in Transition', Leicester, 21–23 April 1992. Birmingham: University of Central England, Faculty of Health and Social Sciences.

Crawford, R. 1977: You are dangerous to your health: the ideology and politics of victim blaming. *International Journal of Health Services* **7(4)**, 663–680.

Crawford, R. 1984: A cultural account of 'health': control, release and the social body. In McKinlay, J.B. (ed.), *Issues in the political economy of health care*. New York: Tavistock, 60–103.

Farley, A. and Hendry, C. 1992: Critical and constructive. *Nursing Times* **88(39)**, 36–37.

Greenwood, J. 1984: Nursing research: a position paper. *Journal of Advanced Nursing* **9(1)**, 77–82.

Hardy, L. 1982: Nursing models and research – a restricting view? *Journal of Advanced Nursing* **7(5)**, 447–451.

Hardy, L. 1986: Identifying the place of theoretical frameworks in an evolving discipline. *Journal of Advanced Nursing* **11(1)**, 103–107.

Jarvis, P. 1992: Theory and practice and the preparation of teachers of nursing. *Nurse Education Today* **12**, 258–265.

Johnson, M. 1986: Model of perfection? *Nursing Times* **82(6)**, 42–43.

Mackay, L. 1989: *Nursing a problem*. Milton Keynes: Open University Press.

Melia, K. 1984: Student nurses' construction of occupational socialisation. *Sociology of Health and Illness* **6(2)**, 132–151.

Melia, K. 1987: *Learning and working: the occupational socialization of nurses*. London: Tavistock.

Mills, C.W. 1959: *The sociological imagination*. New York: Oxford University Press.

Moore, R. 1990: Knowledge, practice and the construction of skill. In Gleeson, D. (ed.), *Training and its alternatives*. Milton Keynes: Open University Press.

Oakley, A. 1984: The importance of being a nurse. *Nursing Times* **80(50)**, 24–27.

O'Donnell, M. 1992: *A new introduction to sociology*. 3rd edition. Walton on Thames: Nelson.

Perry, A. 1987: Sociology in the curriculum. In Allan, P. and Jolley, M. (eds), *The curriculum in nursing education*. London: Croom Helm, 126–148.

Perry, A. 1991: Sociology – its contribution and critiques. In Perry, A. and Jolley, M. (eds), *Nursing – a knowledge base for practice*. London: Edward Arnold, 154–198.

Perry, A. 1993: A sociologist's view – the handmaiden's theory. In Jolley, M. and Brykczynska, G. (eds), *Nursing – its hidden agendas*. London: Edward Arnold, 43–79.

Robinson, K. 1992: Sociological perspectives. In Robinson, K. and Vaughan, B. (eds), *Knowledge for nursing practice*. Oxford: Butterworth-Heinemann, 60–73.

Salvage, J. 1990: The theory and practice of the 'new' nursing. *Nursing Times* **86(4)**, 42–45.

Schon, D. 1983: *The reflective practitioner: how professionals think in action.* New York: Basic Books.

Schon, D. 1987: *Educating the reflexive practitioner: towards a new design for teaching and learning in the profession.* San Francisco: Jossey-Bass.

Seabrook, J. 1985: The fall of the caring classes. *New Society,* **73(1180)**, 190–192.

Smith, P. 1992: *The emotional labour of nursing.* London: Macmillan.

Squires, G. 1990: *First degree: the undergraduate curriculum.* Buckingham: The Society for Research into Higher Education (SRHE) and Open University Press.

Turnbull. A. 1992: A bit of relief after the sciences: teaching sociology on Project 2000. *Medical Sociology News* **17(3)**, 14–17.

United Kingdom Central Council for Nursing, Midwifery and Health Visiting 1984: *Code of professional conduct for the nurse, midwife and health visitor.* 2nd edition. London: UKCC.

United Kingdom Central Council for Nursing, Midwifery and Health Visiting 1986: *Project 2000: a new preparation for practice.* London: UKCC.

Watkins, M. 1991: Nursing knowledge – ultimate objectives. In Perry, A. and Jolley, M. (eds), *Nursing: a knowledge base for practice.* London: Edward Arnold, 308–338.

Witz, A. 1992: *Professions and patriarchy.* London: Routledge.

2 Health care and the new managerialism: policy, planning and organisations

Bridget Towers

Introduction

This is a challenging time for sociologists who are concerned with exploring the dynamics and directional change of health care provision in British society. It is not just the onerous matter of constantly having to redraw maps of the organisational structures and endlessly reformat those genealogical lists of policy and administrative initiatives, nor even the more daunting task of simply keeping up to date with academic literature and research material in the area. It is the more fundamental challenge that is presented in the questioning of the very parameters and core concepts of what had hitherto been a cognisable 'subject field' (health care) with defined 'objects of study' (such as 'health', 'illness', 'disease', 'care', 'therapeusis', 'patients' and 'nurses') (Towers 1992).

In the academic domain this trend towards a sociology of *deconstruction* has its roots in the 1960s, and was strongly developed in the critical approach that sociologists took towards crime and deviance as being social constructions, rather than the ready-made 'objects of study' that earlier generations had taken for granted (Pfohl 1994). Instead of searching for new criminogenic factors to explain rising crime rates, they began to focus on the processes involved in the generation of crime statistics, from the socially situated and negotiated interactions between law enforcers and law breakers to the political and organisational norms governing the administration of criminal justice. Of course this way of looking at high-profile social issues has not endeared sociologists to policy makers; they are often characterised as unhelpful or, even worse, insurrectionary!

Over the last few years health care has become just such a high-profile social issue. At the present time, health policy issues are high on the public and private agendas of political parties, professional associations, trade unions, pressure groups and local associations. Political scientists and policy analysts are using questions of health care decision-making to monitor and evaluate changes in the centre and periphery power relationships of the modern state. Health care is currently a growing specialism within management, as the organisational parameters of the delivery of medical goods and services have become widened and bureaucratised. Health issues are now of major concern to economists and accountants as they try to construct new measurements and forecasts for regulating the demand and supply of a major item of public spending. Within the community of professional sociologists there has been a rapid expansion of medical sociology as a legitimate and funded field of expertise (Stacey 1991).

> In such a context one of the most useful contributions a sociological perspective can make is to do precisely what we have been best at and most unpopular for; namely standing back and studying the process of the construction of 'the object'.
>
> (Towers 1992, p.190)

In this particular chapter we can chart the making of a new community assembled around the discourse on health management.

There is a substantial sociological literature on *discourse* dynamics and analysis. A great deal of it is somewhat impenetrable; a very informative secondary source is Ian Parker (1992). I have also written elsewhere about discourse analysis and screening (Towers 1993). However, for the purpose of this chapter, I would suggest that 'in a rather obvious way it is about looking at who is sitting around what table where, using what kind of language and knowledge claims when something called a "health management issue" is on the agenda for discussion' (Towers 1992, p.190). It is also about identifying which organisations and institutions are reinforced, and which are challenged by, those *situated exchanges*.

From 'health for all' to 'the health of the nation'

Rather than assuming from the start a narrow focus upon the specifically British context, it is useful to recognise that our experience of radically reviewing the management and financing of our system of health care is a common one, not only in Europe but across the developed world.

The importance of using a comparative method, across and between societies, is amply demonstrated in sociology. Indeed, some sociologists would even claim that it is not simply 'one' method but 'the' method of the discipline (Thompson and Tunstall 1971). There are numerous pitfalls in making comparisons between countries without establishing criteria for comparability, and clearly identifying which factors are being identified for study and situating them within contexts which may well be sub-categories of a comparative class. Nevertheless, it can be a helpful and illuminating method of analysis; an easily accessible example can be found in Lyn Payer's comparative study of medical diagnosis and prescribing in Britain, the USA, France and Germany (Payer 1989).

There is no shortage of detailed descriptive material on changes and developments in health care policies in Europe and other continents. Furthermore, it is a useful exercise to practise your data analysis and presentation skills with tables of epidemiological data, per capita spending, ratios of health sector funding, medical manpower or even consultation and referral rates. Comprehensive data for such exercises can be found in the following reports: The Organisation for Economic Co-ordination and Development reports on *Measuring Health Care 1960–83* (Organisation for Economic Co-ordination and Development 1985) and *Financing and Delivering Health Care* (Organisation for Economic Co-ordination and Development 1987); the World Bank's report *Investing in Health* (1993); the World Health Organisation's *World Health Statistics Annual* (World Health Organisation 1988) together with its report on *Health in Europe* (World Health Organisation 1994).

Christopher Hood (1991, p.3) takes an international view of the changes that are occurring in the public service sector, and identifies what he claims are the 'megatrends' associated with newly emerging methods of public management. Lawton and Rose (1994, p.152) have summarised them as:

1 attempts to slow down or reverse government growth in terms of overt public spending and staffing;

2 the shift towards privatisation and quasi-privatisation and away from core government institutions;

3 the development of automation, particularly in information technology, in the production and distribution of public services;

4 the development of a more international agenda, increasingly focused on general issues of public management, policy design and inter-governmental co-operation.

Whilst these are general trends within an increasing pattern of globalisation, there is considerable variation in the ways in which they are being strategically planned by different countries.

Strategic planning is now recognised as being of major importance in the field of health care. This is because the interrelated psychosocial and politico-economic factors which govern health status have made it obvious that tackling one aspect without doing anything about linked factors will not produce optimum results. However, due to the multiplicity of departments, bureaux, boards, agencies and offices who are able to lay jurisdictional claims at some policy or executive level to health matters, if intersectoral co-operation is to be achieved at all, then it has to be based upon a clearly defined and agreed strategic plan. There is an extensive literature on the specific methods of strategic planning and its application to health care (Argenti 1980). It is, however, possible to identify a number of key stages in the formulation of a strategic plan:

1 clarification of objectives and setting of targets;

2 comparing future performance on current strategies with Stage 1 targets (often called a 'Gap' analysis);

3 formulating strategy on the basis of generating 'options' and evaluating them in terms of achieving Stage 1 targets (often called 'Option Appraisal');

4 implementing strategy by drawing up action plans and budgets, and building into the plans monitoring and control mechanisms for evaluating performance against targets.

A very good example of strategic planning at the international level is the World Health Assembly's global strategy of 'Health for All' by the year 2000, led by the European Region of the World Health Organisation (WHO) since 1985. Its central aim is to ensure greater social equity in health. To achieve this aim it has advocated co-ordinated policies in each country directed at:

1 reducing poverty in its widest sense;

2 securing the basic prerequisites for health for everybody – food, safe water, sanitation, decent housing and universal education;

3 ensuring that everybody has access to effective health care (Benzeval *et al.* 1995, p.47).

The strategy was built out of the Alma-Ata declaration of 1977 which located 'primary health care' as the bedrock on which all future health care planning should be grounded. The strategic task was to ensure that by the year 2000:

all the people in all the countries should have at least such a level of health that they are capable of working productively and of participating actively in the social life of the community in which they live.

(World Health Organisation 1986)

The main objectives of the strategy were to promote healthy life styles, to prevent preventable conditions, and to enable rehabilitation of those whose health has been impaired (Ashton 1990). These very broad objectives were clarified as the 'health goals' of health prevention and health promotion, and were further focused into 38 'targets', accepted by all member states, to be achieved by the year 2000.

> The targets cover a wide range of conditions and activities, specifying particular levels of reduction in mortality rates from heart disease, lung and cervical cancer, infant and maternal mortality, and road traffic accidents; also included are reductions in life style risk factors such as alcohol and tobacco consumption. The major emphasis within the targets, however, is the reorientation of medical care towards health promotion, prevention and primary health care and its bearing on the need for community participation and inter-sectoral cooperation.
>
> (Towers 1992, p.191; see also Chapters 6 and 10)

Health care planners have always distinguished between primary, secondary and tertiary models of medical care provision, in terms of emphasis upon specialist hospital, general hospital, and out-patient or community-based treatment services. A further significant difference is emphasised in the document between the medical concept of 'primary medical care', which is individualistic in terms of the patient/practitioner treatment-specific base, and 'primary health care', which is a social concept involving a wide range of health providers in addition to medical personnel, and focused upon whole communities and their general health status (Ashton 1990).

The WHO can claim considerable success in raising awareness of the issues central to 'Health for All', and encouraging policy makers to make commitments to them in their own national health strategies. The WHO, however, has no legal or fiscal powers, and in an ideological and economic climate in which the New Right (Pollitt 1990) is in the ascendancy, international health and welfare organisations, especially United Nations (UN)-based ones, have been regarded with profound scepticism by many national governments. The UK is particularly notable for its lack of enthusiasm for international or European initiatives in health and welfare policies, and has well-rehearsed methods of limiting their impact, usually through bureaucratic and legal delaying procedures presided over by Treasury subcommittees (Towers 1995, p.45).

It is almost 15 years since the Black report (Townsend and Davidson 1982) in the UK stressed the need for wide-ranging action to tackle inequalities in health, and made specific recommendations for interdepartmental machinery in the Cabinet Office to co-ordinate health-related policies (recommendation 36), but the government of the day found the Black report in its entirety unwelcome and took radical steps to marginalise it and minimise its publicity impact (Townsend et al. 1992). However, attitudes have changed markedly in the 1990s, and the government issued a response to the WHO's 'Health for All' with a series of national health promotion strategies drawn up for each of the separate countries within the UK, first for Wales (Health Promotion Authority for Wales 1990), then for England (House of Commons 1992), Scotland (Scottish Office 1992) and Northern Ireland (Department of Health and Social Services, Northern Ireland 1992). (**A useful group project would be to make a comparative analysis of these documents, preferably involving students who have identification links with each of the countries.**)

The 'Health of the Nation' (House of Commons 1992) reviewed the health status of the population in England and set specific targets for reducing the incidence of identified risk behaviours. It also established a ministerial cabinet committee covering 11 government departments, to develop and implement the strategy (Benzeval et al. 1995). There have been no published reports on the work of the groups to date, although in May 1994 a new subgroup of the Chief Medical Officer's Health of the Nation Group was established to look specifically at 'variations in health' (Department of Health 1994).

In contrast to the WHO, the European Union (EU) has considerable legal and fiscal powers to influence member states. Although it did not have an official health focus until 1993, it has a number of well-established strategic approaches which have a direct bearing upon health, such as the EU Poverty Programme, the Social Fund for regeneration in areas of disadvantage, and particularly the Social Chapter of the Maastricht Treaty.

There is considerable enthusiasm from those concerned with problems of equity in health care for the opportunities presented by the Social Chapter (Benzeval et al. 1995). Under article 129 of the Maastricht Treaty, the EU is now legally obliged to encourage the improvement of public health in its member states, and also to assess the health impact of other EU policies and programmes of economic and industrial development, and to incorporate health protection measures where necessary (Benzeval et al. 1995, p.47). It does, however, remain to be seen whether there are strong mechanisms for enforcement, or merely guidelines of encouragement to good practice. There is still a deep reluctance in many member states to link issues such as the transportation of hazardous materials, the regulation of chemical plants, the development of genetic engineering and the use of pesticides to mainstream health policy until after a catastrophe has occurred (Beck 1992).

It has to be acknowledged that global and international policy objectives often command only lip-service application in collaborating countries, and that there are wide variations in the enthusiasm, manner, form and comprehensiveness with which they are implemented at the national level. Nevertheless, it is clear that there has been a radical shift in the direction of health care planning. Until the 1970s, it had been assumed that the best model to be globally pursued was a specialist/hospital-based medical service, and that the task of governments was to focus upon increasing access and utilisation.

Health care and the fiscal crisis

By the mid-1970s health care costs were presenting major problems for developed countries, regardless of the structure of their health services or the methods of financing them, and in the context of what was called the 'fiscal crisis', redirecting spending from other public sectors was not an option that was believed to be available. To understand this dilemma and its particular impact in the UK we need some understanding of the role of economists in the discourse on health care.

From the late 1950s onwards, a long drawn out crisis in the British economy began to break. Despite policies throughout the 1960s to try to stimulate growth, restore profitability and initiate investment, the underlying problems remained unsolved. As oil prices rose and the world boom began to falter, the UK was faced with a fiscal crisis, a crisis of state finance, manifested in a growing deficit of the state budget and increasing borrowing on the capital markets to meet the gap between tax revenues and expenditure.

In 1976, the Labour government was faced with the necessity of cutting public expenditure as a whole rather than, as in the past, cutting some programmes in order to allow a rise in others which had a higher priority. It was no longer possible to raise funds to cover their existing commitments by increasing the burden of taxation, and so the government had urgently to turn to other sources, negotiating a loan from the International Monetary Fund to support the pound sterling. The rather stringent and unpopular conditions attached to the deal required both an immediate major cut in overall public expenditure and also a commitment to a policy of continuous decline in public spending as a proportion of gross national product (GNP). Here was the beginning of what has become over the last 20 years a radical restructuring of UK welfare policies (Conference of Socialist Economists 1979).

In trying to account for this change, it is tempting to have recourse to arguments of economic determinism and certainly, for a time, the dynamic of adjustment and restructuring was characterised as driven by the unfortunate necessities of an economic policy, and the metaphor of the British people 'taking their medicine like adults' was common. However, by the 1980s this explanatory framework had been replaced by the conservative and New Right ideological commitment to reduce positively the role of the state in British society, since it was believed to be taking and spending too much of the nation's income and crowding out the competitive potential of the progressive private sector (Buchanan and Tullock 1962). The rhetoric was now about liberation and the imagery of rolling back the frontiers of the state.

Whilst economic conditions provided the basic operational constraints, these were mediated by political and ideological factors which led to the selection of particular policy choices and the rejection of others. These can be seen very clearly in the experience of the health sector. Until the time when the Departments of Health and Social Security (DHSS) were split up, the DHSS was the biggest spender in terms of government expenditure; its scale dwarfed that of all other departments. The whole of the NHS took a quarter of departmental spending, and the largest component of that (two-thirds) was for the cost of maintaining the hospital and community health services. Despite the belief at the time when the NHS came into being that the call on funds would gradually decrease, the reality was an almost continuous growth in government expenditure on the health service in real terms. It was apparent that, without intervention, this trend would accelerate. Technological developments in treatment methods entailed a massive increase in future costs, and together with a changed *demographic profile* a new heavy demand for medical care for the elderly was projected.

Early responses to the concern over predicted increasing expenditure were focused upon policies of cost containment which involved, amongst other things, restrictions on the training and supply of medical manpower, limiting the purchasing power of providers of health care, and restricting capital expenditure on high technology. These types of policy were still rooted in the model of equating good health care with the consumption of medical goods and services.

> The shift away from this approach was influenced partly by the opposition of the medical profession to any attack upon their autonomy and their resistance to implementing policy, and also by the recognition that cost containment was an inadequate basis for long-term planning in so far as it was purely reactive. In the multi-national context of pharmaceutical companies and medical technology, price controls at the national level were inoperable, and so a major component of the increasing expenditure remained uncontrollable.
>
> (Towers 1992, p.192)

It was the new thinking in Canada which was to have a direct impact on the formulation of the WHO 'Health for All' strategy and an indirect influence on UK health care policy makers. In 1974 a new era of health policy in Canada based on a new agenda of prioritising preventive health care at the national level had been set in motion by the Lalonde report (1974). The real attraction to health economists of the Canadian venture was its frank acknowledgement that the key to past and future advances in health lay not in increasing access to curative medicine, but in focusing upon environmental and personal behavioural factors. Here was clear testament that curtailing the growth of traditional health care systems would not harm health status, and that small increases in the public health care sector would even result in savings on total health care costs (Lewis 1987).

In our attempt to chart a *discourse community*, it has become clear that we need to take an international perspective, and further to look at contemporary history and the key role of economists in establishing the centrality of the problem of financing public expenditure in health care planning. We now need to look at the role of another group of key participants, namely the public sector financial managers and strategists, for whom health care was an integral part of their agenda to reform radically the organisation and management of public services in Britain.

Financial management and the pressures for change

There is a sense in which financial management is now something that clinicians, managers and specialists at all levels and in all types of health service organisations are expected to practise. This means that they are more than likely to be responsible for managing a devolved budget and giving a due account of its spending. This represents a massive change from the way in which resourcing issues were traditionally dealt with, not only in the National Health Service but generally in the public service sector.

After initially making further cuts in public expenditure, the incoming Conservative administration in 1979 turned its attention towards a radical review of the management of the remaining budgets. Sir Derek Rayner, now Lord Rayner, was appointed with a 'roving brief' to look at ways of improving efficiencies in government departments. His position as Managing Director, and later Chairman, of Marks and Spencer was deemed to be particularly appropriate for the task, the more so as he had no background or affiliation with the Civil Service. In a word, he epitomised the sort of 'business ethos' that the Thatcher cabinet wanted to see running through all aspects of national life. His reports, known as 'Rayner Scrutinies', were concerned with investigating all possible ways, within a given programme or project, of achieving savings, increasing efficiency and effectiveness and implementing the resultant proposals. Whilst savings were certainly made, the real significance of his work lay in sensitising senior civil servants to the more widespread and lasting reforms that were set up in the Financial Management Initiative (FMI) (Likierman 1988).

Using the vocabulary and language of business management, the FMI aimed to promote in each government department an organisation and system in which managers at all levels:

1   clearly set out their objectives and the means of assessing and measuring their performance in relation to these objectives;

2   had responsibility for ensuring a critical scrutiny of output and value for money in the use of their allocated resources;

3   had access to all relevant information, guidance and expert advice.

This model of management differed sharply from the traditional bureaucratic system of public service administration, which stressed due process, neutrality, and direct provision. The contrast has been characterised somewhat invidiously as the difference between 'rowing' and 'steering':

The bureaucratic model brought with it a preoccupation with service delivery – with rowing. And organisations that focus their best energies on rowing rarely do much steering. They develop tunnel vision. Because they are programmed to think of government as service delivery by professionals and bureaucrats, they wait until a problem becomes a crisis, then offer new services to those affected.

(Osborne and Gaebler 1992, p.221)

Operationalisation of the new financial management in the NHS came with the Griffiths Report (1983), which established for the first time the principle of general management at regional, district and unit level, and the allocation of budgets to units. There were considerable problems in the beginning, for not only did the managers often lack the necessary financial skills to understand budgetary information, but even less well equipped were the clinicians holding their decentralised budgets (Perrin 1988). It is claimed that this problem has subsequently been dealt with by extensive use of training programmes and packages, but whether these have generated critical and creative understanding of the process or simply given a competency in pro forma budgeting techniques is open to question. Many nurses and doctors are less than enthusiastic about spending their time acquiring these new skills, and claim that this was not the reason why they chose to become medical workers. Why indeed should they be involved? One argument is that claims to clinical autonomy should be tied to an awareness of the financial costs of such activities, and that the new techniques for identifying, classifying and calculating these costs should be an integral part of the repertoire of all health care professionals (Fitzgerald 1992).

Here we need to consider another participant voice in the discourse; that of *Public Choice Theory* (Dunleavy 1991; Hughes 1994; Lawton and Rose 1994). In straightforward terms, this is a political economy theory applied to the bureaucracy. Instead of being motivated by the public interest, bureaucrats – like anyone else – are assumed to be motivated by their own selfish interests. Individual bureaucrats try to maximise their own budgets, for an increase in their share of the budget leads to an increase in their status. Bureaucracies, therefore, have a built-in incentive to expand, constantly seeking to increase their size, staff numbers, finance and scope of operations. Sociologists appeal to a similar theoretical argument when they claim that executive agencies manufacture conditions to perpetuate their own existence (Platt 1969). There is an extensive literature on medicalisation which would tend to support such claims (Conrad and Schneider 1980).

Public Choice Theory has provided the theoretical underpinnings for the strategies of allowing competition and choice through market mechanisms to determine the allocation of health care goods and services, and to return as many health care activities as possible to the private sector. It has also provided the 'intellectual gloss' for crude caricaturing of all government as pernicious and all bureaucrats as self-serving (Hughes 1994, p.262). There is, of course, something of a paradox with respect to the role of health care professionals in the NHS, who are often characterised as behaving in exactly this rational maximising way by health care managers who are, in turn, often characterised by professionals as self-serving bureaucrats.

Markets and contracts

The Conservative government of the 1980s, in political economy terms, is usually characterised as defending the philosophy and politics of neo-liberalism in the central importance it gave to the market system (Butler 1985). The basic tenet of neo-liberalism, as developed in the work of Milton Friedman

(1962, 1980), is the economic and political freedom of the individual to exercise his or her power in the market place. When money changes hands in a direct relationship, people assume that they have some power over the goods or services that they are purchasing. A free market is based on the concept of voluntary exchange where production is governed by the price mechanism, which adjusts supply accordingly; and the self-interest of everyone in the production chain acts as a co-ordinating mechanism, ensuring satisfaction for all concerned. This somewhat idealised view ascribes all positive virtues to the market, namely responsiveness, innovation, flexibility and neutrality. This last quality is often much vaunted in the claim that markets do not discriminate between individuals because it is not to their advantage to do so. However, it is quite clear that markets do discriminate against 'classes' and 'groups' of people and that the prerequisites for participation, information and purchasing power, are not evenly distributed between classes.

By contrast other writers, from a democratic socialist perspective, accept some of the benefits of a market system, such as innovation, freedom of choice and decentralisation. They also acknowledge some very considerable disbenefits (Estrin and Le Grand 1989), the most important being a grossly inequitable distribution of resources resulting from a market system which imposes 'a tyranny of small decisions which, when they are combined, produce adverse outcomes' (Williams 1992, p.32).

If we situate this debate specifically in the field of health care, we can see that those who place a primacy upon the market would stress the efficiency and innovatory role of the market. They might appeal to examples in the USA where highly innovative techniques of medical intervention have been developed and where standardised costings and integrated patient care systems have been initiated by private health insurers (Shortel and Reinhardt 1992). In contrast, those who see the need for an active interventionist role of the state would focus upon persistent and systematic inequalities in access to health care and the resultant inequitable patterns of mortality and morbidity in countries like the USA (Griffith 1987). The role of the state is minimal in the neo-liberal model of society, and it was the ideas of F.A. Hayek, the political philosopher, which attracted attention in the 1980s because they appeared to give theoretical legitimacy to the political programme of 'rolling back the frontiers of the State'. Hayek recognised that the market could only operate within a legal framework to provide protection for individuals in society; the State had the important but minimal function of establishing the rules for resolving disputes and grievances (Hayek 1976). Since the market mechanism was identified as the most efficient and effective allocator of goods and services, it follows that one of the principal ways in which the NHS could be reformed, barring full-scale transfer and privatisation, would be to introduce the disciplines of the marketplace. The concept of 'internal market', first proposed in the White paper 'Working for patients' (Department of Health 1989), and introduced in the 1990 NHS and Community Care Act descriptively, if not theoretically, captures the elements of competition between the self-governing 'service providers' and their trading relations with the 'service commissioners' who hold centrally funded but delegated budgets.

A great deal has been written about the nature of this 'market' and there is considerable debate as to whether it is a 'quasi-market' at all, given the monopoly positions that dominate it on both supply and demand sides (Robinson and Le Grand 1994). This is an important reservation, since two of the necessary conditions for a market to operate efficiently are claimed to be:

1 free competition on both purchaser and provider side;

2 adequate information about costs, prices, quality and other attributes of the goods and services available to all participants.

It appears to be the case, both in practice and in principle, that the health care market has proved particularly susceptible to attempts by participant organisations to limit competition in the following ways:

1 by creating monopolies;

2 by cornering the market by erecting entry barriers to new providers;

3 by exploiting their informational advantage by failing to provide and allow access to accurate and current information on range, type, quality, applicability, availability and efficacy of services (Robinson and Le Grand 1994, p.253).

If *markets* were seen as the best mechanism for the allocation of health care goods and services, then *contracts* were inevitably the means of managing the now formal relationships between the parties involved. A contract is based on the concept of exchange; it may be formal, binding and legally enforceable on both sides, or it may be an informal understanding of promissory intent. A formal contract involving commodities usually stipulates the exact 'quantities' to be exchanged, and is tightly specified in terms of costs, prices, quality and conditions. It is also the case that such contracts operate within a legal system which inscribes and protects the rights of individuals; for example, in the UK there is a substantial body of legislation protecting consumer rights (Williams 1992).

The position with regard to contracts involving health care goods and services is significantly different. This has led some writers to claim that, strictly speaking, they cannot be called contracts at all, and that they are really a form of *'impure contract'* (Hodgson 1988). What has to be acknowledged in the sphere of health care is that the exchange is not reducible to crudely itemised commodities; we are also dealing with sets of normative values and understandings that pertain to our sense of what it means to be a participative member of our society. Contracts are being drawn up by commissioners acting as agents on behalf of patients for services in response to identified 'need', but what is need and how is it defined and by whom? Because health care needs are so difficult to specify, contracts often have to be flexible enough to allow for variation in interpretation, and to take account of the fact not only that needs can change, but also that within the same categorical groupings they can vary greatly in form and content (Williams 1992). Since these contracts for health care services cannot be as tightly specified as other commodities, there has to be a compensatory strong element of trust between the parties concerned. However, 'trust' is a very different kind of basis for reciprocity; it is built up over time on the basis of the knowledge and understanding of both parties.

In an atmosphere of change and apprehension about health care provision there are two likely outcomes. On the one hand, both parties might favour loosely specified contracts with those organisations that they already know well and have had dealings with, and thereby discourage new competitors. On the other hand, there will be a tendency for parties to pursue vigorously tightly specified model contracts, and thereby undermine informal but highly complex and valuable relationships with organisations and service providers that have been built up over a period of years. What has often been forgotten in the heat of enthusiasm for a 'new contracting culture' is the amount of organisational resources (e.g. personnel, funds, time and expertise) necessary to cover the many *transaction costs* involved in the contracting process. These are often most apparent to practitioner staff in those health care organisations which have introduced *Service Level Agreements* as a way of formalising in contract form all those things which had hitherto been in-house services such as photocopying, telephone and computing facilities or 'informal requests' or 'favours'. The result is that the preparation and monitoring of such operations becomes work for a new managerial tier of resource controllers.

It is sociologically interesting that the 'market model', with all of its assumptions about human behaviour and rationality, is the dominant paradigm for both policy makers and analysts at this time. The cruder words and phrases for representing the commercial relationships of the health care market-place have become softened:

> 'Buyers' in the White Paper became with the passage of time, 'purchasers' and then 'commissioners'. 'Sellers' became 'providers'. General Practice 'Budgets' became 'funds'. Drug 'Budgets' became 'amounts'.
> (Robinson and Le Grand 1994, p.22)

However, behind this linguistic change remains embedded a world view of human relationships that is governed by principles of contractual exchange and on which basis not only economic viability but also political, moral and legal authority can be built. Hartsock provides a trenchant critique of this view, which has particular resonance for those whose work in health care plays such an important part in maintaining the bonds of social trust on which public institutions must rest:

> The paradigmatic connections between people on this view of the social world are instrumental or extrinsic and conflictual, and in a world populated by these isolated individuals, relations of competition and domination come to be substitutes for a more substantial and encompassing community.
> (Hartsock, quoted in Kittay and Meyers 1987, p.116)

Evaluation and performance measurement

Nobody – particularly Government – wants to volunteer the material by which they may be judged and found wanting. Nobody wants to set out clearly in advance what they mean to achieve, and then provide the information on results that show how far they have fallen short.
(Sir Gordon Downey, former Comptroller and Auditor General, 1986, quoted in Likierman 1988, p.101)

As we have seen, one of the important dimensions of a market- and contract-based health care service is reliable and up-to-date information about services on offer. Contract managers are urged by the Treasury not only to negotiate robustly to secure the best possible deal, but also to ensure that they have full information about quality, volume, cost, efficacy and reliability. In order to obtain this, the onus falls on those organisations providing health care to set up their own continuous performance-monitoring systems, and to make this information publicly understandable and available. The impact of this on health care practitioners in their everyday work is that they are subjected to an increasing level of surveillance and evaluation as new management information systems become introduced.

Only too often the experience of front-line workers in such situations is to feel that the classifications and categorisations of work tasks, which become the units of efficiency measurement, or costings that are employed by management are out of touch with reality. We may recognise that it is reasonable that in publicly funded services there should be some systematic method of monitoring and evaluating service provision, and indeed even accept the necessity to have some basis for comparative evaluation. We should also be mindful of the caution given by feminist writers on methodology. A set of abstract procedures and conceptual categories imposed on the phenomenon that is being studied too often leads to the continued compilation of an alienated 'male' knowledge that is divorced from the subject 'knower' (Farnham 1987).

There are three core areas in which managers of health care organisations are now most concerned to collect accurate information: finance, manpower utilisation and clinical activity. A heavy investment in new information technology has been justified by health care managers on the grounds that its primary function is to facilitate a meshing together of data for all three areas, and so provide a total picture of *organisational performance* at any one time. In a hospital setting, what this might mean is the linking of *data sets* on patient information (e.g. primary diagnosis, patient's doctor and planned medical procedures), clinical activity (e.g. patients treated in each diagnostic category, drugs used, theatre times) and manpower control (e.g. staff allocation between wards and larger units). Examples of new performance indicators dependent on linked data are diagnostic costings which, although not as well developed as the American diagnostically related groups (DRGs), are used across districts and regions in order to identify average treatment costs for closely defined diagnostic categories (Coombs and Green 1992).

The medical profession has always had a profound antipathy to any attempts to make its work conform to predetermined standards. The following extract comes from an editorial in *The Times* in 1921, in response to the Ministry of Health instruction that all Panel Doctors be required to use the newly agreed International Classification of Diseases (ICD) categories on patient record cards. It was claimed that overworked doctors would be forced to name diseases such as tuberculosis rather than simply to record their own general and often idiosyncratic observations, and that this would generate a whole set of new erroneous policies:

> . . . the new record cards will tell us nothing but untruths, untruths will go to Whitehall and be bound in blue covers. We shall learn again that we are the least healthy nation in Europe or the World and great and costly schemes of regeneration will be submitted to Parliament.
>
> (*The Times*, 5 January 1921)

Here, surely, are the same sort of heartfelt concerns that are expressed today by practitioners and professionals in a broad range of health care work. Despite the drive by health care managers to embrace all sections of their organisation in a *total quality performance evaluation*, the medical profession has still managed to secure for itself an almost insulated niche in which to perform its own *medical audit*. The Department of Health defined this as:

> . . . the systematic, critical analysis of the quality of medical care, including the procedures used for diagnosis and treatment, the use of resources and the resultant outcome and quality of life for the patient . . .
>
> (Kerrison *et al.* 1994, p.155)

In practice, it has become a confidential peer review process that is owned and led by the medical profession.

It is easy to see how these kinds of defensive manoeuvres are often inseparable from the defence of past monopolies, privileges and class/gender power. It is one of the acute paradoxes generated by the Thatcher administration that it targeted professional power which was genuinely felt to be ripe for more accountability, but substituted a new financial managerial hierarchy equally contemptuous of participatory decision-making and democratisation of knowledge. There is a debate amongst sociologists as to whether the origins of this managerial perspective, with its emphasis upon simplistic quantitative output measures, lie in the work of the American F.W. Taylor (Cassell 1993). Pollitt, for example, is clear about the connection:

> The chief feature of both classic Taylorism and its 1980's descendant was that they were, above all, concerned with *control* and that this control was to be achieved through an essentially *administrative* approach – the fixing of effort levels that were to be expressed in quantitative terms.
>
> (Pollitt 1990, p.177)

Writing at the turn of the century, Taylor was concerned to apply the methods and techniques of science to create efficient organisations. At that time, this meant the painstaking observation of working processes and their disaggregation into the most simple discrete tasks that could be precisely defined, timed and controlled; efficiency could then be calculated as a mechanical measure from time and motion studies. He posited a notion of the worker as something of an automaton who would only respond to financial incentives automatically; hence managerial control rested upon a system of piece rate payment, strict job specification and close surveillance (Taylor 1911).

Braverman, writing in the 1970s, looked at how far Taylorist methods had permeated all sectors of western capitalist economies, and had resulted in a progressive but radical *deskilling* of their workforces (Braverman 1974). He claimed that deskilled workforces inevitably result from management's compulsion to assert direct control over workers. He analysed in particular what he called the 'Taylorization' of office and other service work, which led to work becoming fragmented, the skill requirements for the bulk of jobs being lost or progressively eroded, and the holistic integration of 'conception' and 'execution' in work being destroyed. Whilst Braverman has been criticised for failing to recognise the extent of resistance to these measures, and for ignoring the amount of reskilling that accompanied the deskilling, there is broad agreement that the impact of the transformation of the labour process through job design, work study, skill mix and performance monitoring has been profoundly demoralising for the majority of staff employed in health care services.

What this whole section has perhaps failed to acknowledge, which the opening quote from Downey so disarmingly did manage to do, is that most people feel uneasy about having their work monitored and assessed. How do we account for this? Is it because they do not see assessment in terms of 'feedback' but rather as 'criticism'? Is it linked to our educational experience of seeing assessment as 'grading' and ultimately about allocation to the good jobs/things in life/rewards? Is it significant that we have trust in the people doing the evaluation? In which case, surely a disinterested outsider using scientific methods is best placed to be unbiased? Or is it that we prefer to be evaluated by someone who 'really knows us', not only someone within our own peer group but someone we like and trust?

Deskilling and flexibility

There is a large and growing literature on skill mix and the management of labour processes in nursing. The majority of this material emanates from a neo-Taylorist perspective; despite genuflecting at the altar of qualitative factors, it is primarily concerned with simplistic quantitative measures, 'outputs', that have a direct and mechanical relationship to nursing care, the 'product'. Too often writers not only ignore dimensions of process but also iron out complex conceptual and practical strategies that are situation-specific and are intrinsic to the messy business of interacting with human beings on a routine and harmonious basis (Carr-Hill *et al.* 1992).

There is still a tendency amongst work study writers to deconstruct the work processes of nursing into 'tasks', thereby ignoring the whole historical background within which groups and collectivities have negotiated and constructed their 'work knowledge', repertoires, traditions and interpretive schemas, as well as the more straightforward professional codes of practice and occupational ideologies. Sociologists have demonstrated that the work world is a complex cultural system and that perceived threats to any one part of it are interpreted within a network of norms, values and beliefs that involve core senses of the self, as opposed to simple adaptations to a changed work role (Fagin and Little 1984). We can see this articulated most clearly by occupational groups who, through their professional training and socialisation, have a well-developed sense of what it means to be a 'doctor', a 'lawyer', or a 'priest'. It is present and also articulated in different and less public forums by such groups as milkmen and home-helps (Littler 1985).

The problem for health care workers, like nurses, is how to defend those elements of their occupation which they feel to be inviolable in a language and form which will be heard in the new financial planning and commissioning domains (Evers *et al.* 1992). How can this be achieved? First, there is a necessity to set out clearly those elements of the work process, the work role and the occupational ideology which practising nurses think are important, and to take seriously their claim that they wish to be evaluated on their ability to fulfil those elements. The next stage would be to identify precisely where such elements conflict with the new managerial expectations and performance indicators, to explore how far there are irreconcilable differences, and how far the defence of any one element is integral or peripheral.

Perhaps a good way of thinking this through is to imagine how you might evaluate your own work this year. Take some time to identify clearly what you think are the general categories within which you fit your performance, and then identify which of them feel wrong; ask yourself what other categories might cover the aspects that you think are important but do not seem to be captured. Compare what you have constructed with the formal assessment criteria under which you have to operate as a student.

Maybe because contemporary management information systems are almost exclusively computer-based, there is a tendency for those who feel unhappy about the ability of such systems to capture their own working reality and performance to target their hostility on to 'the computer', which rapidly becomes *anthropomorphised* into a managerial archetype, an autocratic, unfeeling figure. There is evidence that district nurses, who as an occupational group have recently been subjected to some intensive performance and work-study evaluations, become extremely antagonistic to the computer and its data-inputting system with its fixed menu of task categories (Towers 1994). They see it as an alien instrument, neither belonging to them nor cast in their own language and everyday conceptual categories. It becomes something to be overcome or outsmarted. There is little evidence of nurses acknowledging that the problem lies with the particular software; its design specifications are often the result of management choices and decisions. Frontline practitioners might potentially have some scope not only to influence codes and categories, but also to make the whole system provide the information and do the work that they want. For instance, the feminist writer Sherry Turkle urges women to view the computer's role as an 'object to think with' rather than bracing themselves for a battle of control over the machine and mastery of the 'correct' programming style (Turkle 1984).

In contrast to Braverman's picture of a general deskilling of the labour force, there is another view which argues that, although there is a radical transformation of work taking place, it is leading to the creation of more *flexible* work situations and segmented work-forces (Atkinson 1988). Atkinson's approach is focused on the explicit strategies employers and managers use to create greater flexibility in their organisations. A flexible organisation is one which extends the amount of work it subcontracts and concentrates on fewer core activities, while in those remaining core areas it introduces more flexible work regimes and employment contracts. We have seen in the earlier sections of this chapter how the health care system in the UK has moved from an early start in subcontracting towards a more radical 'hiving off' of activities and privatisation; it has also made significant moves towards the creation of a 'flexible' labour market. This new structure is characterised by a small *core* of employees and a *peripheral* workforce. The small core is composed of employees

> . . . with full time permanent status central to the long term future of the organisation, enjoying greater job security, good promotion and reskilling prospects, and relatively generous pension, insurance and other fringe benefits, this group is expected to be adaptable, flexible and, if necessary, geographically mobile.
>
> (Harvey 1994, p.150)

There are two main groups in the peripheral workforce. The first group is composed of full-time employees, but they tend to be seen as 'disposable' because their skills are readily available in the labour market. They have fewer employment rights, minimal benefits and no career development opportunities. The second group is composed of part-timers and temporaries, including public subsidy trainees, 'casuals', job sharers and fixed contract staff. Overall, they provide great numerical flexibility but have even less job security and worse remuneration. At the extreme edge of this category, there are temporary agency staff or 'the bank', who have no employment contracts with the organisation at all. There is evidence of a significant growth of both part-time and 'bank' staff amongst health workers, and they are often central to the functioning of many provider units in the UK health services (Walby *et al.* 1994).

Whatever way we evaluate these theories and appraise the empirical studies linked to them, it is clear that the pattern of employment, the work process and the organisational structure of health care work have been radically transformed in the last 20 years (McDowell 1992).

Conclusions

We can conclude that, when we talk about the 'new managerialism' in the context of the management of the UK health service, we are referring to a collection of policies and practices which were triggered by the fiscal crisis of the mid-1970s but had their roots in the ideological platform of New Right theorising. Christopher Pollitt argues that the new managerialism is not a theory but an ideological movement:

> Managerialism is the 'acceptable face' of New Right thinking concerning the State. It is an ingredient in the pot pourri which can attract support beyond the New Right itself. For that wider constituency 'better management' provides a label under which private sector disciplines can be introduced to the public services, political control can be strengthened, budgets trimmed, professional autonomy reduced, public service unions weakened and a quasi-competitive framework erected to flush out the 'natural' inefficiencies of bureaucracy.
>
> (Pollitt 1990, p.49)

Our table of participants in the health management discourse has cut across disciplinary boundaries. Instead of the usual counterbalancing of viewpoints, however, there has been an almost disconcerting unanimity in which the common language of managerialism has had a mesmeric effect upon academics and commentators who would normally be noted for their profound distrust and scepticism of such ideas. However, I would argue that what has arisen is a momentary state of sterile orthodoxy which is already collapsing as it is confronted by the mounting political reality of voices of dissent. What this promises is a return to the more familiar and fertile territory in which sociological and indeed all forms of productive discourse can flourish.

Acknowledgements

I should like to thank David and Alice-Claire Painting for their sustaining assistance with the production of this chapter.

CASE STUDY

All institutions and individuals are fictitious. The idea for using an incident in a cardiac unit came from an American case study 'Malpractice or minor mistake', published in *People in Organisations* edited by Terence Mitchell and James R. Larson, and published by McGraw-Hill (USA) in 1987.

An incident in the cardiac unit at Gainsborough General Hospital

Gainsborough General is a modern general hospital, built in 1978 and with newer additions made in 1984. It is located within the Thameside Regional Health Authority and has held Trust Status since 1992. The hospital acts as a training centre for nurses, and also as a medical teaching centre; it has over 550 acute sector beds.

On 10 January an incident occurred on Samuel ward in the cardiac unit which attracted some media interest and thereby brought the hospital into public view over its handling of complaints of malpractice. At an emergency meeting of the Executive Board, it was decided to appoint a specialist team of management consultants to investigate the incident and to report back to the board with recommendations. Basics Public Sector Management Team (BPSMT) have long experience in working with discretion and sensitivity in precisely these sorts of situations, and they can be relied upon to produce an informed and thorough report within a tight time schedule.

The incident
On 10 January half-way through the afternoon shift on Samuel ward (acute medical ward specialising in cardiology), it was brought to the attention of the charge nurse (Sister 'N') that patient 'X' (a 49-year-old male), who had been well on the road to recovery (planned discharge date 13 January), was in the midst of a serious relapse. The charge nurse made a number of quick enquiries and the following situation emerged.

Nurse 'P' (C grade), a part-time direct employee since 1 January (previously she had been a full-time bank nurse), had set up an IVAC unit (intravenous delivery) at the beginning of the shift to deliver some Inderol to patient 'X', in accordance with nursing procedures governing the administration of medication by intravenous route. Inderol reduces the rate of the heart beat, and the precise delivery dosage is finely specified by the prescribing and attending physician. Later in the shift the patient's pulse was significantly slower and somewhat more irregular than it should have been, and the patient was showing signs of distress. The attending physician (Dr 'Z') was called, and whilst examining the patient, she noticed that the wrong tubing had been put in the IVAC. As a result, the patient was receiving the drug at approximately five times the prescribed dosage. The IVAC was immediately taken down, the patient began to show signs of cardiac arrest and emergency procedures were instituted to save his life. These were unsuccessful, and later that night the patient died.

Sister 'N' was required to submit a preliminary report and to interview Nurse 'P' the following day. Her report sets the context of the incident and is summarised below.

The context
The ward is extremely busy and is persistently running under full staffing levels: sickness and absenteeism rates are high, and at times bank nurses, predominantly lower grades, are the mainstay of the shift. The ward has been the subject of a Work Study exercise, and Skill Mix teams have been introduced since October in order to reduce the skilled nursing manpower needs. The ward design is a modern nuclear one, and the charge nurse exercises a supervisory/managerial role, although at times she might have to spend 75% of her time in patient-centred nursing care. When patient loads are heavy, it is not unusual for A- and B-grade nurses (only a few of whom have ENB qualifications) to take sole responsibility for nursing procedures which should involve more highly qualified, higher grade nurses. Attending physicians are not likely to take undermanning amongst nursing staff into consideration when planning and organising treatment procedures. It

is simply unrealistic to expect double-checking on medication in the present climate, where it is frequently impossible to accomplish all the shift tasks without help and assistance from patients and their visitors.

Most nurses have come to accept a high rate of 'near misses' in their work, and would admit to a sense of trepidation that an incident such as that which happened on 10 January was 'waiting to happen'. They have expressed this through the nursing management channels at the hospital and at the ward level. However, it is also widely believed that, in the event of an enquiry, it is the individual unskilled nurse who will be 'scapegoated', and responsibility will be located at the ward or unit level, leaving senior management relatively untouched by such events, except in their handling of the surrounding publicity.

Morale on the ward and in the unit is now at a perilously low level, and the few remaining long-serving senior nurses on the ward have indicated that they will seek relocation within the Region.

Tasks for BPSMT to be completed in report form

1   What is your initial judgement about the cause of the patient's death?

2   What sorts of additional information will you need to acquire, and how will you set about getting this? Produce a detailed plan of how you propose to investigate. (Draw on comparisons with other hospital procedures.)

3   What sort of recommendations for action are appropriate? Distinguish between short-term and long-term recommendations.

and finally, as an adjunct to the report:

4   Explore, either by way of a focus group or a discussion paper, the implications of this incident for the ways in which a clinical team can handle conflict over issues of professional practice. Identify clearly the different avenues open to members.

References

Argenti, J. 1980: *Practical corporate planning*. London: Allen & Unwin.

Ashton, J. 1990: Public health and primary care: towards a common agenda. *Public Health* **104**, 387–398.

Atkinson, J. 1988: Recent changes in the internal labour market structure in the UK. In Buitelaar, W. (ed.), *Technology and work: labour studies in England, Germany and the Netherlands*. Aldershot: Avebury, 139–145.

Beck, U. 1992: *The risk society: towards a new modernity*. London: Sage.

Benzeval, M., Judge, K. and Whitehead, M. 1995: *Tackling inequalities in health*. London: Kings Fund.

Braverman, H. 1974: *Labor and monopoly capital: the degradation of work in the twentieth century*. New York and London: Monthly Review Press.

Buchanan, J. A. and Tullock, G. 1962: *The calculus of consent: the logical foundations of constitutional democracy*. Ann Arbor: University of Michigan.

Butler, E. 1985: *Milton Friedman. A guide to his economic thought*. London: Temple Smith.

Carr-Hill, R., Dixon, P., Gibbs, I. *et al.* 1992: *Skill mix and the effectiveness of nursing care*. York: Centre for Health Economics.

Cassell, P. 1993: *The Giddens reader*. London: Macmillan.

Conference of Socialist Economists 1979: *Struggle over the state*. London: Conference of Socialist Economists.

Conrad, P. and Schneider, J. 1980: *Deviance and medicalization*. St Louis: Mosby.

Coombs, R. and Green, K. 1992: Work organization and product change in the service sector: the case of the U.K. National Health Service. In Wood, S. (ed.), *The transformation of work?* London: Routledge, 279–295.

Department of Health 1989: *Working for patients*. London: HMSO.

Department of Health 1994: *On the state of the public health: the annual report of the Chief Medical Officer of the Department of Health for the year 1993*. London: HMSO.

Department of Health and Social Services, Northern Ireland 1992: *A regional strategy for Northern Ireland 1992–97*. Belfast: Department of Health and Social Services, Northern Ireland.

Dunleavy, P. 1991: *Democracy, bureaucracy and public choice: economic explanations in political science*. London: Harvester Wheatsheaf.

Estrin, S. and Le Grand, J. (eds) 1989: *Market socialism*. Oxford: Clarendon Press.

Evers, H., Badger, F. and Cameron, E. 1992: Finding the limits. *Nursing Times*, **88 (30)**, 60–62.

Fagin, L. and Little, M. 1984: *The forsaken families*. Harmondsworth: Penguin.

Farnham, C. (ed.) 1987: *The impact of feminist research in the academy*. Bloomington: Indiana University Press.

Fitzgerald, L. 1992: Clinicians into management: on the change agenda or not? *Health Services Management Research* **5(2)**, 137–146.

Friedman, M. 1962: *Capitalism and freedom*. Chicago: University of Chicago Press.

Friedman, M. 1980: *Free to choose*. Harmondsworth: Penguin.

Griffith, B. 1987: *Banking on sickness: commercial medicine in Britain and the USA*. London: Lawrence & Wishart.

Griffiths, R. 1983: *NHS management enquiry*. London: DHSS.

Harvey, D. 1994: *The condition of postmodernity*. Oxford: Blackwell Science Ltd.

Hayek, F. 1976: *The road to serfdom*. London: Routledge and Kegan Paul.

Health Promotion Authority for Wales (HPAW) 1990: *Health for all in Wales: health promotion challenges for the 1990's, Part B*. Wales: Health Promotion Authority for Wales.

Hodgson, G. 1988: *Economics and institutions*. London: Polity Press.

Hood, C. 1991: A public management for all seasons? *Public Administration*, **69**, 3–19.

House of Commons 1992: *The health of the nation: a strategy of health for England*, Command Paper No. 1986. London: HMSO.

Hughes, O. 1994: *Public management and administration*. Basingstoke: Macmillan.

Kerrison, S., Packwood, T. and Buxton, M. 1994: Monitoring medical audit. In Robinson, R. and Le Grand, J. (eds), *Evaluating the NHS reforms*. London: Kings Fund, 155–178.

Kittay, E. and Meyers, D. (eds) 1987: *Women and moral theory*. Maryland: Rowman and Littlefield.

Lalonde, M. 1974: *A new perspective on the health of Canadians: a working document*. Ottawa: Ministry of National Health and Welfare.

Lawton, A. and Rose, A. 1994: *Organisation and management in the public sector*. London: Pitman.

Lewis, J. 1987: What has become of public health? Past patterns and future prospects in England, Ontario and Quebec. *Public Health* **101**, 357–368.

Likierman, A. 1988: *Public expenditure: who really controls it and how.* London: Penguin.

Littler, C. 1985: *The experience of work.* London: Gower.

McDowell, L. 1992: Gender divisions in a post-fordist era: new contradictions or the same old story? In McDowell, L. and Pringle, R. (eds), *Defining women: social institutions and gender divisions.* Milton Keynes: Open University Press, 181–192.

Organisation for Economic Co-ordination and Development 1985: *Measuring health care 1960–83.* Paris: Organisation for Economic Co-ordination and Development.

Organisation for Economic Co-ordination and Development 1987: *Financing and Delivering Health Care.* Paris: Organisation for Economic Co-ordination and Development.

Osborne, D. and Gaebler, T. 1992: *Reinventing government: how the entrepreneurial spirit is transforming the public sector.* Reading: Addison-Wesley.

Parker, I. 1992: *Discourse dynamics.* London: Routledge.

Payer, L. 1989: *Medicine and culture.* London: Gollancz.

Perrin, J. 1988: *Resource management in the NHS.* Wokingham: Van Nostrand.

Pfohl, S. 1994: *Images of deviance and social control.* New York: McGraw-Hill.

Platt, A. 1969: *The child-savers.* Chicago: University of Chicago Press.

Pollitt, C. 1990: *Managerialism in the public services: the Anglo-American experience.* Oxford: Basil Blackwell.

Robinson, R. and Le Grand, J. (eds) 1994: *Evaluating the NHS reforms.* London: Kings Fund.

Scottish Office 1992: *Scotland's health: a challenge to us all: a policy statement.* Edinburgh: HMSO.

Shortell, S. and Reinhardt, U. 1992: *Improving health policy and management.* Ann Arbor: Health Administration Press.

Stacey, M. 1991: Medical sociology and health policy: an historical overview. In Gabe, J., Calnan, M. and Bury, M. (eds), *The sociology of the health service.* London: Routledge, 11–35.

Taylor, F. 1911: *Principles and methods of scientific management.* New York: Harper.

Thompson, K. and Tunstall, J. 1971: *Sociological perspectives.* Harmondsworth: Penguin.

Towers, B. 1992: From AIDS to Alzheimer's: policy and politics in setting new health agendas. In Bailey, J. (ed.), *Social Europe.* London: Longman, 190–215.

Towers, B. 1993: Politics and policy: historical perspectives on screening. In Berridge, V. and Strong, P. (eds), *AIDS and contemporary history.* Cambridge: Cambridge University Press, 55–73.

Towers, B. 1994: Holism and fragmentation: directions of change in District Nursing. In Lomax, P. and Darley, J. (eds), *Management research in the public sector.* Bournemouth: Hyde Publications, 45–61.

Towers, B. 1995: Red Cross organisational politics, 1918–22: relations of dominance and the influence of the United States. In Weindling, P. (ed.), *International health organisations and movements 1918–1939.* Cambridge: Cambridge University Press, 36–56.

Townsend, P. and Davidson, N. 1982: The Black Report. In Townsend, P., Davidson, N. and Whitehead, M. *Inequalities in health: the Black Report and the health divide.* London: Penguin.

Townsend, P., Davidson, N. and Whitehead, M. 1992: *Inequalities in Health: The Black Report and the Health Divide*. London: Penguin.

Turkle, S. 1984: *The second self: computers and the human spirit*. London: Granada.

Walby, S., Greenwell, J., Mackay, L. and Soothill, K. 1994: *Medicine and nursing: professions in a changing health service*. London: Sage.

Williams, C. 1992: 'Contracts or community investment' (unpubl.). M.A. dissertation, Kingston University, Surrey.

World Bank 1993: *World Development Report 1993: Investing in Health*. New York: Oxford University Press.

World Health Organisation 1986: *Evaluation of the Strategy for Health for All by the Year 2000, vol. 5*. Copenhagen: World Health Organisation.

World Health Organisation 1988: *World Health Statistics Annual*. Geneva: World Health Organisation.

World Health Organisation 1994: *Health in Europe: The 1993–1994 Health for All Monitoring Report*. Copenhagen: World Health Organisation.

3 Social symbolism of health: the notion of the soul in professional care

Paul Barber

Introduction

This chapter questions the conventional notions with which professionals address health and plan care. Health, I suggest, is professionally approached in an ill way which does not respect the individual as an integral whole. This text explores the various reality orientations that influence professional socialisation and the carer–client relationship in hospital. Finally, I argue that health must be approached in an holistic way, and that disease should be seen as an expression of disharmony between the soma and the psyche.

Themes and issues raised in the discussion are supported by personal observations of medical and nursing practices. My vision of health is informed by experiences gleaned while a psychiatric nurse, a recipient of surgery, a visitor of others in hospital and as a researcher, supervisor and psychotherapist. The perspective I hope to introduce is essentially a humanistic one, alive to symbolic interactionism and attentive to the transpersonal.

'Humanism' puts a high value on human experience. It is alert to the uniqueness of each individual and our ability to learn from experience. It emphasises the authority of personal relationships whereby feelings, emotions and intuition become recognised tools of enquiry (Hillman 1975). Symbolic interactionism raises awareness of the fact that people respond to meanings rather than actual events. It suggests that what we conventionally term 'reality' may be no more than a social creation (Giddens 1989). The transpersonal (phenomena above and beyond the person) helps us to entertain the unknown and unknowable. It also opens our eyes to paradox and to the possibility that there are powers deep within the person with a potential for healing and growth (Hayes 1994).

> Men do not understand how to see the invisible through the visible. They do not realise the arts they employ are reflections of their own natures. For all things are like and unlike, compatible and incompatible, communicating and non-communicating, intelligent and without intelligence. Each is a paradox.
>
> (Hippocrates, quoted in Elliott-Binns 1978)

I present quotes at the beginning of each section to alert the reader to the paradoxical nature of things, and to offer an unusual view of the world. By this means I hope to have challenged professional knowledge claims of purity, certainty and the benefits of impartiality. My arguments will be introduced and discussed in the following order:

1   an holistic approach to health, with reference to oriental medicine and the notion of the soul as the vital essence or energy of the person;

2   I accuse current medicine of having lost its soul, and I draw on its ancient roots to show a time when medicine was holistic and attentive to the divine nature of human beings;

3   how growth and expression of the soul is hampered by socialisation, and all too often educated out of professional care givers through a belief in the dictates of science;

4   how a traditional perspective in health and disease mechanises care, and blinds us to our intrinsic potential for growth; leaving us akin to 'ghosts trapped in a machine';

5   I show how various levels of perception or value orientations influence the way in which we construct 'reality' and effect the dynamics of care. I examine the professional carer–client relationship and how this becomes laden with personal and symbolic material drawn from our earlier social and family history;

6   I end with a consideration of the intrapersonal and transpersonal influences within illness and hospital care, and how disease, though a painful and lonely process can house a potential for spiritual growth;

7   in the final section, I review and draw together the above strands and argue for an integrated approach to the training of care professionals.

Holistic health: recognising the soul in the soma

> The individual unit of evolution is the soul (. . .) In our religious thoughts we acknowledge what we call the soul, but we have not, until now, taken it seriously enough to consider what the existence of the soul means in terms of everyday experience, in terms of the joys and pains and sorrows and fulfilments that make a human life.
>
> (Zukav 1990)

To all intents and purposes I was healthy, mobile, free of discomfort and open to the joys and sadness of human existence, and felt myself to be in good psychological shape. I reasoned, however, that if I was to write a chapter critical of traditional approaches to health and addressing the nourishment of the soul – the essence that sparks to life our mind and body – it was only proper for me to investigate this within myself experientially.

Initially, I was at a loss as to where to start, until I remembered times within 'personal growth' and psychotherapy workshops, when an 'inner me' had felt touched. This usually happened after a period of struggle – when my intellect had given up its attempt to make sense of what had been preoccupying me and my body released emotional energy which catapulted me from the outer world to a place I felt better able to witness myself, deep within. At times like these I felt whole and healed, as if my soul was being nourished. A sense of integration would follow, of being at one with the whole universe, rather than being a self apart.

> I study an ant within the grass (. . .) The planet is alive with life. The ant, the grass, myself are one breath existing singularly yet together; links in the universe's web of feeling (. . .) My emotions and thoughts are no longer locked in isolation. My being moves and feels and thinks as one.
>
> (Barber 1990)

Experiences such as these transform the perceiver and what is being perceived; they are nearer to an appreciation of a divine form, a superreality that underpins and interrelates the whole. From the above stance, splits of intellect and feeling heal, and everything starts to integrate. Many students, clients and colleagues have shared with me experiences similar to my own. Such events appear common to the species, although unique to the person. They are times, I suggest, when you witness the world from the vantage point of your soul.

One Saturday morning I entered a local church hall to browse within the closing moments of a fête. In a remote dark corner was a book stall to which I felt intuitively drawn. I went over and picked up the first book that caught my eye, *The Kung Fu Exercise Book* (Minick 1975). Opening the cover I scanned the first page:

> Some of the most advanced forms of therapeutic exercise ever developed by man have been practised for years in mainland China, almost unbeknownst to the whole Western world (. . .) The system I am going to describe is far more than just a pattern of exercises. It is an integral part of Chinese medicine.
>
> (Minick 1975)

In the following pages some 18 exercises were described. There were warm-up exercises to loosen the sinews, and some to help lower the body's centre of gravity and focus the mind. Some exercises were seen to expand the chest cavity, some to develop internal organs such as the spleen and stomach, while others were aimed at the endocrine glands, sympathetic and parasympathetic nervous systems. Others were stated to boost, stir and direct inner energy, to correct nausea, diarrhoea and breathlessness.

These exercises, said to be some 6000 years old, were similar to Tai-Ch'i. They demanded no strain, indeed quite the contrary, they asked me to move slowly, to breathe deeply and relax. The main feature, however, was not of a physical but of a meditative nature. They had to be performed 'mindfully'. To rush through them or to be mentally distracted was to defeat their purpose. Mindfulness was encouraged by the pattern of breathing they required. They demanded not only deep abdominal breathing but an act of creative imagination, for they required me to visualise my inward breath as entering through my nose, circulating to the back of my head and passing down to the base of my spine, and my outgoing breath as running up the front of my abdomen and out via my mouth.

It all seemed very complex and I was not sure what it was about. However, in the spirit of enquiry I began the 15-minute programme suggested, involving slow stretching movements accompanied by the breathing form described. It took some time before my breathing and visualisation began to synchronise with my movement, but when it did, I felt focused and exercised all over. Mentally, I concentrated upon co-ordinating my movements and breathing; physically, I strove to relax while moving gracefully and breathing deeply; imaginatively, I attempted to visualise the circulation of my breath.

After the first few days I began to experience myself as breathing more deeply, feeling more physically supported and psychologically calm. A month later, I noticed I was working longer hours without my usual fatigue, and observed that my concentration was improved; a newly acquired sense of alertness and peace accompanied all I did. Six months later I noticed that my abdomen muscles, which for some 7 years – following surgical intervention – had bunched together unevenly in an 'S' shape when I bent forward, were now even and co-ordinated again. So what was happening?

The oriental explanation was that these exercises developed Ch'i, a term which translates into 'breath', 'air' or 'energy', the vital force or spirit within each of us. This is roughly equivalent to the western concept of the soul. We shall find later in this chapter that pantheism, a respect for the divine in nature such as this, was integral to the classical roots of medicine. Theory aside, I had begun to feel more fully integrated, as if the cement holding me together was being strengthened and revitalised.

I reasoned that my abdominal muscles changed position because I had revitalised the energy blueprint which shaped me. This rationale is also cited for the change obtained from acupuncture, holistic massage, shiatsu and other energy-focusing, body-orientated therapies. The holistic integration of the spiritual with the physical challenges the western 'scientific' orientation where one thing is isolated from another, in order to be studied and understood (see Chapter 4). In health, as with the soul, the sum of the parts does not equal the whole.

Interestingly, the notion that we have an energy or *etheric* body connecting the physiological and spiritual aspects of existence is not totally alien to western thought. It is to be found in the tradition of spirit healing:

> Energy (sometimes called 'primary' or 'etheric energy') is the substance and the medium. There is no dividing line between any state of matter, force or life.
>
> (Edwards 1976)

In this perspective, the concept of the 'spirit body' is taken to be an exact replica, or counterpart, of the physical. 'It reflects good health or any disharmony shown in the physical state' (Edwards 1950). Nowadays, many of us find it hard to believe in a spirit body, yet we may readily subscribe to scientific notions of a most fantastical nature, e.g. belief in an atom requires the same act of faith as belief in a spirit body.

Personally, I take the stance of a phenomenologist, in that I attempt to accept everything but believe nothing absolutely. To me everything is an approximation of the truth. This phenomenological view of the world places emphasis upon what I experience rather than what I conceive. In other words, it strongly suggests that beyond data drawn from physiological sense-experience there are other reality orientations such as dreaming, lucid dreaming, meditative and spiritual states in which one is intuitively guided.

While the western scientific attitude to disease has become increasingly secular and pragmatic, Chinese medicine retains a spiritual orientation to health. It cites natural laws within the universe to which we can attune, through heightened consciousness and imaginative intent, to revitalise our body, mind and spirit (Chang 1978). In this context, disharmony brings disease. Conversely, western medicine tends to see disease as a result of infectious agents. While westerners exercise their muscles and try to prevent illness through modification of the external environment, people of the east exercise the internal organs and try to fine-tune the spiritual infrastructure which holds the body together.

Six questions are commonly asked by oriental physicians in order to ascertain a person's physical/spiritual health.

1 Are you free from fatigue?
   (Fatigue is taken as a sign that the person is not functioning properly or

fighting disease; healthy people are seen to be joyful, interested and bring a zest for life to all they do.)

2   Do you sleep soundly?
    (A fully engaged person as described above is seen to sleep deeply and soundly, free of disturbing dreams and able to awaken on time at the hour visualised prior to sleeping.)

3   Is your appetite good?
    (A healthy appetite is taken as a sign of vitality and internal harmony, not that being overweight is in any way natural; a man or woman unable to be satisfied runs counter to the laws of nature.)

4   Are you good humoured?
    (To lose one's temper quickly, to harm others or harbour a grudge is taken to be a sign of being out of touch with humanity.)

5   Is your memory good?
    (A failing memory is seen to be a sign of declining physical and emotional stability; a healthy memory is taken to grow, not decline, with age.)

6   Are you precise in thought and action?
    (The inability to respond to the environment instinctively is seen to show disharmony, for in the natural process of things you adapt to the environment rather than it adapting to you.)

The first three questions are physical guidelines, and are allocated something of the order of 10 points apiece. The fourth and fifth questions focus upon psycho-spiritual health and are deemed to be worth 20 points each. The sixth question, also psycho-spiritual, is worth 30 points. How would you score within the above dimensions?

Holistic health necessitates harmony between the body, the mind and the spirit. The questions shared above are designed to explore the health of the cement holding these together. Holistic health may be taken to be a good indicator of the robustness of one's soul.

How western medicine came to lose its soul

So often western thought separates the soul from the body and the body from the mind. Consequently, we lose sight of the interrelatedness that defines the whole:

The body is the instrument of the soul. If the piano player is sick, does it help to repair his or her piano? (. . .) The body needs rest, and it needs care, but behind every aspect of health or illness of the body is the energy of the soul.

(Zukav 1990)

Western medicine has evolved into a science too often isolated from its art. If it were a person it would be busy in thought and attuned to its senses, hard-working and conscientious, but generally impoverished in imagination, denying feeling, and consequently unskilled in developing empathy or managing intimacy in interpersonal relationships. When you adopt this stance, you move towards the position of the analytical scientist who believes that:

> To know is to be certain about something. Certainty is defined by the ability to 'phrase' or enumerate the components of an object, event, person, or situation in a precise, accurate, and reliable fashion. Therefore knowledge is synonymous with precision, accuracy, and reliability. Any endeavour that cannot be subject to this formula or line of reasoning is either suppressed, devalued, or set aside as not worth knowing or capable of being known.
>
> (Mitroff and Kilmann 1978)

Homage to the scientific model is the cost which society has extracted from medicine in exchange for its respectable reputation. Some medics have become critical of this non-dialectical, split, and strictly logical approach to medicine:

> If one takes the 'disease' first and thinks about it carefully one will come to the conclusion that there is no such thing. The word 'pneumonia' for example is hypothetical. There are patients with pneumonia and there are lungs affected by pneumonia, but pneumonia itself is a fiction. In other words disease only exists officially if given a name by a doctor. The disease, patient and doctor are inextricably woven together.
>
> (Elliott-Binns 1978)

Pneumonia is not an entity, but rather a working label. The purely rational tradition to which medicine has come to belong, in distancing disease from its psycho-social and spiritual context, perpetuates its own myths (Harre 1981).

Science claims to be bias-free, but is often anything but pure in its assumptions. Its superficial view looks to logic to replace emotional and/or spiritual meaning, and substitutes 'the world as seen' for 'the world as experienced and felt'. Scientific methodology is, therefore, heavily biased towards rationality, emotional neutrality and impartiality. But what do these qualities imply?

Rationality suggests that everything is understandable through logical reasoning and deduction, a classic error of mistaking the map for the territory. Emotional neutrality implies that emotions are less useful tools of enquiry, calling into question human experience and experiential enquiry. Impartiality denotes a scientist concerned only with the production of new knowledge, rather than the consequences of its use. This, I suggest, is an irresponsible and immoral stance which has caused much evil in the world.

These values call for you to suspend judgement of non-rational phenomena such as intuition and love, and 'put your head before your heart'. In short, they call for an act of faith. This 'scientism' has enriched the material world, but it has led to the creation of a spiritual wasteland. Are such values really conducive to the practice of health and care? Many of my medical friends think not, and have begun to incorporate homeopathy, acupuncture and psychotherapy to enrich their practice of the healing arts. In this way, they return to the artist-healers of old, men of the spirit to whom the founders of medicine, Aesculapius and Hippocrates, belonged:

> . . . the followers of Aesculapius, known as the Aesclepaides, must be regarded as having been a priestly caste who, we know, were bound by the oath of the Hippocrates jusjurandum not to divulge the secrets of their profession, such mysteries, to be sure, having a psychic as well as a physical base.
>
> (Desmond 1956)

Hippocrates, like homoeopaths of our day, advocated giving the patient 'a draught made from the root of mandrake, in a smaller dose than sufficient to induce mania', or as Antiphones had it, 'Take the hair, it is well written, of the dog by which you were bitten' (Desmond 1956). We learn that Galen, another great name in early medicine, was a genuine psychic. In his professional life he attached great significance to dreams, and believed himself influenced by the spirit of Aesculapius. He was the author of 83 treatises on medicine; his *De Usu Partium Corporis Humani* ('Of the use of the parts of the human body'), was written not only with acute scientific knowledge but with deep religious feeling (Desmond 1956). It would appear that medicine and science were not always disciplines unattentive to the sacred and to the soul. No doubt Pythagoras, who employed gymnastics as part of his treatment, would have sympathy with Chinese medicine and its use of healing exercises.

This historical vignette suggests that we are, in the twilight hours of the twentieth century, in the midst of a medico spiritual dark age of our own making. We need look no further than our own small island to see where scientific materialism has taken us. Cost accounting has seemingly replaced a striving for excellence. A colleague holding a senior position in a newly formed health trust tells me of a manager who, against nursing advice, reduced the frequency of air exchange within an air-conditioned operating theatre in order to save money; this increased the risk of cross-infection, and people died. Yet the system remained in use until the statistics of deaths upon the operating table began to look suspicious and drew attention. Deaths were a cheaper alternative to the increased circulation of ventilated air. Other health professionals I supervise have reported that, although money is saved, lives are being put at risk. Has our society lost contact with its communal soul?

Do we really have faith in those who value emotional neutrality, objectivity and intellect to care for us? I think not. There can be no care without love and respect. Critical (rather than nurturing) parenting emanates from a culture without these qualities. Medicine has seemingly lost its soul in the process of becoming scientific. Nursing is treading a similar path, as are schools of psychotherapy which thirst after social acceptability and professional recognition. Interestingly, this process has similarities to socialisation when, as a child, we surrender our personal power in order to belong.

The social entrapment of the soul

If circumstances are bad and you have to bear them, do not make them a part of yourself. Play your part in life, but never forget that it is only a role.

(Yogananda 1974)

Freedom is a concept often spoken of but rarely experienced or respected. But why should it be otherwise? Freedom threatens control, and control is at the heart of politics, professionalism, education, health care and other forms of social order.

When are we really free? I know what 'relaxed' feels like and I have sampled the feeling of release when I work through, or put down, something that is burdening me, but am I free? When I felt 'free' as a child I usually found myself in trouble. When I ran or played with boisterous freedom, I was told to 'be careful', 'stop getting excited', or threatened by such negative fortunes as 'it'll all end in tears'. Being free with my feelings, be they joy or rage, or giving free expression to my physical energies, did not seem to be what growing up was all about. When there were others around – especially grown-ups – I never felt free. Freedom in this context appeared to be a treasure I had to steal. Isolate freedom and you alienate health.

Health is an adventurous state of mind, where problems are seen as challenges, symptoms are guides to lifestyle and emotions are energies which vitalise us. Preoccupation with health is not, in itself, healthy. Health is dynamic, something to be lived rather than defined. Siphon off freedom and you kill it.

A sense of freedom and health grows not so much through achieving extra territory, greater skills or mobility, but rather as a consequence of 'letting go', loosening the 'social scripts' and injunctions previously taught, freeing ourselves of the 'shoulds' and 'musts' that drive us. In my experience, an ill-at-ease mind soon manifests a diseased body.

In certain phases of my life, 'shoulds' and 'musts' have crowded in on me so much I have felt near to suffocation. At such times, I was trying so hard to think well of myself, and so wanted others to do the same, that I lost touch with the inner core of me. This is not to say that I forgot who I was and where I came from, but rather that I remembered my history all too well and felt hemmed in by it. I guess at these times I feared rejection and conformed, wanting to belong and to be loved. My period as a student nurse especially epitomised such times.

When we over-identify with one portion of ourselves we energise this part and withdraw energy from the rest of ourselves. When these parts atrophy, due to a general lack of exercise or nourishment, our options become depleted. To do other than what we are doing now begins to feel like an impossibility. The workaholic is a sobering example. Professional training has been seen to breed practitioners who are very 'head-centred', intellectually stuck in issues of being right or fearing being seen to be wrong, with accompanying fears of losing control or respect, and of failure (Menzies 1960; Barber 1991). So primed, individuals readily flee from their feelings and seek refuge in causal determinism, where problems are approached along:

> (. . .) an invariant cause–effect structure which is translated into a strictly determinable theory. Entirely predictable.
>
> (Southgate and Randall 1981)

And where behaviour and enquiry are regulated by:

> Manuals. Rules and formulae. Experimental testing. Deductive reasoning and logic. Aims at objective, reproducible knowledge.
>
> (Southgate and Randall 1981)

Striving for perfection while containing their own anxiety and vulnerability, professionals thus prepared are prone to adopt the roles of authoritative and/or critical parents, and to enact parent–child relationships with their clients (Moscato 1976). They also have a tendency towards burnout.

Care professionals, akin to other human beings, start from a base of wanting to feel loved, while desperately needing to experience a sense of belonging and achievement. They bring these needs with them to the profession. Fears of rejection, as generated in the family, now become attached to professional life. There is often little time or space to address frustrations of the job, and outlets for distress are usually blocked by the working culture. The person within the professional role learns to cope by splitting emotions off from the intellect, thus repressing painful experiences. However, repression does not work forever; eventually stress becomes acted out symbolically within relationships. Our relationships mirror our health. Displacing personal distress into work is the route the workaholic takes. Strategies such as 'fighting bad feelings upon the inside with good works on the outside', trying to 'work off tensions', 'obsessionally adhering to rules' or 'getting excited about being right or becoming successful', do not take the core hurt away. Stressed out, dis-eased people, attempting to comply with the tenets of scientific positivism in a professional training, do not have enough of themselves available to provide good quality care.

Socialisation (and subsequent 'enculturalisation') is a two-edged sword. At root we have little choice but to belong; we are social at heart and have hungry social needs. Yet it is as if in becoming social we lose integrity, for the 'I', our sense of self and the view we have from the driver's seat, is fragmented into a configuration of interlocking cultural images. As a result, in adulthood we end up with a multi-faceted self-image that has been socially negotiated and co-created via interaction with a multitude of others. With so many significant others in our lives and so many social references of 'how we should be', our sense of who we are becomes confused and crowded. The more crowded and confused we are, the more we are at the mercy of the loudest voice around us. In childhood, the loudest voice is often that of our parents, in adulthood, that of our peers or partner, and in illness, the nurse or doctor. Sometimes we confuse health with being akin and alike to others, and look to them for reference. When we engage in the role of a carer, the profession to which we belong has a very loud voice indeed.

Parents and care professionals share much in common. They both see their charges as in need of education, control and regulation. When we meet with such power and symbolism whilst in the patient role, we all too easily infantilise ourselves and end up feeling disempowered.

In these troubled and threatening times, control does not appear too bad a thing, but too much control, together with the 'machine', may displace the 'ghost' or soul within humankind. The over-conformist who leaves unquestioned the social mores he or she is driven by is arguably as damaged and damaging as the sociopath who has not internalised a workable social model and strikes out at society. Both are alienated from the greater whole of themselves. This said, there are socially acceptable and unacceptable forms of alienation. Talk to God and you are perceived to be praying; say that God talks to you and you will be deemed to be mad (Laing 1967).

Society draws the boundaries, and as individuals we are relatively free within such confines to be the authors (the authority-in-charge) of our own lives. However, when we fall out of the social frame by becoming mad, bad or ill, we meet with professional parents empowered to hold sway over us until we again conform to the required norms. Social norms are different in quality and kind from health, but they have a significant say in its definition. Social norms define health; step outside them and you will be caused to experience considerable dis-ease. It is a sobering exercise to consider how we acquired our 'social genes'.

The social creation of the self

> The people we are in relationship with are always a mirror, reflecting our own beliefs, and simultaneously we are mirrors, reflecting their beliefs.
>
> (Gawain 1978)

In order to develop, human beings need to share. Wipe out a nest of ants, leaving just the unhatched eggs, and ant society with all its structures, roles and strategies will recreate itself in a generation. Wipe out an isolated community of humankind, leaving just babies, and should these survive they will need to largely re-invent what it is to be human. Culture carries our social genes and racial memory, the primordial foundation on which we stand.

Individual action momentarily peaks out of the backdrop of an historically framed and dynamically evolving present. In action we define ourselves; at rest and out of engagement we surrender to the cultural milieu (McLeod

1993). Relationships describe an organismic social dance, in which consciousness and selfhood peak as two selves in movement contact and through action re-define each other. At rest, or when we let our rituals do our thinking for us, we can revert to our socio-cultural history. This is the social blueprint we adhered to before we were able to define our own boundaries and sense of self, and it has a very strong influence indeed.

In the beginning we are born to parents who assume responsibility for and ownership of us, teach us their values and train us in the culture of the community to which they belong. We have little choice in these matters. Unless we have awareness prior to conception and make choices on the astral plane, we do not choose our parents or our culture. Our parents stand in a long social tradition with a particular world view, which they take for granted, realising no other way or orientation to the universe. Reality as they know it, and as we are taught to see it, emanates from this social construction, which colours all that we do and everything we see. It is said that when you give a child the name of a bird, it loses the bird. It never really 'sees' the bird again but only a sparrow, thrush or swan (Cary 1961). Perception is all too often bound up with applying labels rather than appreciating things for their own quality.

Looking through our own socially ground, individually tailored spectacles we are distanced from all other orientations to reality. If we over-identify with the socially constructed world, nothing else is seen to exist; if we under-identify, we risk being diagnosed as deviant and cast out as mad or dangerous. The true patriot, for instance, is often a blinkered social being with little appreciation of the rights or freedoms of cultures other than his or her own. However, give any of us free choice and it is doubtful if we would choose other than our present family and culture of origin. The pull of the familiar remains very strong, while change is synonymous with loss and disorientation.

In our socially defined world, we obviously need relevant skills and the appropriate cultural spectacles in order to survive. Initially, it is our parents' job to provide these. They invest their dreams in us, build us up in their ideal image, teach us and train us in the customs they hold dear and encourage us to be like them. When they trust us to cope, and not to tear the social fabric to which we belong, they set us 'free'. By the time we enter nursery school, we can no longer distinguish between where we end and where the socio-cultural world begins. At this age, our parents are like gods, they are omnipotent and we willingly surrender to their authority. It takes us a long time to realise that they are not gods, and when we do, we feel a powerful sense of being let down, seeing the world as a much more fearful place. However, our need to depend on authoritative others is none too easily removed. Even when we rebel against our parents, we cannot cast them out; their influence lingers and they remain a powerful reference for ever.

Rebelling against, meeting and tussling with others is part of the process of becoming human:

(. . .) far from becoming a self as an organism that takes in what it needs from the environment, we become a self only through meeting

other selves in an I-Thou relationship (. . .) I become a self in order to
go out and meet others. I become a self with others.

(Friedman 1989)

In fully contacting our environment, we are changed by it and take it with
us. Interpersonally, both the person doing the contacting and the person
contacted, are changed. The 'I' and the 'other' undergo mutual exchange.

Having drunk deeply of the social well, we are no more free than a
goldfish in a bowl. Our survival comes to depend upon the cultural medium
surrounding us. We ingest and incorporate good, bad, healthy and damaged
parts of our social environment. Indeed, these very terms are socially defined
word symbols. Just as the fish is the last to see the water, so too we are the
last to perceive the social sea in which we swim. It is no use fretting about
this; it is the way of the world. There are gains in our surrender to all things
social. We have support, we are able to align ourselves to a greater whole,
and we acquire a common language and identity. What is lost in terms of
immediacy and freshness, is compensated by an ability to predict, and hence
to relax. By the time we become adults, we are the cultural system within
which we interact, for self and social system have become intimately related.
Our social chains have, by now, insidiously merged to become us; we now
meet our needs within an intricate social system.

As a social organism, we digest the social worlds of others. Loosening the
'I' in order to become a 'We' causes us to link others to our sense of self (Perls
1969). For every expectation or duty, each person or deity you seek to please,
you apportion a part of yourself to them. Pleasing an audience, such as our
parents internalised and carried as activating memories within, or a current
person without, is the essence of what entraps us. Let us consider the nature
of this internalised audience within. For each of these 'references', a phantom
'puppeteer' is symbolically created within your psyche. There is one string
to your mother, another to your father, other strings for your profession,
country, religion, class and peer group, another for the reputation you strive
to maintain, and so on. As you focus energy upon one or more of these
puppeteers or reference groups, a string is pulled and a portion of you
springs to life. With so much happening, we readily lose sense of who we
are. We vacate the driver's seat and allow space for one or more of our
internal puppeteers to take the wheel. Sometimes we invest so much of
ourselves within our social mask and the puppeteers within us that we
forget how to drive. With so many strings being pulled and so many parts
to play, our life may be lived in a whirl. At this stage we may experience
ourselves as ghosts trapped in a social machine. Our health and the welfare
of our soul fares poorly in a mechanistic social climate. Yet, as we will
discover, this is so often the norm or rule, rather than the exception.

Professional sleepwalking and experiential levels of reality

To see your drama clearly is to be liberated from it.

(Keyes 1975)

As a student nurse within a busy surgical ward I often lost track of who I was and where I was going. There was a host of needy clients before me, a demanding list of tasks and routine duties to perform. With one eye upon the clock to tell me when to check the flow rate of blood and saline drips, or to perform observations of pulse-temperature-respiration rates, and another eye looking out for deterioration in clients recently returned from theatre, there was less a person present than a bio-social professional machine. I had been programmed with the necessary professional 'shoulds' and 'musts' and 'got to's' to function as a nurse, but had lost touch with the more subtle aspects of my humanity. The cost of over-investing in 'the world as we are socially and professionally taught it to be' is that we become unbalanced. We lose touch with other aspects of ourselves which relate to feelings and imagination, 'the world as felt and imagined' and 'the world as we discover it to really be'.

In Fig. 3.1 the orientations to reality are presented, supported by each of these phenomenological world views. What do these experiential levels of awareness imply in terms of health care? Carers who act primarily from 'the world as taught' follow the rules but can fail to research into or find out how things really are – 'the world as we discover it to be'. They are out of touch with 'the world as felt and imagined'. The quality of the care they give suffers, for their capacity for empathy is severely diminished.

When a profession fails to construct strategies whereby appreciation of 'the world as felt and imagined' is accounted for, it loses contact with all things spiritual. I celebrate the worthwhile gains the nursing profession has made in transferring cognitive knowledge, awareness of psychology and care rationale to its trainees. These intellectually awakened nurses with research-mindedness are in touch with 'the world as taught' and 'the world as we have discovered it to be', and alert to 'the world as felt', but they appear little the wiser about 'the world as imagined'. They seem no better able to engage empathetically than I was in my own training some 20 years earlier. They appear to be trapped in a professional globe. Health care is alive with social defences and professional ritual, processes which distance practitioners from the mess and emotional chaos that arise from contact with disease and death (Barber 1991). This is not healthy and does not make for good practice.

In order to become social, we have to inwardly isolate a great deal of ourselves. In Jungian psychology, this equates with the concept of *'the shadow'* – the parts of ourselves we assign to shade, all those qualities that we have been socially schooled to be put away. Contained in the shadow is everything we were told 'not to do', 'not to say' and 'not to

---

FIGURE 3.1 THREE REALITY ORIENTATIONS

Reality as socially and professionally taught
(an intellectually construed view)

We live life and operate by reference to our social scripts, follow cultural rules and norms without undue question and walk in the authoritative footsteps of our parents and teachers. At this level, we show that we have learnt our lessons well and protect ourselves from rebuke and rejection by conformity. Traditions guide us. Professional authority and power also operate at this level. When overused, this world view can cause us to be robotic, obsessional, unadventurous and mechanical, yet appropriately used it makes us aware of the social contract we operate within. Fear of rejection and dependence may cause us to remain at this level.

Reality as we discover it to be
(an experientially derived view)

Our world view is empirically created. Values and strategies are refined by the self and life is lived as enquiry. Research and reality testing emanate from this place and nothing is taken for granted before it is checked out or experientially proven. Personal authority is acquired by this means. When overused, this world view can lead to a cold scientific approach which dismisses subjective experience and emotional meaning. An inability to trust others or a fear of losing control may keep us stuck here.

Reality as felt and imagined
(an emotional and imaginative view)

We are attuned to our emotional needs and expressions as they emanate from within. We are able to engage with imaginative pursuits and to free ourselves in order to entertain new ideas and to create new things. From here emanate subjective skills such as empathy, awareness of things spiritual and a larger picture of life and existence. Sexual fulfilment also radiates from here. This world view may overwhelm us when we spiral down into negativity and experience depression, or lead us into realms of delusion, neurotic anxiety or fantasy if we become ungrounded or fly too far from the mundane/practical concerns of living. Overuse of this world view may leave us feeling out of touch and unsupported in our daily activities; its underuse leaves us grey and dry.

---

be'. To learn self-discipline and emotional containment is a worthy lesson, but our socialisation does not stop there. What is seen as unwanted or unlovable is also put aside. By the time we are adult, the shadow seems a mile long and weighs a ton. Therapists speak of the 'baggage' we carry. As we often consign to the shadow the best of us (spontaneity and creativity) as well as the worst, it is often necessary to unpack and sift through what we have previously put away. By the time we get round to this intra-psychic 'spring cleaning', what we originally put in shadow may be so alien to us as to be terrifying, for it threatens all we have become. Individuals who embark on such work in therapy often feel that they are in danger of becoming unglued. It takes courage to reframe yourself and your world. Most people do not bother until an emotional crisis happens, and then they have to do this. Until we have gone some way towards understanding our shadow, we walk on thin ice. Questing for the light, we may all too easily consign the best of ourselves to shadow. Health care is largely a story about creatures of the shadow who skate on thin social ice. They believe they are the authors of their lives, but are moved by forces below the social ice, of which they have little or no knowledge.

Akin to our biological parents, professional ones contain and mould us to the hospital's social order. As with our earlier parents, care professionals are steeped in social tradition, and on society's behalf are prescribed legitimate power to lord it over us. It is small wonder then that as clients of professional carers we may find ourselves regressing back to earlier phases of our lives. Professional carers themselves may indeed encourage this; a dependent 'regressed' client is much easier to manage and presents fewer problems all round.

I recently had cause to visit a relation in hospital. She is generally furiously independent and vociferously wilful. Quickly in hospital so many internal strings were pulled that her free-spiritedness was confused. It seemed as if care staff triggered off her parental strings, and she responded to them as if they were indeed parents, even though most were half her age. She effectively surrendered her independence and 'freedom' and forgot herself, the 'I'. In terms of world views, the staff were empowered and very much in touch with 'the world as taught' and 'the world as we discover it to be', while my relative was immersed in 'the world as felt and imagined'. Both parties thus remained isolated from the value orientation and world perspective of the other.

I have attempted to illustrate the dynamics I encountered in Fig. 3.2. Carers were clearly aware of the professional requirements of their role. They knew what was expected of them and were given social power and status within the hospital environment. They were also engaged in a formal and purposeful existence, enjoyed role security, and had the means, rights and strategies to acquire information and to manoeuvre empirically in the world before them. Conversely, my kin, the patient, was unfamiliar with the professional world into which she was propelled without a formal role or purpose, and was thus compelled to interpret imaginatively what was happening to her. Ungrounded and detached from her usual environment, she was cast adrift in a world informed by feelings and fantasy. Not knowing the rules, and not wishing to be a problem, she refrained from asking questions, and awaited instructions regarding what was expected of her.

Figure 3.3 shows that hospital reality has many layers. Sensory data may overwhelm us on admission. We are often in the throes of acute physical distress, disorientated by the profusion of sights, sounds, smells and tactile investigations that bombard us, and we may be dulled by the chemotherapeutic agents administered to us. Socially, we form a contract with health professionals whereby they undertake to diagnose, problem solve and treat us. Money is exchanged for this service, either indirectly through tax/

FIGURE 3.2 STAFF–CLIENT PERSPECTIVES

Staff perspective

Professional theories, rules, rituals, routine understood and seen as friendly; familiarity with environment causes much to remain unquestioned

Task vision and demands of the ward cause people to become secondary to the immediate jobs at hand

Nurses and doctors have high status in this environment; professional jargon used to speed things up; mechanical routine of hospital system demands attention over and above time spent with patient

Feelings may be denied as they get in the way of task efficiency and the functional reality at hand; little time to educate the patient to hospital ways; fears of life and death and personal blame or responsibility for this

Client perspective

Client of care unable to perceive with clarity what unfolds around; feels lost and strives to orientate to an alien and unfriendly world

Business of staff interferes with the development of relationships; clients thrown together in self-supporting allegiances

Little meaningful activity to be engaged in; general lack of purpose, isolation from decision-making process, long hours of waiting for results, investigations, visits by consultants and duty doctors

Disorientation through unfamiliar smells, noises and surrounding events, difficult to relax deeply; effects of drugs may further isolate a client's sense of self.

Reality orientations supported

Dominating view of 'the world/life as socially and professionally taught' with reference to 'the world/life as it is discovered to be'

Tendency to be detached from 'the world/life as felt and imagined'; to preserve professional distance and functional clarity, own distress is bracketed off along with empathy; little managerial recognition of the need for emotional support; own emotions may be denied

Dominating view of 'the world/life as felt and imagined', hopefully informed in time by evidence of 'the world/life as it is discovered to be'

Tendency for 'the world as socially and professionally taught' to veer towards an archaic/regressive view akin to childhood when parenting was to the fore; client may be constantly on the look-out for cues as to how they should be to avoid rejection and gain acceptance

Behavioural roles stimulated

Staff play out the role of professional parents; sometimes nurturing but more often than not controlling clients

Clients play out the role of adapted child; uninformed, needy and dependent, without a meaningful or useful role

---

FIGURE 3.3 THE VARIOUS REALITIES AT PLAY IN HOSPITAL CARE

Sensory level (sensate reality)
The hospital as a whirl of smells, noises, sights, pains and sensations that we strive to adapt to, seek medication for, or escape from so that we may find peace and rest.

Social institutional level (conventional reality)
The hospital as we are generally encouraged to see it in its conventional task-fulfilling role as an institution for the care of the sick, staffed by all-knowing professionals, highly trained to look after the needy on society's behalf.

Familial level (transferential reality)
The enactment of family dynamics and roles, where staff act out their need to parent – controlling and nurturing others – and clients all too often fulfil this expectation by obligingly acting out regressive and/or childlike dependent behaviour. As both carers and clients bring with them earlier behavioural scripts or role models of how parents and children behave, these may now inform their actions. Within the staff group and client group, peer relationships may echo earlier unresolved sibling rivalry and/or competition. For example, rivalry for the attention of special others; the ward sister's or consultant's affection may be played for by staff or client group alike.

Ego mirroring level (projective reality)
In order to relate and/or identify with the surrounding environment, individuals may project their own internal world outwards, to better identify with and feel supported by the external world. An individual client in pain and distress may seek out a persecutor to give meaning to their suffering and to vent their anger upon. A caring member of staff may be motivated to care for others in an effort to redress the care they felt that they were earlier denied or presently seek in their lives. An individual may acquire high status and position in order to counterbalance the deep sense of inferiority or inadequacy they feel within themselves.

Transcendental level (transpersonal reality)
The hospital's powerful symbolic holding of the mysteries of life, in the form of birth and death, may trigger a whole new perspective or enable the working through of unresolved personal issues relating to pain, neediness and disease. Altered states of consciousness may be evoked due to physical disorder, medication, anaesthesia or confrontation with one's own mortality. In the throes of disease many individuals meet with a part of themselves they never before recognised, make renewed contact with a spiritual aspect of the self, or gain new clarity and/or vision. Sometimes a deeper level of the unconscious comes to the fore to spur personal development; flashes of intuitive insight may come to the practically minded, passion might arise in the cold intellectual, or a peace of spirit in one who is busy and restless. Such is the power of the hospital to evoke, release and work upon aspects of 'the shadow' of ourselves that we carry within us.

---

insurance or directly by hand. We pay respect to the service we receive, consent to be helped and offer ourselves up for treatment. Transferentially, we are restimulated by what happens within the care setting to reconnect with feelings and dramas from the past; family dynamics are revisited, and authority figures such as the ward sister and consultant evoke those behaviours we engaged in with our parents of old.

Projectively, we re-create ourselves in the world. The way in which we conceive of the self influences how we perceive others, for we project parts of ourselves on to them, in order to make them appear known and knowable. When we project out and connect through others with the parts of ourselves we like, we call them friends. When we project an unwanted or disowned part of ourselves on to another, we reject them. When we meet new routines and people, e.g. on admission to hospital, a great deal of projection occurs. Transpersonally, we engage with the universe imaginatively and symbolically, meeting with a deeper thread of ourselves. Such a soulful meeting as this is particularly stimulated when we find ourselves confronted by death. The hospital is a powerful symbol of the fragility of the human condition.

Contractually, we are familiar with the social rituals involved when we engage medical help. We see a doctor, most often a general practitioner (GP), who intercedes on behalf of the socially verified 'god of medicine'. The god 'medicine', acting through the GP, may label us as healthy or diseased, sane or insane. By recourse to a consultant, the GP draws on powers capable of hospitalising us, if deemed necessary against our will, thereby isolating us from our community and the usual props whence we nourish our self-identity. What freedom society gives, it may likewise take away. Those who treat us and those who teach us, legislate for us and govern us, are powerful agents of social control:

> Traditionally, nursing has evolved in the shadow of medicine and has adapted a similar 'authoritative' approach to care. Patients who are already isolated behind hospital walls, were until comparatively recently further estranged from themselves and their potential social reality by nurses who assumed responsibility for them on their behalf. When nurses act as agents of control, they run the risk of perpetuating those very behaviours they seek to correct therapeutically, namely dependence, depersonalisation and regression. Such behaviours, when encouraged by nurses, lead to the syndrome of learned help-lessness known as institutionalisation.
>
> (Barber 1987)

The clients are not the only sufferers; the carers are often wounded by the social system within which they find themselves professionally entombed. For example, note the nurse's story below:

> Stress is a much abused word today, used by most people to give some meaning to the unpleasant feelings they experience such as anxiety, anger, frustration, fatigue and restlessness due to the excessive physical and psychological demands being thrust upon them. But I, like most people, used words such as stress without ever really understanding their meaning or how it was actually affecting my mind and body. I never gave myself the time or opportunity to try to understand my feelings and anxieties, but went along with them without realising how they were changing me and without evaluating my coping methods – or lack of them, and found it difficult to ventilate my feelings for fear of embarrassment and a feeling of being a weakling.
>
> (Barber 1990)

Socially, we accept the contract that special others whom we invest with 'heavy duty' respect, such as doctors, know what is best for us. We believe in the advice of these 'professional parents'. It is well to remember the patient's position at this time:

> The patient does not know what his illness is nor what causes it, neither does he know what to expect. He is given orders, suffering his illness at the time and afraid of the future: hoping for immediate relief rather than long term health: frightened of death but unable to endure his illness.
> (Hippocrates, quoted in Elliott-Binns 1978)

At this level the patient is very much dependent upon the doctor's professionalism:

> First he needs to know what is wrong with him and what to expect. Doctors often fail to perceive this and send the patient away with no explanation or, worse still, too complex an explanation (. . .) The second reason for the patient's visit to the doctor is the obvious one, the relief of symptoms. A patient with severe gout, acute heart failure, or retention of urine does not want an explanation of what is wrong. He wants relief first, explanation second (. . .) The third reason is the deeper one of fear of death which affects almost everyone over the age of forty, and many much younger. A cough may be the first sign of cancer of the lung, a stab of pain in the chest the precursor of a fatal heart attack, a slight irregularity in the periods the opening burst of gunfire in a long war of attrition ending in cachexia and death. Patients know this and something more than simple reassurance may be needed. It is what I call a sub-phobic state.
> (Elliott-Binns 1978)

Society bestows 'professional status' on those who parent us on its behalf, but not until it has subjected them to long years of intensive enculturalisation. Some entrants to the professions never recover from this; it is as if they can no longer relate anything to other than 'the world as taught', and are forever driven by rules. Entombed within a social role, they may never use their talent to benefit the client fully. Look into their eyes, and they look right through you, without engagement. They live in their head, intellectually removed from the world of senses and feelings. Talk to them about 'freedom' and the 'soul' if you dare. Just as the goldfish does not recognise its imprisonment within the bowl, such professionals are oblivious to their actions and to what has snatched their minds. The doctor quoted below was lucky; he became aware that his professional socialisation was a rite of passage whereby he had surrendered a portion of himself in order to belong:

> I am a forty-year-old white male doctor. My background is working class and I had the misfortune to go to a London teaching hospital. The traditional medical education I received was my first introduction to the profession. Initially it was frightening and disturbing, but I learned to adapt and, on qualifying, the workload left little time for questioning what I was doing.
> (Reason 1988)

Later, he awoke to the realisation of what he provoked and socially created in his practice:

> Several years ago I began to feel ill-equipped to deal with the problems presented to me. My consultations had a 'warlike' quality about them, a battle between the person trying to convince me they were ill and myself trying to slot them into rigid categories, giving advice and talking too much (. . .) I became aware of a growing anger towards doctors based on their attitude towards their patients. How angry were my patients when they came to me? They had come, they were ill – how did I use my power? I began to look critically at myself in a three-piece suit giving an air of confidence: if not actually behind my desk, then across the corner of it. I was surrounded by my instruments, stethoscope often around my neck. I was fully dressed and the patient often undressed. I kept control, dispensing knowledge, advice, and prescriptions.
>
> (Reason 1988)

In this context, care professionals make decisions for us and re-create a parent–child relationship with powerful symbolic overtones. Our general practitioner, an elder of our community tribe, has power to refer us to a specialist, a 'wise one' steeped in even more arcane knowledge, and invested with even greater social status – a professional parent of immense proportions. In tribal terms, we meet a chief amongst village elders.

At this stage, the social or tribal level of our everyday reality begins to wear thin. A further dimension of experience enters into the field of our interactions with the world, namely, *'transference'* – an emotional level of reality as evoked by patterns of the past. While the social layer of reality relates us to a conscious, conventional view of the world, the transferential level refers to all the semi-conscious, emotional patterns we bring to present relationships, based on those in the past. These emotional influences are seen to colour everything we do now. Transference is a way of explaining why we so readily engage in child-to-parent relations with care professionals, idealising them perhaps, and surrendering ourselves to their will. In other words, there is a sufficient emotional 'fit' in the patient–carer relationship to evoke emotionally the child–parent one:

> I was aware in the next minute after his refusal to change his tablets that he was probably going to attack me if I persisted. I remember thinking, 'Well, at least this is going to be interesting! . . .' He grabbed me by the collar saying he was going to (. . .) kill me, that all doctors were the same. They'd done this to him to begin with and now they just treated him like a little kid (. . .) He let go of me and began to cry. I gave him a 'scrip and phoned the psychiatrist. Later I cried too – a mixture of shakiness, fear and melodramatic exhalation.
>
> (Reason 1988)

When we are driven by our earlier social patterns (responding to others as representatives of people we have so engaged within our past), we act as if we are blind to our surroundings. Such behaviour may be the result of an unconscious desire to fulfil a behavioural 'loop' previously left unfinished or incomplete, an unaware re-creation and working through of relationships that we left unresolved with significant others from our past. Unresolved psychosocial crises which hold negative feelings for us can all too often become re-stimulated, surface, and demand address in later life. I am reminded of how many people seem to re-create specific problematic events in their lives in an effort to re-live or re-engage with what torments them, hoping that this time around their resolution will be successful. Viewing Erikson's (1995) developmental model of human growth (*see* Table 3.1), we begin to glimpse what this 'unfinished business' may be.

In the hospital, clients may find themselves confined to bed. As such, they are out of touch with their own authority and purpose, dependent on carers in a similar manner to being dependent on parents, and likely to revisit psychosocial crises and traumas of early childhood. They may be re-stimulated into wrestling with 'trust versus mistrust' and 'autonomy versus shame', in an attempt to re-establish or maintain their 'drive and hope' and 'self-control and will power'. Conversely, staff may deal in their professional family with 'initiative versus guilt' as they strive for 'direction and purpose'. I find adolescent and childhood behaviour patterns commonplace within hospitals, and, likewise, repressive parenting to counter this. The revisiting or acting out of transferential relationships will differ from person to person, depending upon the unique stimuli they are prone to and the extent of their unfulfilled needs.

Socially, we respond intellectually to the world as taught, while transferentially, we respond to the world as we have emotionally experienced it before. For example, when we visit our parents after a long gap, we may find ourselves acting as if we were many years younger and still living at home. There is always a 'small child' within us, an earlier emotional self, who is not so much left behind as carried along inside in silence. When emotionalised events occur, this part may reassert itself, causing us to act out of character. Dealing simultaneously with the past in the present is the essence

Table 3.1 The nature of unfinished business

Age appropriate stage	Psychosocial crises	Significant relationship	Favourable outcome
Birth – 1st year	Trust vs. mistrust	Mother	Drive/hope
2nd year	Autonomy vs. shame	Parents	Self control/willpower
3rd–5th year	Initiative vs. guilt	Family	Direction/purpose
6th year – puberty	Industry vs. inferiority	Neighbourhood and school	Method/competence
Adolescence	Identity vs. diffusion	Peer groups/leadership	Devotion/fidelity
Early adulthood	Intimacy vs. isolation	Partners/cooperation	Affiliation/love
Young to middle adulthood	Generativity vs. self-absorption	Divided labour vs. shared labour	Production/care
Later adulthood	Integrity vs. despair	Mankind my kind	Renunciation/wisdom

Source: (Erikson 1995)

of transferential reality. At times of transferential re-stimulation, emotional reality can swing either way:

> In the ambulance, on a narrow bed with the cot sides up, earlier memories were triggered of a similar ride when I was seven and had broken my leg. I had spent a discomforting night then also. I was surprised by how vivid these earlier memories were and how readily they had been restimulated by current events. It was difficult for a few moments to recollect if I was aged forty or seven.

> (Barber 1991)

Entering hospital, we are severed from our usual functional self and coerced into following routines. We do not know what to expect or what is going to happen to us. We wait for long hours feeling powerless and dependent on what appear to be all-knowing others. Everything seems to conspire to stimulate regression to earlier dependent times, nor are the carers immune from transferring in patterns of their own. They may feel driven to indulge in parenting, to re-enact how their own parents were, emotionally working out their own need to control others. Maybe this time they can get it right, feel fully in control, remain powerful, and be adored and loved for what they do. Compulsive caring often disguises a compulsive need to be loved (valued for oneself). This 'dance', client-to-carer, symbolic child with symbolic professional parent, has many forms. When in full swing both partners appear as if sleepwalking, engaged yet strangely out of contact with each other, unaware of the interactive ritual, one saying 'I am in need and want to be helped', the other saying 'Please let me in I want to help you'. Does either communicate, in a contactful way?

'*Projection*' is a process whereby we deal with unacceptable parts of ourselves by splitting them off and attributing them to others. It runs riot in the emotional climate of the hospital. We do not perceive merely with our senses. Perception is a dialogue between what we believe and what we see. Here the 'world as imagined' and the 'world as it is found out to be' are in direct communication. Too much of the former and our vision and communication are ungrounded, idiosyncratic and inattentive to evidence; too much of the latter and we see without an attributed meaning or deeper internal effect. Professional perception often suffers from this latter malady.

> The moment we say the word 'I', we immediately cut ourselves off from everything we experience as 'Not-I', or 'you' – and with this step become prisoners of polarity. Henceforth our 'I' shackles us to the world of opposites, which is divided not only into 'I' and 'you', but also into inner and outer, man and woman, good and bad, right and wrong, and so on.

> (Dethlefsen and Dahlke 1990)

Polarisation and splitting are common enough in those who have been socialised to the usual degree. For individuals who submit themselves to many extra years of enculturalisation in order to become a professional these processes are greatly magnified. As personal identity becomes bonded to 'the world and life as socially and professionally taught' (*see* Fig. 3.1), this becomes the predominant and all too often rigidly held world view. Professionalism and the ego it fosters kill an appreciation of what is integral and whole, severely limiting the breadth of our perceptive field. All knowledge bases are narrow, but their power and social influence, as in the case of medicine, may be widespread. Professional vision, as previously noted in Fig. 3.2, has a tendency to be intellectual and littered with splits. Such vision is unwholesome.

> Our intellect does nothing but constantly cut up reality into ever smaller pieces ('analysis') and then distinguish between the resultant bits (the 'power of discrimination').
>
> (Dethlefsen and Dahlke 1990)

Medical diagnosis takes this flight into polarisation and analytic thinking further, reducing the client from a whole to a diseased part. It also projects upon them the world view of logical positivism (as described in Fig. 3.1). This process is not, however, totally exclusive, for what is denied and held in shadow also informs professional vision.

We may think of ourselves as confident, competent, independent and knowledgeable professionals, but to do so we must hold back the anxious, vulnerable, dependent and insecure parts of ourselves. Such qualities may all too easily end up projected onto and attached to clients. The more we suppress the message of the shadow the louder its voice becomes, and the more likely we are to act contrary to our conscious intent. The news media is alive with such anomalies of behaviour as abusive parents, lewd clergy, corrupt policemen or cruel nurses. It is not by accident that custodians of the moral order end up breaking the very rules that they rigidly enforce. Rejected parts of one's psychological reality, out of sight, grow in power and turn upon one unexpectedly to influence behaviour; it is best to accept and keep the whole of oneself in sight.

In the care professional, such shadowy elements have been identified as depersonalisation, denial of the individual, detachment, ritual task performance and an avoidance of change (Menzies 1960). Do carers generate such behaviours as a result of denied aggression, cruelty, fears of vulnerability, illness and death, I wonder?

> The law of resonance states that we can only ever come into contact with that with which we ourselves resonate.
>
> (Dethlefsen and Dahlke 1990)

It is a truism that they who raise the shadow are invariably rejected and cast out. After all, segregation from the community is the norm for those deemed to be diseased, psychologically distressed or deviant in behaviour. It is well to remember that hospitals were originally places of incarceration and reform for vagrants, the feeble-minded and the mentally ill (Giddens 1989, p.293).

A transpersonal view of disease and reality

> A man must elevate himself by his own mind, not degrade himself. The
> mind is the friend of the conditioned soul, and his enemy as well.
>
> (Bhagavad-Gita, vi, p.5)

Illness and hospitalisation exert a powerful symbolic effect upon individuals. Illness puts you in touch with your mortality; you can no longer deny your vulnerability or impermanence within the universe. You are confronted with the fact that your time in the world is finite. In illness you face yourself without veils, your body cannot be forgotten, your emotions can no longer be denied, and you face the world and others with a thin skin. Illness also transports you into altered states of consciousness.

One face of illness is frightening and alive with primordial fears of your past, feeling vulnerable with a tentative hold on the world, shaken to your core and discomforted by pain. The other face is one of a personal spiritual journey in which the individual wrestles with feelings and awareness beyond the self, a meeting with things transpersonal. Sometimes it is not until long after the event that transpersonal insight surfaces. As with most experiential learning, the full gain takes time to integrate. It is as if whatever happened stirs an unaware part of oneself first, and the conscious part takes time to catch up. When this finally occurs it feels as if a very deep part of oneself has been touched:

> Post surgery I feel in one way completed. As if nothing is left to instil
> fear in me again, I know I can stand pain and work my way through it.
> Likewise I can rely on my own store of courage; I feel tested and
> somehow relieved. I am no longer the least bit afraid of death and,
> in my saying of this, conversely, feel I love life the more; as if this time 'I
> choose to be here' rather than 'find myself born'.
>
> (Barber 1991)

In this light, the ill and diseased are to be respected for undergoing a spiritual rite of passage, but I wonder how much of nursing and medical care attends to 'spiritual meaning':

> Life (. . .) is a constant path of dis-ill-usionment, in that one illusion
> after the other is stripped away from us until we can finally hear the
> truth (. . .) those of us who are prepared to risk and tolerate the
> realisation that illness, morbidity and death are essential (. . .) eventually discover that this (. . .) ends not in hopelessness, but (. . .) helps
> us find our true, our healing path.
>
> (Dethlefsen & Dahlke 1990)

Illness is seen here as an ally directing us towards personal development, but for this to happen we must put aside our vain and rigid thinking and develop sensitivity to our still small voice within. The body never lies. Illnesses force us to be honest with ourselves and tell us that the time for delusion is past.

A review

> The unconscious mind contains priceless resources that can be mobilised for personal growth and healing (. . .) Freud was the first to call it the unconscious (. . .) Jung gave a different quality to the essence of the unconscious, proposing that an individual was not only driven by the unconscious but led by it to increased personal growth and a sense of well being.
>
> (Simonton *et al.* 1978)

The unconscious communicates to us through our feelings, dreams and intuitions. These messengers are often undervalued in our culture in favour of external events and objects, material and logical things. Through this process we lose contact with our inner guide, our energy blueprint or soul. The body manifests our unconscious. Patients and those who care for the ill must learn to listen to the inner self, the voice that speaks bodily to us in a language of symptoms. When we listen and our body feels truly heard, symptoms become superfluous. Instead of investigating illness and disease, we should be studying life. When we face up to what we are resisting there is often no longer a need for illness. This is akin to the working of dreams; when you face the message of the nightmare it ceases to haunt you again. Our own resistance in both nightmare and illness keeps distress to the fore.

If symptoms are messengers, conveyors of a wisdom that we consciously resist, then illness is a path to becoming whole. In the throes of illness we face ourselves, drop our social guard and see our bodily, social and psychic splits for the nonsense that they are. Put simply, we are drawn back from outer illusion and propelled to our core to stand face-to-face again with the self behind the mask and the vulnerable balance of our existence.

Socrates said, 'If we are to know anything absolutely we must be free from the body and behold the actual realities with the eye of the soul' (quoted in Elliot-Binns 1978).

We have seen in this chapter that, at its most mundane, healing/caring is a mechanistic act performed by professionals trained to do a job, while at its most enlightened it can become a mindful act of respectful service which allows a healing of the soul:

> In brief, the object of healing is to touch the sufferer's soul so that it can begin to come into its own. Sickness should be the means of making that individual aware of what lies beyond the physical senses. That is the prime objective of the healing.
>
> (Miller 1975)

Caring and curing are sacred acts; whether you administer drugs, surgically remove a diseased part, or nurse or counsel another person, you draw near to their soul, and in so doing define the quality and worth of your own.

In this chapter I have argued for an holistic and qualitative approach to health which recognises personal experiences and spiritual development along with biological repair. In order to emphasise why our approach to health must change, I have highlighted deficiencies of practice. We have seen that caring often appears to be a routine act performed by professionals trained to do a job. I have tried to show that this is not the whole story, for at its most enlightened it can be a mindful act of respectful service which allows a healing of the soul.

I neither expect nor wish western medical practice to consign itself to the dustbin. I might invite it to question itself instead, and to re-examine its ancient origins. Industrialisation caused medicine to grow more mechanical in its heart and mind, and modern medics are often far from the developed, spiritually alert individuals of old of whom we read. Machines do not care – they do. Care is more about a quality of relating and being.

In becoming an applied science based on pure science principles, medicine lost touch with philosophy and its art, and blinded itself to 50 per cent of what it is to be human. The art of relating and the openness of mind necessary to speculate on non-physical phenomena need to be reinvested into the professional preparation of nurses and doctors. An orientation to the differing levels of reality – especially the transpersonal level – presented in this discussion (Fig. 3.3) could well help to initiate this process.

Postscript

A short period after completing this chapter I was plunged into a life event which tested my beliefs to the core. My robust 23-year-old son, Marc, was diagnosed as having cancer. Six months following this diagnosis he died. In hindsight, writing this chapter seemed to be a preparation for what was to come. As a postscript to this work and as testimony to the human spirit, to 'care' as an intimate relationship and in celebration of the development of the soul, I share the experience below.

Throughout his illness Marc was supported by healers of the spirit, vitamin supplements, massage, self-healing and psychological counselling. All contributed immensely to his clarity and comfort right to the final moment. I remember sitting with Marc when his medical consultant first informed us that the options were running out. Marc's first thoughts were of me. 'It must be really hard for you, dad, to watch your son die'. This says masses about his quality and nature. Later, when we heard that there was nothing more to be done, we discussed the options, shed our tears together and moved to a place where the present moment was far more important than the past or future. We did much work to prepare ourselves. I remember watching Marc play with the young son of a patient next to him. Soon after we worked together upon letting go of the future and mourning the family he would never have. Marc did much growing during his last 2 weeks. He told one nurse he had 'learnt to love the executioner', he was no longer angry with his tumour. He told another he was 'moving to a new level'. Spiritually, Marc really began to fly. His desire to be free from pain, free from drug-induced haze and mentally alert to the end was achieved through excellence of nursing and medical care. He made one request of me, not to wake up alone. I am indebted to the nursing staff who enabled Marc to spend his last days in a private room – usually reserved for fee-paying patients – so that I might sleep alongside him. During our final days together we meditated upon 'what was', 'what had been' and 'what we meant to each other'. Marc shared his love and thanked me for all I had done. He also acknowledged that he would without hesitation have done the same for me. He could never understand why he was so loved by all who met him. I remember asking him if he felt worthy of being loved yet. He said 'he was getting there'. Shortly before he died I guided him through several meditations from which he returned with powerful symbolic images of what he took to be earlier lives. There was one in which he was in a Celtic tunic, a warrior in a metal helmet resting on one knee with his short sword drawn. Having repulsed one wave he was preparing himself for the final battle as the light faded. He returned from another journey having been taught breathing exercises by a man in white. Earlier, Marc's mother had been visited in a dream by his great grandfather who told her 'not to worry – everything would be alright'. Marc's great-grandfather felt very present for me as I held Marc's hand, encouraged him to relax, to go with love and to depart gently in his own time. Although he was as much a friend as a son, in the final days he became my teacher. Four qualities especially summarize him at this time: courage, humour, compassion and joy.

The ward community who cared for Marc also shared in mourning for his death. They shed their professional shackles so as to meet and share with him fully. A few of these doctors and nurses were little older than Marc himself; they related together as friends. You cannot truly relate to or care for another until you come out from behind the professional veil, but the cost of this is that you walk alongside your clients and feel their full reality. Carers need preparation for this act, and personal and professional support to enable them to meet with others in distress. The Tibetan god of death, Yama, holds a mirror up to you and invites you to look within into the depths of your soul. Disease and death invite us via our shared mortality to touch each others' souls.

If you have not lived through something, it is not true.

(Kabir 1977)

References

Barber, P. 1987: Preparing the way for nursing models. In Barber, P. (ed.), *Mental handicap: facilitating holistic care.* London: Hodder & Stoughton.

Barber, P. 1990: 'The facilitation of personal and professional growth through experiential groupwork and therapeutic community practice.' PhD thesis, Department of Educational Studies, University of Surrey.

Barber, P. 1991: Caring: the nature of a therapeutic relationship. In Perry, A. and Jolly, M. (ed), *Nursing; a knowledge base for practice.* London: Edward Arnold, 230–270.

Bhagavad-Gita 1987: 'Song of God': principal Hindu philosophic text (translated by Prabhavanda, S. and Isherwood, C.). Hollywood: Vedanta Press.

Cary, J. 1961: *Art and reality.* New York: Doubleday and Co.

Chang, S.T. 1978: *Chinese yoga: internal exercises for health and serenity of body and mind.* Northants: Turnstone Press.

Desmond, S. 1956: *Healing, psychic and divine.* Essex: Anchor Press.

Dethlefsen, T. and Dahlke, R. 1990: *The healing power of illness.* Shaftesbury: Element.

Edwards, H. 1950: *A guide to spirit healing.* London: Spiritualist Press.

Edwards, H. 1976: *A guide to the understanding and practice of spiritual healing.* Shere: The Healer Publishing Co.

Elliott-Binns, C. 1978: *Medicine: the forgotten art.* London: Pitman Medical Publishing Co.

Erikson, E. 1995: *Childhood and society.* London: Vintage.

Friedman, M. 1989: Dialogue, philosophical anthropology, and gestalt therapy. A panel discussion on Dialogical Gestalt; 11th Gestalt Conference. *Gestalt Journal* **13(1)**, 7–40.

Gawain, S. 1978: *Creative visualisation.* San Rafael: Whatever Publishing.

Giddens, A. 1989: *Sociology.* Cambridge: Polity Press.

Harre, R. 1981: The positivist-empiricist approach and its alternative. In Reason, P. and Rowan, J. (eds), *Human inquiry: a sourcebook of new paradigm research.* Chichester: John Wiley & Sons.

Hayes, N. 1994: Alternatives to the medical model. In *Foundations of psychology: an introductory text.* London: Routledge.

Hillman, J. 1975: *Revisioning psychology.* New York: Harper and Row.

Keyes, K. 1975: *Handbook to higher consciousness,* 5th edition. Kentucky: Living Love Centre.

Kabir 1977: In Bly, R. (ed.), *The Kabir book.* Boston: Beacon Press.

Laing, R. 1967: *The politics of experience.* Harmondsworth: Penguin Books.

McLeod, L. 1993: The self in gestalt therapy theory. *British Gestalt Journal* **2(1)**, 25–41.

Menzies, I. 1960: *The functioning of social systems as a defence against anxiety.* London: Tavistock.

Miller, P. 1975: *The science, art and future of spirit healing.* Shere: Healer Publishing Co.

Minick, M. 1975: *The Kung Fu exercise book.* London: Corgi Books.

Mitroff, I.I. and Kilmann, R.H. 1978: *Methodological approaches to social science: integrating divergent concepts and theories.* San Francisco: Jossey Bass.

Moscato, B. 1976: The traditional nurse-physician relationship: a perpetuation of social stereotyping. In Kneisl, C. and Wilson, H. (eds), *Current perspectives in psychiatric nursing.* St Louis: Mosby.

Perls, F. 1969: *Gestalt therapy verbatim.* New York: Real People's Press.

Reason, P. 1988: Whole person medical practice. In Reason, P. (ed.), *Human inquiry in action: developments in new paradigm research.* London: Sage.

Simonton, O., Matthews-Simonton, S. and Creighton, J. 1978: *Getting well again.* London: Bantam Books.

Southgate, J. and Randall, R. 1981: The troubled fish: barriers to dialogue. In Reason, P. and Rowan, J. (eds), *Human inquiry: a sourcebook of new paradigm research.* Chichester: John Wiley & Sons.

Yogananda, P. 1974: *Autobiography of a yogi.* California: Self Realisation Fellowship.

Zukav, G. 1990: *The seat of the soul.* New York: Simon & Schuster.

Sociological methods: health services and nursing research

Ann Pursey

Introduction

Sitting down to write this chapter I found myself faced with a common dilemma; should I write in the first or the third person? As a qualitative researcher I have always felt that the use of the third person passive ('the researcher'/'the author') to denote the views, ideas and findings contained in my writing denied the necessarily interactive and human component of sociological interpretive research. Indeed, during my doctoral research (Pursey 1992) I had struggled with the arguments of my supervisor that academic protocol demanded I call myself 'the researcher' when writing my thesis. Contained within my work were findings which said as much about my world view as that of the interviewees. Why then was I encouraged to reflect the notions of impartiality and objectivity by using the third person whilst discussing my work? Reading a recently published article by Sam Porter (1993), I was interested to note his experience of having an article refereed by the *Journal of Advanced Nursing*, a respected and reputable research publication. The referees had commented on Porter's use of the first person in the article, claiming that it implied a 'lack of objectivity' (Porter 1993). Use of the first person in descriptions of academic and health services research is uncommon (exceptions being Swanson-Kauffman 1986;

Webb 1989; Reid 1991; de la Cuesta 1992) and, whilst it may appear at first to be a trivial point and one only worthy of passing mention, the tradition of using the third person passive is in fact underpinned by a set of assumptions about what constitutes 'good research' and the pursuit of an 'objective truth'. I shall return to this issue of objectivity later in the chapter.

The aim of this chapter is to provide an overview of the main traditions of sociological research enquiry and to examine the contribution of sociological methodologies to nursing and health services research. Many textbooks deal with the theoretical aspects of research without relating methodology to specific research examples. It can then be difficult for the reader (particularly the novice researcher) to integrate the theoretical aspects of a methodology with their application in 'the real world'.[4.1] This chapter is divided into sections which examine the theoretical basis of the popular approaches to sociological research (quantitative/scientific research, phenomenology, grounded theory and feminist research) and their practical application in turn. By linking theory with specific examples I hope to demonstrate that the sociological tradition of research has much to offer nursing and health service researchers at all stages of their careers.

Research in nursing and health care

Historically, nursing and health services research has had a strong tradition of quantitative methods (Melia 1982). In the case of the nursing profession this is perhaps partially due to its attempts to gain credibility in the predominantly 'scientific' world of the medical profession, which has a history of research in the natural scientific method. It is readily assumed that the world of nursing research still shares with medical and other health services colleagues a view of research, which values 'objective' quantitative research over more qualitative interpretive work. Certainly during my research training there appeared to be a lack of clarity regarding the relative contributions and importance of 'scientific' as opposed to interpretive research.

In order to ascertain whether there was any basis for this assumption, I undertook a content analysis of research published in the *Nursing Times* and the *Journal of Advanced Nursing* during the 5 month period from January 1993 to May 1993. In order to categorise research articles and research reports, I divided them into four sections:

1   those which used a predominantly qualitative research methodology and analysis;

2   those which used a predominantly quantitative research methodology and analysis;

3   those which used a combination/mixture of qualitative and quantitative methodologies and modes of analysis;

4   those articles which consisted of a review of literature about a particular subject, or concerned a critical analysis of research methodology.

The *Journal of Advanced Nursing* generally publishes 20 reviewed articles per month, ranging from full research reports to comprehensive literature reviews and critical analyses of research methods. It has a circulation of over 2500 subscribers, and its main readership consists of senior nurses, midwives and health visitors, advanced nursing students and nurse researchers (Blackwell Scientific Publications 1994, personal communication). During the period January to May 1993, this journal published 100 articles (excluding editorials and book reviews). The *Nursing Times*, by comparison, is a weekly publication which publishes a wide range of articles, from topical news items to detailed research reports. It has a wide readership within the nursing profession, and the largest circulation of any UK nursing publication. During the period January to May 1993 the *Nursing Times* published the findings of 10 research articles per week on average; the presentation of these included full and short reports, and clinical update summaries of research.

A preliminary examination of the research contained within the two publications revealed a difference in the nature and style of research that was being published. Table 4.1 shows the proportion of research reports in the four categories described at the beginning of this section for each of the publications.

The *Nursing Times* published the findings of a wide range of research, but the vast majority of it (92%) was in the form of short reports or short clinical updates. There was a heavy emphasis on the reporting of clinical/medical research pertaining to specific diagnoses, conditions and treatment, usually sourced from work published in more academic journals. For example, one edition (*Nursing Times*, 24 March 1993) contained clinical updates on blood sampling, the link between dental disease and coronaries, the aetiology of AIDS and HIV–1, the safety of implantable catheters and paediatric resuscitation. These were synopses of original research published in the *Lancet*, the *British Journal of Surgery* and other medical journals. The same edition contained short reports on post-venepuncture haemostasis (originally published in *Quality in Health Care*), post-surgery pain relief (originally published in the *British Medical Journal*), and circadian rhythms in student nurses (not published elsewhere). There was a small number of full reports of original research contained within the *Nursing Times* during that period.

The *Journal of Advanced Nursing*, by comparison, published a range of

Table 4.1 The types of research reported in two nursing journals

	Qualitative research	Quantitative research	Mixed methods	Literature review/ analysis of research methodology
Nursing Times	15%	67%	13%	5%
Journal of Advanced Nursing	17%	39%	8%	36%

research, most of which was conducted by nurses. There was a high proportion of research concerning conceptual issues in nursing, the review of theories of nursing, developments in nursing practice and some articles pertaining to nursing intervention for specific clinical conditions. In addition, there was a high proportion of articles which reviewed published literature on a specific nursing topic and/or presented a critical analysis of research methods in nursing. Within the two publications, research in the 'qualitative' tradition represented a small proportion of the total (15% in the case of the *Nursing Times*, 17% in the case of the *Journal of Advanced Nursing*).

The findings from my small review are verified by evidence from a recent analysis of nursing research published[4.2] in 1992 (Smith 1994). This shows that quantitative and 'survey' research methods continue to dominate published nursing research, although the nursing journals contained more 'qualitative' research than the *British Medical Journal*. I found myself asking whether this was because fewer researchers were undertaking funded qualitative research and/or whether there were more problems encountered in getting qualitative research published. Recent experience has led me to believe that both are probably true.

If we take funding, for example, many funding bodies and committees (which identify the proposals to be financially supported) are dominated by academics with a track record of 'scientific' quantitative research, who may lack a clear understanding of qualitative research methods. My own experience of membership of such a committee has been that it is difficult to judge the relative merits of a randomised controlled trial as against a proposal, say, for a piece of theoretical, exploratory research. On the face of it, when reading such proposals, the randomised controlled trial appears to have more rigour, a greater clarity of aims and methods and measurable outcomes. The qualitative research proposal often appears vague and uncertain in its potential utilisation, and seems to lack clarity in methodological terms. Arguing the case for funding of qualitative research becomes difficult when committees are dominated by biomedical scientists who are unconvinced of the need for qualitative research to be flexible and developmental in nature.

Publishing the findings of qualitative research can also present problems. Most qualitative research consists of small study samples (unlike 'scientific' research, where the sample size is generally determined by statistical viability). Reviews of papers frequently criticise the findings as 'ungeneralisable' and 'subjective', suggesting that they are not worthy of publication because of this, and ignoring the fact that rigour, whilst different in nature, may still have been upheld. So long as committees of funding bodies and review panels of academic journals continue to be dominated by researchers who have a long tradition of work of a quantitative nature, there will be problems in getting funding for and publishing qualitative research.

Decisions about methodology

The decision-making process concerning which methodology should be used in research begins essentially with the formulation of the research question. The general position I have adopted in this chapter is that all sources of data may have some use, and that there is no one 'correct' method for doing research. What we require in health services and nursing research is an acceptance of methodological pluralism. This position is particularly applicable, I believe, to health services research, which frequently has to encompass the beliefs and value systems of a huge range of political, professional and client groups. We must articulate the research question(s) more clearly, and find appropriate methodologies for collecting and analysing data to help us to answer those questions.

Methodological pluralism has been discussed within the field of sociological research for some years. In 1962, Townsend wrote:

> The future of sociology may depend, more than anything else, on the question of whether statistical and survey techniques can be married to the complex but often inexplicit techniques of personal observation and description. As yet there are relatively few signs of earnest courtship, let alone betrothal and consummation.
>
> (Townsend 1962, p.15)

Whilst this was written over 30 years ago, the debate about the relative value of qualitative and quantative research continues. I believe that both quantitative and qualitative research methodologies have their place within health services research, and the choice of one approach over the other is essentially linked to the theoretical assumptions and aims of the study under consideration. In order to make decisions about appropriate methodology, therefore, it is important to understand the theoretical bases of the various approaches to sociological research, which are overviewed in the following section.

Sociological research methodologies

It is possible to identify two broad traditions within sociological research. The tradition of 'scientific' quantitative methodology was predominant during the 19th century, when sociologists considered the production of 'objective' knowledge to be of paramount importance. During the 20th century, however, sociologists began to pose questions regarding the existence of an 'objective truth' about social situations. During the latter part of this century sociology has had a growing tradition of qualitative research. The question is not, however, solely one of methodology, but combines the issue of methodology with the belief systems that underpin our understanding of how individuals operate within the context of society. This section considers the variety of approaches to research methodology in sociology, and their application in recent health services and nursing research.

Quantitative research methodology

'Quantitative' research methods are essentially those which attempt to attach numerical significance to the study of phenomena. Quantitative research methodology is largely represented by the 'scientific' approach to gathering, analysing and reporting information. Emphasis is placed on empirical measurement and control of variables, whereby observations are quantified and analysed in order to permit numerical comparisons, the calculation of statistical probabilities and the certainty of a particular outcome (Duffy 1985). The assumption behind quantitative methods is that the world can be described by objective forms of measurement that are grounded in a logical, deductive form of reasoning. Quantitative researchers emphasise the replicability and uncontaminated nature of the findings, and may be correspondingly sceptical about the rigour and reliability of qualitative research (Cook and Campbell 1979).

Perhaps the most extreme version of the quantitative approach in sociology is associated with 'positivism'. The positivist approach to sociological enquiry was advocated primarily by Comte (1986) and Durkheim (1938) in the late 19th and early 20th centuries. Positivist sociologists advocate that the belief systems, customs and institutions of society are 'social facts' (Durkheim 1938) that can be directly observed and objectively measured in the same way as the objects and events of the natural world. Society, therefore, is viewed as a collection of individuals who are directed by collective beliefs, values and laws (social facts) which have an existence (or reality) of their own. Positivists therefore aim to classify the world in an objective way and to count sets of observable social facts. Through the use of statistical analysis, correlations between variables or facts (tendencies for two or more things to occur together) can be sought, and the relative influence of particular variables on the phenomena under study can be described. Finally, positivist sociologists seek to establish causal connections between social phenomena, i.e. to establish that one social fact is the cause of another.

Positivists believe that there are laws of human behaviour, and that individuals therefore have little or no choice about how they behave. This could be termed an 'objective science of society' (Taylor and Ashworth 1987). It should be noted, however, that positivism is essentially an 'inductive' methodology. This means that the researcher starts by collecting data and analysing it in order to develop a theory. This theory is then tested against other data sets in order to determine whether it is confirmed. If it is repeatedly confirmed then it can be considered to be a 'law' (Durkheim 1938).

Another type of 'quantitative' methodology stems from the writings of Karl Popper (1959) who advocated a 'deductive' approach to research. The logic of the deductive approach is, in many respects, similar to that of 'positivism', but there are large practical differences. Popper (1959) argued that scientists should start with a 'hypothesis' or statement about what is to be tested. The development of a hypothesis stems from a theory about the relationship between variables or phenomena. The purpose of any data collection, therefore, is to prove or refute that theory (that there is or is not a link between the two phenomena). Popper (1959) argues that it does not matter how the theory is developed. It may be on the basis of instinct or inspiration; what matters is that the research study tests the existence of the theory in an objective and measurable way. What makes the theory scientific is its ability to make precise predictions. Doll and Hill's (1964) seminal work on the relationship between smoking and mortality in a cohort of general practitioners is an example of this.

That study (Doll and Hill 1964) involved sending a questionnaire on smoking behaviour to a cohort of British doctors and following the cohort for subsequent death. By statistical analysis of the variables, the researchers concluded that there was a clear relationship between smoking behaviour and death from a variety of diseases, most notably lung cancer. However, the study examined only one risk factor (smoking), and did not take other lifestyle information into account. Subsequent studies have demonstrated that the causal link between smoking and lung cancer is in fact more complex than it appeared to be at the time. More recent studies have demonstrated that the risk of developing lung cancer is increased by various other factors, such as the position of households near busy roads where traffic pollution is high.

The value of quantitative research in examining the causal links between different variables or behaviours should not be underestimated. What the research does not tell us is why people choose to smoke in the first place, and why they may find it difficult to quit. Quantitative scientific research is not concerned with the meanings behind the behaviour of individuals, but instead focuses on the consequences and associations between particular behaviours and particular outcomes. In order to plan, for example, a comprehensive strategy for health promotion which aims to reduce the incidence of smoking, we may need more information about the meaning of smoking to individuals living within our society, and the context in which their smoking behaviour takes place. There may be (for particular individuals) some fairly pragmatic reasons why they smoke, such as stress, boredom and social pressures. Giving up smoking may therefore have knock-on effects for people's psychological or emotional health which are not easily measurable quantitatively, although this may be productively investigated using an interpretive, qualitative approach.

Perhaps the most highly valued form of research in the natural sciences is the experimental (or controlled trial) method (see Chapter 8). Widely used in pharmaceutical and biochemical research, an experimental study involves comparison between a 'control' group and an 'experimental' group. The control and experimental groups are matched as closely as possible so that they are as similar as possible. The experimental group is then exposed to a particular phenomenon (e.g. it is given a particular drug) to which the control group is not exposed. The effects of this variable on the experimental group can then be monitored and evaluated. In the natural sciences these experiments are generally carried out in a laboratory setting where the environment can be easily controlled. The advantage of a laboratory study is that, so long as the precise nature of the experiment and the environment is recorded, other scientists can reproduce identical conditions in order to determine whether the findings are replicated. Laboratory conditions are often used in disciplines such as psychology, but sociologists rarely use them because the study of 'society' is not easily undertaken in a laboratory setting.

Sociologists do, however, carry out 'field experiments' which involve intervening in the social world so that hypotheses can be tested by isolating particular variables. A problem encountered with field experiments is the difficulty in controlling variables as closely as can be achieved in a laboratory setting. One example of a field experiment is a study by Brooker (1993), part of which examined the educational impact of psychosocial interventions by Community Psychiatric Nurses (CPNs) on relatives of people suffering schizophrenia. Brooker compared the knowledge scores for a control group (families receiving standard CPN care) with an experimental group of families who received specific psychosocial intervention from the CPNs who visited them. Attempts were made to standardise the criteria for selecting the families so that the control and experimental groups were fairly comparable. The findings of the study indicated that there were statistically significant improvements in 'experimental relatives' functional knowledge about schizophrenia . . . (and) no changes in control group relatives' (Brooker, 1993). It should be noted, however, that the number of families studied was very small (a total of 30 families in the control and experimental groups combined), and consequently any statistical analysis should be treated with caution.

Another area of health care in which controlled trials are advocated as the 'best methodology' is the study of clinical outcomes of rehabilitation for stroke patients (Nuffield Health Institute 1992). There has been a large increase in the number of units/wards specifically catering for stroke patients, despite limited evidence that admission to a specialised stroke unit (as opposed to a medical or general rehabilitation ward) makes any difference to the short- and long-term health outcomes for stroke patients. In the bulletin 'Effective Health Care' (Nuffield Health Institute 1992), the authors conclude that the only research method that can evaluate the effectiveness of stroke units is a randomised controlled trial. Conducting a randomised controlled trial on a subject such as this is fraught with methodological and ethical difficulties. First, it is very difficult to 'match' individuals in control and experimental groups unless the sample is large enough to reflect the range of variables considered to be risk factors for stroke (e.g. age, smoking behaviour, general health status and fitness). Secondly, comparing the outcomes for patients on a specialist stroke rehabilitation unit with outcomes for patients on other wards would mean denying the control group of patients access to a specialist stroke rehabilitation unit. This has ethical implications in terms of equity of access to services. Although health care professionals often have to make ethical decisions about access during the course of their work, they are not doing this for the purposes of research. Whether researchers have the right to manipulate the opportunities of individuals should be taken into consideration.

Quantitative approaches to research give pre-eminence to systematic, 'objective' means of gathering data. 'Objectivity' in this sense implies that the researcher is 'neutral' and 'value-free' in the research process, and detached from the area of study. In the scientific tradition of research enquiry the notion of 'objectivity' is highly valued. However, some writers have claimed that, even in 'scientific' research, objectivity is a misnomer as the selection of variables, structuring of hypotheses and application of statistical tests is influenced by scientists' personal beliefs, values and decisions (Webb 1992).

Social survey methodology

Survey methods have an important place in the development of research about nursing and health care provision, and deserve a special mention for the contribution they have made to the body of knowledge about populations and sub-groups within populations. In many ways the social survey has become the 'typical hallmark of British sociological enquiry' (Fennel et al. 1988). There are many different types of survey, but the main aim is to 'establish the facts' by enumerating the distribution of certain characteristics in a population. Social surveys tend to be descriptive in nature, the main aim being to describe the incidence of particular characteristics within a population, not to analyse statistically the associations between variables. One form of survey is the 'census' method, which aims to achieve maximum coverage of the population under study rather than 'sampling' (i.e. studying a specified proportion of that population).

A recent example of this type of survey is the National Census of Practice Nurses (Atkin et al. 1993), carried out by the Social Policy Research Unit at the University of York and funded by the Department of Health. The reasons for commissioning this survey were twofold. First, there had been a huge increase in the number of practice nurses employed in general practice during the period between September 1991 and March 1992, and secondly there was anecdotal evidence that these 'new practice nurses' were undertaking a variety of new tasks within the GP surgery as a consequence of the recently introduced General Practitioner's contract (Health Departments of Great Britain 1989). From a policy perspective there was a clear need to develop a national profile of practice nurses, the work they undertake, their professional training and experience and their training needs. However, there was a related need for 'an understanding of how practice nurses' work stands alongside that of other community nurses and how that work can best be managed and developed' (Atkin et al. 1993, p.3). If we examine these two requirements for information it is clear that different methodologies were appropriate. The first part (developing a national profile) was most easily conducted using a postal questionnaire of all practice nurses employed in England and Wales. The questionnaire was designed to collect 'easily quantifiable data' (Atkin *et al.* 1993) such as biographical, demographic and professional characteristics of practice nurses. With regard to the second requirement for information, that of a detailed understanding of the role of practice nurses, a more in-depth (qualitative) study of fewer nurses was required. This part of the study (not yet published) will enable the researchers to understand more about the context in which practice nursing operates and the processes involved in the day-to-day work of the practice nurse. The postal survey merely enabled the identification of the basic similarities and differences between individuals and groups of practice nurses, and facilitated the gaining of knowledge of what the population of practice nurses was like. However, this was very important given the unknown nature of the 'new practice nursing'.

Many studies that fit into the 'quantitative' category collect data by means of a questionnaire (mainly because this is the most pragmatic way of capturing a large data set required to produce meaningful numerical comparisons). Population surveys such as the National Census and the General Household Survey have provided invaluable information about the characteristics of the total population and groups within it, and some basic information about behaviour, lifestyle and health. However, they do not provide us with detailed information about the lives of individuals or the contexts in which their lives are set. To obtain such information we require a different type of methodology, which enables us to examine the meaning of behaviours and lifestyles within the broader context of society.

Qualitative research methodology

Interpretive or qualitative research rejects the notion of 'objective' numerical measurement of social phenomena. Essentially, qualitative research is that which

> attempts to uncover the sense of given action, practice or constitutive meaning; it does this by discovering the intentions and desires of particular actors . . . and by elucidating the basic conceptual scheme which orders experience.
>
> (Fay 1975)

For several years, powerful arguments have been put forward for increasing the involvement of health services researchers in qualitative methods, rejecting the idea that the paradigm of the natural sciences is the only truly scientific methodology (Duffy 1985). The argument parallels a change of focus in other disciplines such as sociology and social psychology, but stems from the fact that the philosophies of measurement, prediction and causal inference (which underpin quantitative methods) do not sit easily with a subject in which the variables under study are frequently concepts such as 'care', 'health' and 'participation' (Corner 1991).

Qualitative methods are being seen as increasingly important in the development of nursing and health care service knowledge. Essentially they seek to examine phenomena in context. Unlike quantitative methods, which attempt to minimise or eliminate researcher 'bias' as far as possible, the researcher and the researched in qualitative methodologies are considered to be participants in the process of data collection and analysis. The researcher and the 'subject' are seen as part of a two-way process: this adheres to a principle of 'subjectivism'. Unlike quantitative methods, no attempt is made by the researcher to control extraneous variables; the natural context in which the phenomenon under study occurs is considered to be an essential part of the phenomenon itself. Qualitative research is a process whereby theory is built inductively from the perspective of the participants in the research study. The main purpose is to *understand the meaning* of human action rather than to *predict* it.

There are several different sociological methodologies which are considered to be 'qualitative' in nature. For purely pragmatic reasons I have chosen to discuss three main approaches (phenomenology, grounded theory and feminist research) and their utility in, and relevance for, health services and nursing research.

PHENOMENOLOGICAL RESEARCH

The phenomenological approach to research is possibly the most radical departure from 'scientific quantitative' methodology that there is. In phenomenological research, the researcher and the researched are seen as interacting with each other in order to explore the meaning of the lived experience through the eyes of the researched and the researcher (Bergum 1989). It is a methodology which intends to facilitate the uncovering of meaning in everyday, taken-for-granted life situations. The founder of phenomenology is generally accepted as the existentialist philosopher Husserl, who suggested that phenomena cannot be separated from the experience of them. Husserl advocated that 'lived experiences' must be studied through the words and actions of those individuals who have experienced the phenomena (Cohen 1987). Husserl's phenomenology followed the tradition of regarding human beings as 'subjects' in a world of 'objects'. He viewed human behaviour as the product of intentional action by human beings towards particular objects. However, a more recent phenomenologist, Heidegger (1962), reconsidered the nature of phenomenology by questioning this basic tenet. Heidegger argued that people are primarily 'in' and 'of' the world, and that they frequently interact with 'objects' in an unconscious but expert way. This belief, that human beings are so immersed in the world that they often do not realise the complexity and expert nature of their interactions with the world around them, means that many interactions are taken for granted. This is really the purpose of Heidegger's phenomenology (called hermeneutic), namely to uncover the significance of the world, including that which is taken for granted.

Phenomenological researchers believe that there is no 'objective reality' beyond the subjective meanings of a given situation to individual human beings, and they reject the possibility of producing causal explanations of human behaviour. Therefore the validity of any data generated in a phenomenological study can only be confirmed or refuted by individuals themselves. Phenomenologists are not really concerned with validity and generalisability, as they view individuals as essentially unique and not generalisable. The job of the researcher using this approach is merely to understand the meanings from which social reality is constructed, rather than to attempt to classify behaviour or action. 'Social reality' is therefore made up of the meanings and classifications that human beings impose on the world in order to make sense of it, and is necessarily subjective. The acknowledgement of subjectivity in terms of both the individual's descriptions and the researcher's interpretations of them is crucial to the success of the method. Phenomenology offers a means of accessing the 'real life' experiences of individuals, and is therefore particularly attractive to health service and nursing researchers.

One of the most influential and popular studies of health care which has used a phenomenological approach to research is Benner's (1984) study *From novice to expert: excellence and power in clinical nursing practice*. Benner used a phenomenological approach to investigate the notion of expertise in clinical nursing. Inspired by Heidegger, Benner asked nurses working in acute care settings to describe 'critical' incidents or real-life events in which they had been involved in making decisions about patient care using a semi-structured interview schedule. These incidents were specific situations that were identified by the nurses as being important or significant in some way. Benner analysed these incidents, looking for evidence of expertise and knowledge in decision-making, and concluded that experienced nurses possessed a high level of skills and expertise, particularly in the area of making quick assessments and judgements about the health status of individuals and the input required from nurses. These skills and the knowledge underpinning their actions were often not realised by the nurses themselves, Benner (1984) suggested.

A later study (Reed 1994) attempted to use the same methodology to study the notion of expertise in long-stay care settings, again asking nurses to identify specific incidents in which they were involved with patients. Reed (1994) aimed to conduct 12 interviews (with some semi-participant observation beforehand), but eventually collected data from three nurses who worked on a ward for the long-term care of older people. She found that there were problems in identifying the notion of expertise in long-stay care using this methodology, partly because the nurses had difficulty in identifying discrete incidents. Because of Benner's (1991) suggestion that one of the marks of expertise is the ability to identify incidents (to know where they begin and end), Reed (1994) began to question whether nurses in long-stay care had any expertise, or whether it was the nature of their work that prevented them from describing discrete incidents. Long-stay care is an area of work which requires continuity and a flow of human interaction and experience, and Reed concluded that it was the context in which long-stay care work occurred that made it difficult for nurses to articulate their experiences in the form of incidents. Nurses placed heavy emphasis on the establishment of relationships (which have a time dimension) and on the affective domains of nursing interaction, rather than on the technical skills that we associate with high levels of expertise. Phenomenological studies tend to concentrate on the process of articulation (the study of phenomena as people immediately experience them), rather than incorporating the other notions of past and future phenomena in a chronological flow of events (Reed 1994). In Benner's (1984) study this did not appear to be an issue, as she studied acute and critical-care settings where life events (or incidents) can often be discretely divided. However, there will be problems utilising this method in areas such as long-term care unless researchers are careful to incorporate the three dimensions of phenomenology (past, present and future). Reed (1994) concludes:

> . . . the fundamental tenet of phenomenology, to examine behaviour and events in context, still remains central, but researchers need to clarify the nature of this context . . . These observations indicate that phenomenology is an extremely complex undertaking. The complexity of this was well appreciated by Heidegger, who recognised that full understanding of the world . . . might well be impossible to achieve.
>
> (Reed 1994)

The suggestion that full understanding of the world might be impossible to achieve will not be surprising to anyone who has undertaken sociological qualitative research. As interpretive researchers, we find ourselves frequently frustrated in our attempts to understand other people's mind-sets, value systems and behaviour. The humanistic values and beliefs of a phenomenological approach sit easily with an occupation such as nursing, which focuses on the unique nature of human beings as individuals. Used carefully and thoughtfully, phenomenology can provide nursing with a research approach which focuses on a client's and a nurse's lived experience of the care that they receive and deliver, respectively. In this way it can be used to reflect historical and current care provision, and also to plan future care (see Chapter 3).

GROUNDED THEORY

The grounded theory approach to research is rapidly gaining popularity in this country. Grounded theory provides a method for investigating previously unresearched areas (Stern 1980), and its current popularity in nursing research is probably due to the fact that researchers are attempting to develop their knowledge of the theories that guide nursing practice. Well used and tested in the USA, a grounded theory mode of enquiry involves a progressive building up from data to substantive theory to grounded formal theory (Glaser and Strauss 1967). In other words, rather than testing an already established theory, the grounded theory researcher begins with an area of study and allows the issues pertinent to that area to emerge during the course of data collection. Strauss (1987) states that grounded theory is not really a *specific* method or technique, but rather a *style* of conducting qualitative analysis and of generating theories in a natural context (Glaser and Strauss 1967).

Grounded theory is derived from the symbolic interactionist social science perspective. Symbolic interactionism requires a naturalistic approach to research, i.e. the examination of life events as they occur in their usual social settings (Blumer 1986). Emphasis is placed on understanding human behaviour by attempting to understand social actions in terms of the meanings that individuals give to them. Symbolic interactionism acknowledges that change over time is an important aspect of the way that individuals learn from society and also modify that society (Cuff *et al.* 1979). Interaction is therefore seen as emergent and negotiated, and it is 'symbolic' because of the words, languages and meanings that are used in any interaction.

Two broad principles guide grounded theory from this perspective. First, events are considered to be changing continuously as the conditions within society change. Secondly, individual people have the ability to control their own destinies by their responses to conditions. Therefore grounded theory seeks to uncover relevant conditions of the phenomena under study, to determine how the individuals/groups being studied respond to changing circumstances, and to explore the consequences of their actions (Corbin and Strauss 1985).

Grounded theory seeks to uncover the basic socio-psychological problems and processes inherent in a given situation. A theory is built around the social process in which the research findings constitute a theoretical formulation of reality (Glaser and Strauss 1967). There are three pivotal issues in grounded theory research:

1   data is collected in a naturalistic way;

2   analysis focuses on processes;

3   analysis aims at discovering and building theory.

(Strauss and Corbin 1990)

In grounded theory, data is collected by a process of 'theoretical sampling', where decisions are made during the course of the study as to how and where to collect data. In general, data is collected by means of observation and interviews. Theoretical sampling is frequently used in qualitative research. Antle May (1989) states that:

Selection of the informant must also be determined initially by the research question and availability of informants and then modified as needed, based on experience gained in the field about who or what is the 'natural unit' of analysis.

(Antle May 1989)

This way of sampling for data collection has been pioneered by proponents of the grounded theory method (Glaser and Strauss 1967; Chenitz and Swanson 1986), where events are sampled on the basis of concepts that are relevant to evolving theory (de la Cuesta 1992). The term theoretical or purposeful sampling refers to a system in which the researcher selects 'key' respondents (or informants) as the research progresses, i.e. respondents who are thought to be most capable of clarifying aspects of the research question. The difference between this and the type of sampling commonly associated with surveys and quantitative methodology is that:

> rather than selecting a sample using criteria based on typical or representative population characteristics, such as age . . . (in theoretical sampling) the sample is selected according to the informants' knowledge of the research topic.
>
> (Morse 1989)

There are similarities with the phenomenological approach here, in that the informants are considered to be 'experts' as opposed to the 'subjects' of research scrutiny (as is the case with much quantitative research). However, grounded theory differs from phenomenology in several respects. Grounded theorists believe that it is possible to explain human behaviour and that there are theories and perspectives that guide groups of people in a similar way. In addition, the mode of analysis in grounded theory is highly specific (for more detail, see Strauss and Corbin 1990), and involves procedures that must be worked through in order to build the theory. The strategy for generating theory using this method is comparative analysis. Data is coded and categorised through a process of open-coding (coding all data collected) to selective-coding (actively seeking out particular categories or themes in the data). The guidelines for coding, categorising and linking themes are quite specific in grounded theory, and it is not appropriate to discuss them in detail here. Basically, during the course of analysis, grounded theory researchers are examining the data, looking for the conditions, strategies and processes that guide human action.

There is a plethora of studies using grounded theory that have implications for nursing practice and health services in general. For the purposes of this chapter I shall discuss the findings of three studies that utilised a grounded theory approach to research, and their relevance to nursing practice.

One of the main aims of a grounded theory study is to uncover the processes that relate to the phenomenon under study. Melia (1981) used grounded theory to study the occupational socialisation of student nurses in Scotland during the late 1970s. In this study the process was identified as the means by which students manage the two worlds of 'education' and 'service' during their training. Melia undertook informal interviews with 40 student nurses, and considered herself a participant in the interviews, stating that 'the close involvement of the researcher in the production of the data is as true of the informal interview method of data production as it is of participant observation' (Melia 1981, p.362). From the data generated, she demonstrated that students used various strategies, such as 'getting the work done', 'fitting in' and 'just passing through' in order to cope with the transient nature of their training and the often competing demands of the education and service segments of nursing. In addition, Melia demonstrated that the 'technical/medical' aspects of nursing work were highly valued by students, while 'basic nursing care' was low status, uninteresting and could be done by anyone. The study contributed to a body of knowledge about nurse training which had implications for its organisation. Some of the issues highlighted in Melia's research have been addressed by the introduction of Project 2000 (in which students are theoretically supernumerary during the service segment of their training).

In a later study, also using a grounded theory approach, Smith (1987) demonstrated that more experienced (third-year) student nurses associated technical acute nursing with a good learning environment, whereas long-stay care was considered to be an area of work where there was little requirement for 'nursing' expertise, although it provided good 'basic care' experience. Smith (1987) demonstrated that student nurses did not think they needed to be taught how to operate in the affective domain of nursing (what she termed emotional labour), but felt that they could meet patients' affective needs through the interest in people that had brought them into nursing. She argues that, unlike technical nursing, affective aspects of nursing care are taken for granted as women's natural work by nurses and other health care professionals.

What are the implications of these studies for nursing? If we think back to Reed's (1994) phenomenological study of long-term care, we can see that there are threads of similarity here. There is a clear indication of difficulty in acknowledging skill and expertise in areas of nursing where technical tasks are not a major part of the work. These studies demonstrate that if 'therapeutic' nursing is ever to become a reality, then we have to re-think the values that we place on particular types of skill and expertise. Primary nursing, which was developed in the USA, can be seen as an attempt to develop therapeutic nursing where nurses and patients work in partnership with one another, and where 'the relationship' between the nurse and the patient is highly valued.

Another recent study using a grounded theory approach to research is de la Cuesta's (1992) investigation of health visiting practice. She attempted to uncover basic social processes in health visitors' interactions with their clients. Data was collected by means of 20 formal interviews and 41 days of participant observation. De la Cuesta concluded that the process by which health visitors introduced their services to the client was one of 'marketing the service' (de la Cuesta 1992). By further analysing the components of this marketing strategy, she was able to reflect on the tactics that health visitors use to make their services acceptable, relevant and accessible to clients.

Grounded theory studies have a significant contribution to make to our understanding of the processes that take place in human interaction. In nursing (particularly in British nursing) we have very few theories that are grounded in the reality of practice. Many of the theories we are encouraged to use have been created to *inform* nursing practice, not to *reflect* it (see

Chapter 1). This may be one reason why practising nurses find it hard to use theories created by nurse academics such as Orem (1985), Rogers (1989) and Roy (1984) to guide their care of patients.

FEMINIST RESEARCH

There has been an increasing interest in feminist approaches to research methodology over the past 20 years, particularly in the study of nursing. The development of feminist sociology has made a significant contribution to sociological and nursing research. Within health care research there is interest in two particular areas:

1   the experiences of women as receivers of health care services;

2   the experiences of women as providers of health care services.

Within nursing, feminist research holds particular attractions, perhaps because women represent the largest proportion of the profession. Feminists advocate an eclectic approach to research methodology where methods are selected for their suitability for investigating the subject under scrutiny, rather than claiming 'privileged status for any particular method or methods' (Webb 1993). Methodological purists who have a strong belief system embedded in a theory about the way in which society is constructed would criticise feminist researchers for this pragmatic viewpoint. However, feminist sociological research is not just interested in specific research questions which pertain to women, or situations in which women are present; it also challenges conventional 'male paradigms' of research (Oakley, 1981). Feminist research, therefore, involves 'a set of principles of inquiry: a feminist philosophy of science' (McCormack, 1981).

The emphasis within feminist methodology is on the critique of 'women's traditional place within society (and a) call for research relationships to be non-hierarchical' (Webb 1993). Oakley's (1981) seminal work on interviewing women who were having babies has been highly influential in emphasising a non-hierarchical relationship between interviewer and interviewees. Oakley (1981) suggested that the notion of reciprocity was of paramount importance when undertaking feminist sociological research; in this sense, interviewer and interviewees should be seen as equal participants in the pursuit of knowledge about a particular issue. However, more recent authors have criticised Oakley for not acknowledging the inevitability of a power relationship between interviewers and interviewees (Ribbens 1989; Webb 1993). Webb (1993) suggests that researchers pursue a theoretical direction for their research, whereas participants in the research may only be aware of their own experiences and may not put those experiences into a theoretical framework. This creates an imbalance; the researcher interprets the data collected during a particular study, not the participants themselves (see Chapter 5).

Recently, feminist researchers have called for an acknowledgement of the value basis of research enquiry and a recognition of the power base that exists between the researcher and the participants in research (Webb 1993).

Research methods should therefore be used in 'ways which attempt to reduce the power inequalities within research relationships . . . and to include within the analysis the role and influence of researchers themselves' (Webb 1993).

Because feminist research recognises the value of many methodological approaches, it offers great scope to researchers concerned with nursing and health service provision. Smith's (1987) grounded theory study of student nurses and the emotional labour of nursing drew on the writings of feminist sociology in order to make sense of the gender basis of the provision of nursing care. Using a feminist perspective, she tried to make sense of what she described as 'women's work' within the broader context of nursing work. In the concluding section of the book which arose out of her research, she writes:

> Nursing leaders exhort nurses to care but . . . they do not consider the way in which care is stereotyped as women's 'natural' work, nor the gender division of labour and the power relations between doctors and nurses within the health service which marginalise care to 'the little things' . . . One important question is whether the predominant image of nursing as women's traditional work will have to change.
>
> (Smith, 1992, p.135)

This quotation highlights the recognition within her research of the gendered basis of health service and nursing work, seen through the eyes of a woman researcher.

Another study conducted in Australia concerns the social construction of the menopause, and has highlighted the issues of knowledge construction, power and control of women's bodies (Seibold *et al.* 1994). The researchers suggest that, until recently, studies of the menopause have been conducted by male members of the medical profession. They claim that this has led to an oversimplified and narrow perspective of the menopause based on the 'norms of men's development and experience' (Seibold *et al.* 1994), and that it is only through feminist research methodology that this perspective can be challenged.

The acceptance of the value of a wide range of methodologies is an appealing aspect of feminist research methodology. Certainly there are areas of health service provision which merit scrutiny using research which acknowledges and seeks to challenge the gendered basis of health care. As Smith (1992) suggests, the notion of caring as women's work has important implications for the nursing profession. However, feminist research is a relatively new area of work in this country (the first account of its methodology was published by Webb in 1984), and it is acknowledged that there are paradoxes and dilemmas which have yet to be resolved (Webb 1993).

MIXING METHODOLOGIES

It should be recognised that not all sociological and health services research fits neatly into 'quantitative' or 'qualitative' paradigms. There are divisions within the two paradigms as well as between them. The rapidly changing nature of health care provision has resulted in a situation where there is more to be discovered about the way in which health services are constructed and provided.

In the section on social survey methodology, I briefly described a National Census of Practice Nurses (Atkin *et al.* 1993). It was clear that a National Census was required at the time because of the changing nature of practice nursing work. I went on to describe how, in order to gain insight into the specific roles of practice nurses, a more qualitative in-depth approach to research was required. Many authors have suggested that qualitative and quantitative research methodologies sit at the pole ends of a continuum of approaches. Whilst there are epistemological differences (i.e. differences in the belief systems underpinning various methodologies) between the quantitative and qualitative paradigms, perhaps one of the most outstanding differences is the mode of analysis. As we have said, quantitative analysis involves attaching numerical significance to the study of variables, while qualitative research is essentially that which derives findings in a non-mathematical way, without any attempt at quantification (Strauss and Corbin 1990). In order to demonstrate this, I have drawn on my experiences of conducting research on community nurses' constructions of work with older people (Pursey 1992).

The study was funded by the Department of Health and conducted in two phases. The first required practice nurses and health visitors to describe incidents, using Flanagan's (1954) critical incident technique, in which they had been involved in nursing and health-visiting work with older people. When I came to analyse this written material I realised that I had not thought about the specific mode of analysis I wanted to use. There were two fundamental options open to me. The first was to group together the incidents that shared common characteristics (as Flanagan suggested), and to use statistical analysis to reflect the significance of particular approaches to work with older people. However, contained within the incidents was a large amount of detail about the issues and contexts in which these incidents took place. I felt that reducing this to a number would result in the loss of the detailed descriptions that my respondents had written. The alternative approach was to undertake a thematic content analysis of the data (Holsti 1969; Altheide 1987), looking for themes that emerged from the data and possible links between phenomena. This would enable me to retain and reflect the detail contained in the written descriptions, avoiding reducing them to numerical values. The dilemma for me in doing this was that I would be unable to come up with any 'hard facts' about the approaches nurses used in their work with older people. As a compromise, I decided to use both forms of analysis. I grouped the incidents together according to their common characteristics and was able to reflect associations between key variables by using statistical analysis. I also analysed the content of each incident using qualitative thematic content analysis. This allowed me to reflect more closely the intricate nature of nurses' work with older people and the differences between individual situations. I felt that this was the only way in which I could satisfy the requirements of my funding body to make some generalisations about nursing work with older people, whilst also reflecting the complexities involved in nurses' interactions with older people. As a relatively novice researcher, I found this a helpful way of discovering the pros and cons of different types of analysis and approaches to research.

An appreciation of the value and place of different methodologies is a vital issue for the development of health services research. Before concluding this chapter I would like to describe some recent studies that, for a variety of reasons, have adopted an eclectic approach to data collection and analysis.

One example is a study by Ferlie *et al.* (1993) of the construction of the management boards of health authority purchasing authorities. In order to investigate the process of change in 'new' NHS purchasing organisations, Ferlie *et al.* (1993) adopted a case study methodology. Case study methodology is 'longitudinal, processual and comparative' (Pettigrew *et al.* 1992) and involves a detailed analysis of a variety of data sources. The methodology involves an in-depth study of organisations (in this case District Health Authorities), and draws on both secondary and primary data. Secondary data is information that has been collected other than for the purposes of research (e.g. routinely collected statistics, archival material in the form of minutes of meetings), which is then analysed with reference to the research question. In case study methodology, primary sources of data include interviews and formal and informal observation.

By comparing data collected from case study sites, Ferlie *et al.* (1993) were able to reflect on the differences and similarities between the construction and functions of various UK District Health Authorities. The study revealed variations in the rate and pace of change in the purchasing function. The roles of, for example, nurse executives at board level were questioned, as it appeared that purchasing authorities had not clearly delineated the function of nurses in purchasing.

Case study methodology is quite regularly used in sociological research. Whilst case studies make no claim to be representative, they do provide fascinating insights into the complexities of an organisation, a society or a social group. A study by Wilkin and Hughes (1987) used this approach to examine institutional life in residential care from the perspective of the consumer. Six residential homes for older people were selected, and a variety of approaches to data collection were employed. Residents were assessed using a behavioural rating scale, and a broadly representative sample was interviewed using a semi-structured interview schedule. The researchers carried out a period of fieldwork in each of the case study sites, which involved formal and informal observation, to assess the social and interactive environment. Structured interviews were also carried out with staff.

A large amount of data was generated during the course of this study. The researchers used a variety of approaches to data analysis, which included quantitative analysis of issues such as time spent in social activity and the characteristics of residents, in addition to a more qualitative analysis of the interview and observational data. In this way the researchers were able to state numerically, for example, the amount of time residents spent in social interaction with staff and other residents, whilst also reflecting the content and context of that social interaction. Although the research was only able to demonstrate the issues pertinent to the six residential homes involved in the study, the findings had implications for many residential care settings.

Conclusions

I have looked at current approaches to sociological research and their application within the broader context of nursing and health services research. The trend within sociological research is for methodological pluralism; this is particularly appropriate for an evaluation of health care provision. Health services research as a discipline enjoys a relatively short history. Much of what we currently do in researching the health service is influenced by the theoretical underpinnings of the natural or applied 'sciences' (for example, bacteriology, pharmacology, physiology, biology) or the social sciences (in particular, sociology). Perhaps this is because we have very few 'theories' about health care provision that have been generated by health professionals and health service researchers themselves. Nursing 'theories' have been developed to be applied in practice, but the relationship between theory and research has only recently enjoyed the attention that it merits.

Whilst the knowledge base of *what* we do in the health service is reasonably developed, knowledge of the reasons *why* we do particular things or the *consequences* of what we do is sadly lacking. The political thrust from the National Health Service Management Executive and the Department of Health is focusing attention particularly on the outcomes of health service intervention, but the expectation is for health services research to focus on scientific, measurable outcomes. However, interpretive qualitative research has much to offer in developing our knowledge of the processes involved in the delivery of health care. In addition, the current focus on 'measurable outcomes' is very egocentric in that the outcomes considered to be of value are generally defined by professionals working within the health service. Research examining the consumer's (or patient's) perspective of acceptable outcomes following health care intervention is sadly lacking. In order to understand the NHS from the consumer's perspective, we need research methodologies which enable us to see the world from their point of view. In this respect, too, interpretive qualitative research has much to offer.

I believe that a pragmatic approach to research in the area of health services provision is required. Research is constrained by issues such as time, ethics and financial resources. What is needed is a 'best fit' between the research question and the methodologies used to investigate that question. Sociological research has, increasingly, an important place within health services research where investigation of the reasons 'why' things happen is often more important than merely accepting that they occur. Meaning and context are vitally important considerations in the improvement of health care provision. The health service does not operate in a social vacuum; most 'caring' activities are social activities in themselves. The debate about the relative values of the different approaches as exclusive categories is proving less and less productive, particularly in the area of health services which enjoys a relatively short tradition of examination by research. Time might be better spent by concentrating our attention on developing coherent and realistic research questions, and considering the methods best suited to the collection of data which would answer those questions.

Endnotes

4.1 Care should also be taken not to confuse 'methodology' with 'methods'. Methodology is the 'science of methods', as opposed to 'method', which is the specific procedure carried out. Hence methodology refers to the belief systems underpinning various approaches to research, and methods are activities such as interviewing, questionnaires, observations, etc.

4.2 The journals used in the review included the *Journal of Advanced Nursing*, the *International Journal of Nursing Studies*, the *Journal of Clinical Nursing* and the *British Medical Journal* (Smith, 1994).

References

Altheide, D.L. 1987: Ethnographic content analysis. *Qualitative Sociology* **10(1)**, 65–77.

Antle May, K. 1989: Interview techniques in qualitative research: concerns and challenges. In Morse, J.M. (ed.), *Qualitative nursing research: a contemporary dialogue*. Rockville: Aspen Publishers.

Atkin, K., Lunt, N., Parker, G. and Hirst, M. 1993: *Nurses count: a national census of practice nurses*. York University Press: Social Policy Research Unit (SPRU).

Benner, P. 1984: *From novice to expert: excellence and power in clinical nursing practice*. California: Addison-Wesley.

Benner, P. 1991: *Caring: nursing's mandate for the future*. Conference Plenary Paper, Glasgow Polytechnic.

Bergum, V. 1989: Being a phenomenological researcher. In Morse, J.M. (ed.), *Qualitative nursing research. A contemporary dialogue*. Rockville: Aspen Publishers.

Blumer, H. 1986: *Symbolic interactionism: perspective and method*. Berkeley: University of California Press.

Brooker, C. 1993: Evaluating the impact of training CPNs to educate relatives about schizophrenia: implications for health promotion at the secondary level. In Wilson-Barnett, J. and McLeod-Clark, J. (eds), *Research in health promotion and nursing*. Basingstoke: Macmillan Press.

Chenitz, W.C. and Swanson, J.M. (eds), 1986: *From practice to grounded theory: qualitative research in nursing*. Wokingham: Addison-Wesley.

Cohen, M.Z. 1987: A historical overview of the phenomenologic movement. *Image*, **19(1)**, 31–34.

Comte, A. 1986: *The positive philosophy.* London: Bell & Sons.

Cook, T.D. and Campbell, D.T. 1979: *Quasi-experimentation: design and analysis issues for field settings.* Chicago: Rand McNally.

Corbin, J. and Strauss, A.L. 1985: Managing chronic illness at home: three lines of work. *Qualitative Sociology,* **8(3),** 224–247.

Corner, J. 1991: In search of more complete answers to research questions. Quantitative versus qualitative research methods: is there a way forward? *Journal of Advanced Nursing,* **16(6),** 718–727.

Cuff, E.C., Payne, G.C.F., Francis, D.W., Hustler, D.E. and Sharrock, W.W. 1979: *Perspectives in Sociology.* London: Allen & Unwin.

de la Cuesta, C. 1992: 'Marketing the service: basic social processes in health visiting.' Unpublished PhD thesis, University of Liverpool.

Doll, R. and Hill, A.B. 1964: Mortality in relation to smoking: ten years' observation of British doctors. *British Medical Journal* **1,** 1399–1410.

Duffy, M.E. 1985: Designing nursing research: the qualitative-quantitative debate. *Journal of Advanced Nursing* **10(3),** 225–232.

Durkheim, E. 1938: *The rules of sociological method.* New York: Free Press.

Fay, B. 1975: *Social theory and political practice.* London: Allen and Unwin.

Fennel, G., Phillipson, C. and Evers, H. 1988: *The sociology of old age.* Milton Keynes: Open University Press.

Ferlie, E., Fitzgerald, L. and Ashburner, L. 1993: *The creation and evolution of the new Health Authorities: the challenge for purchasing.* Working paper, Centre for Corporate Strategy and Change, Warwick Business School, University of Warwick.

Flanagan, J.C. 1954: The critical incident technique. *Psychological Bulletin,* **51,** 327–358.

Glaser, B.G. and Strauss, A.L. 1967: *The discovery of grounded theory: strategies for qualitative research.* Chicago: Aldine.

Health Departments of Great Britain 1989: *General practice in the National Health Service.* London: HMSO.

Heidegger, M. 1962: *Being and time.* 7th edition (translated by Macquarrie, J. and Robinson, E.). Oxford: Blackwell.

Holsti, O.R. 1969: *Content analysis for the social sciences and humanities.* London: Addison-Wesley.

McCormack, D. 1981: *The research process in nursing.* Oxford: Blackwell Scientific Publications.

Melia, K. 1981: 'Student nurses' accounts of their work and training: a qualitative analysis.' Unpublished PhD thesis, University of Edinburgh.

Melia, K. 1982: 'Tell it as it is' – qualitative methodology and nursing research: understanding the student nurse's world. *Journal of Advanced Nursing* **7(4),** 327–335.

Morse, J.M. (ed) 1989: *Qualitative nursing research: a contemporary dialogue.* Rockville: Aspen Publishers.

Nuffield Health Institute 1992: *Effective health care.* Leeds: Nuffield Health Institute Bulletin.

Oakley, A. 1981: Interviewing women: a contradiction in terms. In Roberts, H. (ed.), *Doing Feminist Research.* London: Routledge and Kegan Paul, 30–61.

Orem, D. 1985: *Nursing: concepts of practice.* 3rd edition. New York: McGraw-Hill.

Pettigrew, A., Ferlie, E. and McKee, L. 1992: *Shaping strategic change: making changes in large organizations: the case of the National Health Service.* London: Sage.

Popper, K.R. 1959: *The logic of scientific discovery.* London: Hutchinson.

Porter, S. 1993: Nursing research conventions: objectivity or obfuscation? *Journal of Advanced Nursing,* **18(1),** 137–143.

Pursey, A.C. 1992: 'A comparison of health visitors' and practice nurses' constructions of work with older people in the community.' Unpublished PhD thesis, University of Liverpool.

Reed, J. 1994: Phenomenology without phenomena: a discussion of the use of phenomenology to examine expertise in long-term care of elderly patients. *Journal of Advanced Nursing,* **19(2),** 336–341.

Reid, B. 1991: Developing and documenting a qualitative methodology. *Journal of Advanced Nursing,* **16(5),** 544–551.

Ribbens, J. 1989: Interviewing – an 'unnatural situation'? *Women's Studies International Forum,* **12(6),** 579–592.

Rogers, M.E., 1989: Nursing: a science of unitary human beings. In Riehl-Sisca, J.P. (ed.), *Conceptual models for nursing practice.* Norwalk: Appleton & Lange, 181–195.

Roy, C. 1984: *Introduction to nursing: an adaptation model,* 2nd edition. Englewood Cliffs: Prentice-Hall.

Seibold, C., Richards, L. and Simon, D. 1994: Feminist method and qualitative research about midlife. *Journal of Advanced Nursing,* **19(2),** 394–402.

Smith, L.N. 1994: An analysis and reflections on the quality of nursing research in 1992. *Journal of Advanced Nursing* **19(2),** 385–393.

Smith, P.A. 1987: 'Quality of nursing and the ward as a learning environment for student nurses: a multi-method approach.' Unpublished PhD thesis, King's College London.

Smith, P. 1992: *The emotional labour of nursing.* Basingstoke: Macmillan Educational.

Stern, P. 1980: Grounded theory methodology: its uses and processes. *Image* **12,** 20–33.

Strauss, A.L. 1987: *Qualitative analysis for social sciences.* New York: Cambridge University Press.

Strauss, A.L. and Corbin, J. 1990: *Basics of qualitative research: grounded theory procedures and techniques.* London: Sage.

Swanson-Kauffman, K.M. 1986: A combined qualitative methodology for nursing research. *Advances in Nursing Science* **8(3),** 58–69.

Taylor, S. and Ashworth, C. 1987: Durkheim and social realism: an approach to health and illness. In Scambler, G. (ed.), *Sociological theory and medical sociology.* London: Tavistock, 37–58.

Townsend, P. 1962: *The last refuge – a survey of residential institutions and homes for the aged in England and Wales.* London: Routledge and Kegan Paul.

Webb, C. 1984: Feminist methodology in nursing research. *Journal of Advanced Nursing* **9(3),** 249–256.

Webb, C. 1989: Action research: philosophy, methods and personal experiences. *Journal of Advanced Nursing* **14(5),** 403–410.

Webb, C. 1992: The use of the first person in academic writing: objectivity, language and gatekeeping. *Journal of Advanced Nursing* **17(6),** 747–752

Webb, C. 1993: Feminist research: definitions, methodology, methods and evaluation. *Journal of Advanced Nursing* **18(3),** 416–423.

Wilkin, D. and Hughes, B. 1987: Residential care of elderly people: the consumer's views. *Ageing and Society* **7(2)** 175–201.

A world without illness? The 'thinking away' of the chronically sick

5

Patricia de Wolfe

Introduction

When people fall ill in a way which removes them from their normal life for any length of time, they feel as though they have entered a different world. Not only does their body behave in unfamiliar and alarming ways, making ordinary, taken-for-granted actions problematic or impossible, but they move into what seems to be uncharted territory, a space that they never knew existed, and in which the rules for behaviour are unknown. If the illness persists, and resists diagnosis or medical treatment, the sense of strangeness increases. This is partly due to the inability of sick people to continue their accustomed lives, but that is not the whole story. It is as though nobody had ever fallen ill before, and what has happened to them is quite unaccountable. Friends and acquaintances may avoid them, or avoid mentioning the illness, or may suggest that they have in some way brought the illness upon themselves. Sick people may consider these suggestions and may be uncertain as to whether or not they are true.

My aim in this chapter is to bring what feels like the very private experience of chronic illness into the realm of the social, and to explain why this experience – which is after all not unusual – feels so remote from ordinary life. I shall first examine the way in which the sociology of health and illness has constituted the experience of chronic illness, arguing that it has generated a discourse of private suffering which reproduces the sense of isolation from mainstream life characteristic of the experience of chronic illness itself. As an alternative approach, I shall outline several discourses on illness, all of them in common currency, and examine their implications for the way in which chronic illness is experienced by those undergoing it, and viewed by those who are not. These discourses are important because they combine (although not necessarily consistently) to create, shape and limit the possibilities – open to the sick and the healthy alike – for attributing meaning to the experience of chronic illness and for evaluating the behaviour of the chronically sick.[5.1] I shall suggest that, despite their diversity, the discourses share a common feature in that they render chronic illness invisible or portray it as anomalous, as something which is inexplicable and ought not to occur. Before examining these discourses, however, I shall comment briefly on the category of people under discussion in this chapter, namely the chronically ill.

In a sense, it seems strange that chronic illness should be experienced as remote from normal life, because its increasing prevalence, relative to acute illness, is often cited as one of the main features of the nature and pattern of disease in the industrialised world of the 20th century (Turner 1992, p.155; Corbin and Strauss 1985, p.224; Beck 1992, p.204). This alleged increase is viewed in different ways by a variety of commentators. It may be seen positively as an effect of medical success, resulting from the capacity of modern medicine to cure acute disease and to keep alive patients who would previously have died (Gerhardt 1990, p.1149). On the other hand, it can be regarded negatively as a consequence of the pathogenic quality of modern life and a polluted environment. From a different perspective, it may be asked whether the growing prevalence of chronic illness is apparent rather than real, a result of new ways of classifying disease. Writing from a Foucauldian point of view, Armstrong (1990) suggests that chronic illness should be seen as a new category which emerged out of population surveys in which people were questioned about their health, and which were then used to recruit these individuals to the medical enterprise, in an extension of

medical power from the clinic to the community. Beck (1992) also a
the increase in chronic illness, at least in part, to the definitional rathe
the curative powers of the medical profession. He alleges that, hav
monopolised illness and deprived people and institutions of the capacit
to deal with it, the medical establishment diagnoses as sick those people
whom it cannot treat, and then leaves them to cope (Beck 1992, p.205).
However, as will be seen later, the drive towards medicalisation is not a
one-way process; sick people may clamour for their condition to receive
medical recognition and attention. The emergence of chronic illness as a
category may also be attributed to factors other than medical imperialism;
these factors would include institutional and cultural changes which enforce
strict boundaries between the sick and the healthy, such as patterns of work
and social security and the equation of identity with occupation (Parsons
1951; Herzlich and Pierret 1984).

These questions of whether chronic illness can be said to be 'really' on the
increase and, if so, why, are beyond the scope of this paper. From an
empirical point of view the question is vastly complicated, partly because
there is no clear-cut boundary between chronic and acute illness (Gerhardt
1989, p.155) – or indeed between the chronically sick and people with a
multitude of 'everyday' aches and pains – and partly because the term
'chronic illness' covers so much. It extends, for example, from people who
achieve a more or less normal working and social life, even if this is
complicated and occasionally disrupted by pain, disability or medical procedures, to those who are permanently housebound, from people who
require constant medical treatment and monitoring to those for whom
medicine can do little or nothing, and from those whose condition is more
or less stable to those who face almost certain deterioration. The difference
between those individuals who are able to continue in work and those who
cannot, and who therefore lose both their income and their place in society, is
particularly marked. What these very diverse people have in common is that
they are not expected to recover quickly – or indeed at all – and that they are
not expected to die quickly either. They also share the fact that all illness in
western industrialised societies takes place to some extent under the aus-
pices of the medical profession, whether or not the latter can offer relief. This
is because it is almost always the medical profession to which people turn for
help, hope and explanation, but also because the medical profession is
sanctioned by the state to certify that these people are sick. This certification
is essential not only economically, for the purposes of sick leave, sick pay
and state benefits, but also socially, in order to legitimate illness behaviour in
the eyes of family and friends. Much more will be said about the medical
profession later on.

Qualitative research on chronic illness

The importance of the medical profession in defining and so shaping the
experience and social meaning of illness is reflected in the traditional pre-
occupations of the sociological study of illness, which has to a large extent

i medical practice. On the one hand, under the heading
:ine, it has applied a sociological approach to medically
ich as compliance with doctors' orders (Turner 1992,
hand, the sociology of medicine has, from a variety of
a more critical stance towards the medical profession,
e, to its power to create and impose definitions and
ss, and to the resultant disparities of power between
n medical encounters (e.g. Oakley 1980; Freidson 1988).
Chronic illness is, however, lived to a large extent outside medical settings;
even people who require frequent medical supervision usually bear the
brunt of managing the disease at home. The project of studying the experience of chronic illness has accordingly led sociologists to look at the impact
of illness in a variety of non-medical contexts (Conrad 1990, p.1260).

The predominant trend within the sociology of chronic illness is based in a
tradition of 'insider' sociology which came to prominence in the 1960s, and
which gives a voice to marginalised groups; the emphasis in these accounts
is accordingly on the definition of the situation as held by the actors, i.e sick
people themselves (Gerhardt 1990, p.1153). From the 1970s onwards, studies
of the experience of illness outside patienthood began to emerge (Conrad
1990, p.1260) and, after initial reservations amongst sociologists about the
wisdom of studying specific medical complaints (Bury 1991, p.457), there has
been a proliferation of studies of the lived reality of a range of chronic
conditions.

The literature on chronic illness experience is extensive, and a diversity of
themes has been explored.[5.2] Many studies focus in some way on identity
and self-image, stressing, for instance, inevitable loss of self, as valued
activities are foregone and control over one's life is eroded (Charmaz 1983;
Gerhardt 1989, p.141), on the unstable nature of adjustment (Yoshida 1993),
or on different aspects of adaptation to illness (Bury 1991). One common
topic is the effect on illness experience of labelling and stigma, whether
anticipated or actually encountered (Scambler and Hopkins 1988, 1990).
Another theme is the way in which people explain illness to themselves
and reconceptualise their lives in order to account for it (Williams 1984). The
practical and emotional work of illness management is a further important
issue (Wiener 1975; Corbin and Strauss 1985); the process of balancing these
types of work to allow sick people to hold on to life emerges as precarious in
the extreme (Corbin and Strauss 1985). Studies have also highlighted the
physical and social difficulties of dealing with and presenting oneself to
others with conditions whose day-to-day symptoms and long-term outlook
are unpredictable (Wiener 1975; Robinson 1988), and have charted the effects
of illness on family relationships (Anderson and Bury 1988).

Most of the studies in this field are based on data gathered in unstructured
interviews, although some use written accounts solicited from respondents
(Robinson 1990), or the personal experience of the writer (Jobling 1977). Most
also rely on some form of grounded theory (Glaser and Strauss 1968;
Gerhardt 1989, p.140; Charmaz 1990), with occasional variants such as
narrative analysis (Riessman 1990; Robinson 1990). Overall, it can be said

that the approach adopted in these studies is an interactionist one, with an emphasis on process and change (Conrad 1990, p.1258), and that this type of investigation of chronic illness aims to generate theory on the basis of spoken (or occasionally written) experiential accounts given by sick people to researchers.

Critique of the sociology of chronic illness

This literature on the experience of chronic illness has brought to light many aspects of illness experience which had not previously been explored, and which are largely unknown to people who have not themselves been ill. However, the knowledge which this research has generated remains in some respects incomplete and problematic. My criticisms fall into two categories. First, I would claim that the gathering of material by means of interviews produces a discourse which conveys the experience of illness in a partial way. Secondly, the sociological discourse tends to posit the experience of illness as timeless and removed from any social context. It is rarely clear, for instance, except in the sense that frequent references are made to the role of the doctor, that being ill today must feel very different from the experience of being ill 200 years ago.

Some problems of interview research

Before turning to the first set of criticisms, it is necessary to note very briefly that there is debate amongst social scientists about the epistemological status of interview data. Some would argue that there is some essential reality in people's lives to which social scientists can gain access; others would claim that the only level of reality accessible to us consists of the multiple accounts given by different informants at different moments in time, all of which are equally 'true' in their own terms (Silverman 1985, chapter 5). For those who eschew the latter, relativist position, problems remain regarding the inter-pretation of data, for instance, whether and under what conditions inter-pretation can be said to distort the data and its relationship to reality. These are immensely complex issues which it is impossible to explore further here. For the purposes of this chapter, I will only say that I, in common with most researchers in the field of chronic illness, am assuming the possibility of accessing some sort of reality through the accounts which emerge in inter-view situations, although I am less sanguine than they about the possibility of accessing this reality solely by gathering and interpreting interview material. The discussion which follows concentrates more on problems of what is and is not said in interview situations, than on problems of inter-pretation of data. The discussion is couched primarily in terms of interviews with chronically sick people, although many of the points could be applied to interviews more generally.

A characteristic of interviews with chronically sick people is the almost inevitable difference in status between researcher and respondent. The researcher will have a good job and the prospect of future work, and above all be in reasonably good health. A respondent whose occupational prospects and general standing in the world may have been undermined or totally ravaged by illness may respond to this situation of inequality by attempting, consciously or unconsciously, to establish some sort of moral parity with the researcher. This might entail presenting him or herself as someone still aware of, and living according to, the work ethic and, therefore, valiantly and uncomplainingly striving to make the best of difficult circumstances. On the other hand, the respondent might accept the inequality and attempt to exploit it, for example by viewing the researcher as someone who has the power to make resources available.

Another factor likely to affect the self-presentation of the respondent is the interest shown by the researcher. For a person who is housebound and isolated, whose friends may have drifted away, the advent of someone eager to listen to them and find out about their life may be uniquely exciting. Respondents may genuinely cheer up in this new situation, or they may feel obliged to behave in ways that sustain the unaccustomed pleasure of the conversation. This may include protecting the interviewer from the knowledge of the full horror of the disease. Goffman (1990, p.140) graphically describes the convoluted games that people with disabilities may have to play in order to shield normal people not only from the pain of the disability, but also from the difficulty that they – the normals – would have in accepting this pain if they were made aware of it. Goffman suggests that these convolutions are the precondition for the limited and precarious acceptance which the disabled may hope to achieve. Able-bodied researchers may in fact want reassurance that disabled bodies can be coped with (Anderson and Bury 1988, p.251) and, sensing this, their subjects may offer a sanitised version of their experiences. Attempts by respondents to conceal aspects of their condition occasionally come to light, more or less by accident, in the research. Pinder (1988, p.83) describes how a Parkinson's sufferer, absorbed in his conversation with her, forgot to take his regular pill, and shortly afterwards collapsed on the floor in a state which, it later emerged, he usually went to great lengths not to reveal to outsiders. Putting on a show, he explained, was one of the few strategies left to him, whatever the cost to him afterwards. The researcher does not comment on the implications of this strategy for her project of discovering the 'reality' of illness by means of interview.

However, even in cases where respondents strive to tell the truth as they see it, an incomplete picture may still emerge, for feelings associated with the body, whether pleasurable or painful, may be amongst the hardest to put into words. We inhabit our bodies; they are not simply objects, amongst others, whose breakdown we can describe dispassionately. Moreover, we may be resistant to listening when another person attempts to convey an experience of bodily disintegration. The assumption implicit in interview research, that language is a medium into which all experience can be translated, and which can be unproblematically grasped by the person to whom it is directed, may not be valid in this context.

These considerations are liable to affect the nature of the data which can be gathered, and the claims that are made about the experience of illness. It is not possible, for obvious reasons, to state with certainty in what direction the research has been influenced. However, when one looks at the results, certain themes stand out, while others are conspicuously absent. The research reports convey hard work, deployment of a range of strategies to maintain everyday life and relationships with others, and, on an emotional level, depression, a sense of loss, and a need to make sense of an arbitrarily disrupted life. However, some of the more unruly emotions associated with long-term illness are missing. Where, for example, is the rage, the despair, and the wish to die? Where is the sheer terror associated with the onset of a new disabling symptom which will perhaps never go away again? Concepts such as loss of self (Charmaz 1983) do not express the violence of these feelings. Other concepts, too, seem tame; those of adaptation (Bury 1991), or the management of emotions (Conrad 1990, p.1261), for example, even if not intended to denote a happy or stable outcome, have a eufunctional ring about them, which may, at least for some sick people and for some of the time, belie an experience of pain, frustration, disbelief, and physical and emotional 'muddling through'. Obviously anyone who does not opt for suicide will somehow go on living, and to that extent can be said to have 'adapted'; anyone who does not have a mental breakdown can be said to have 'managed' their emotions – but terms which suggest that the sick person adjusts to circumstances, feels in control of them, or even ceases to be surprised by them may be misleading.

Thus important elements of the bodily and emotional experiences of illness are absent from the sociological discourse because they cannot be articulated verbally, or because the subjects of research do not wish to express them and/or the researchers to hear them. It should also be noted – and this is also relevant to the section on causes and context which follows – that we are virtually never given the transcript of the interviews on which the studies are based. It is therefore impossible for the reader to know how interviewees were invited to speak, and to what extent the expectations and fears of the researcher structured the accounts of experience given by the subjects. Similarly, we do not know how the transcripts were edited and interpreted to produce the final published version.

Causes and context

I suggested earlier that in many of the sociological studies the experience of illness is presented as existing in a social vacuum. Here I shall briefly examine the reasons for and the implications of this limitation, before going on to explore the impact of wider social forces on the experience of chronic illness.

The nature of the discourse produced by qualitative research on the chronically ill is partly attributable to its notion of theory and explanation. The grounded theory approach adopted by most writers in the field (see Chapter 4) depends on an inductive logic to create theoretical categories from the data and then to analyse relationships between these categories (Charmaz 1990, p.1162). This produces a version of theory as generalised description; in other words, the questions which the theory is designed to answer are 'what?' and 'how?', but not 'why?'. Thus examples of questions which arise within this framework include: how people first notice something is wrong, how they come to seek medical care, what impact diagnosis has on them, how they cope with formal and informal disfranchisements based on a diagnosis, how they adapt to physical discomfort, and what strategies they use to 'get by' in their lives (Conrad 1990, p.1260). The theoretical categories which emerge in an attempt to answer these questions organise descriptions of experience; they do not, however, attempt to explain it.

The consequences of taking this view of theory become evident if one thinks about those aspects of illness which stem from social attitudes rather than from physical problems. For example, stigma attaching both to illness in general and to specific symptoms is a recurring theme in the literature. However, the reasons for stigma are rarely discussed; indeed the 'covering up' of symptoms that are seen as discreditable is sometimes presented together with strategies such as pacing oneself as simply another aspect of illness management (e.g. Wiener 1975, p.99). But a difficulty arising from the attitudes of others is not, theoretically, of the same order as one which stems from an immutable physical condition, even if both seem, in the mind of the sufferer and in a given context, to present a similar type of problem. The failure to ask why illness, or particular aspects of it, should be stigmatised, and whether we live in a cultural and political milieu which fosters this stigma, makes it impossible to consider whether attitudes might be susceptible to change, and the experience of illness thus made easier to bear.

Even when theorists do depart from their data to discuss the cultural context of illness, they take it fairly much as given. For instance, in his account of psoriasis Jobling (1988) talks about the connotations of shame and guilt carried by skin disease in many cultures (p.226). Anderson and Bury (1988, p.252) refer to the 'performative' ingredient of contemporary cultures and the importance attached to bodily restraint and control; they suggest, therefore, that attempts to integrate the chronically sick into public life could prove a mixed blessing for those they are intended to benefit, and should be undertaken with caution. There is no suggestion here that cultural trends which deny important aspects of many people's experience – indeed, since physical decay is part of the human condition, they arguably deny aspects of everybody's experience – should be challenged rather than accepted as inevitable.

What at least a section of this literature advocates, rather than a change in the cultural or institutional context of illness, is something more modest: an improvement in communications between chronically sick people and their medical advisers. Some contributors both to medical journals (Bury and

Wood 1979; Williams and Wood 1986) and to sociological publications (Wiener 1975; Scambler and Hopkins 1988; Charmaz 1990; Gerhardt 1990; Strauss 1990) see their work as instrumental in bringing about this improvement. An understanding of patients' concerns, in particular their need to make sense in biographical rather than medical terms of the disruption caused by the disease, is sometimes proposed as a solution to the problem of non-compliance with medical instructions (Williams and Wood 1986, p.1435). More often, however, improved doctor/patient communication is advocated simply so as to enable the doctor to play a counselling role, helping chronically sick patients to deal with their feelings (MacDonald 1988, p. 200; Scambler and Hopkins 1988, p.175; Locker 1991, p.91; Scambler 1991, p.194).

This proposal clearly has practical difficulties, for few doctors could find time to act as counsellors, even if they were equipped by training and temperament to do so. However, practical considerations aside, this suggestion for alleviating the distress and isolation of chronically sick people fails to address the question of why emotional support for the long-term sick should, when not carried out within the family, be relegated to the consulting room, rather than being more widespread in society as a whole. The sociology of chronic illness, by failing to link the experience of illness to specific social circumstances, constitutes chronic illness as private suffering, and so offers no way of challenging the terms in which people, sick or healthy, think about their bodies and the propensity of these bodies to decay. It is accepted within this discourse that anyone whose body has failed will be removed both from public activity and from public consciousness, and must be dealt with in private.

The discourse also fails to question the conditions of its own existence. Why should it be necessary for sociologists to investigate and report on the experience of the chronically sick at all? Why is the experience of illness not common knowledge? Sick people are not, after all, a remote tribe, nor are they, like some other subjects of 'insider' sociology, such as drug users, in breach of the law and therefore unable to speak openly. Moreover, many people move in and out of illness; it is not a state beyond everybody's ken. The discussion which follows aims to address these issues by examining various ways in which chronic illness is constituted as a freak occurrence.

Chronic illness as anomaly

In this section, I shall examine three discourses which stress the possibility of averting or overcoming disease. These are the discourse of medical progress, the discourse on stress and the discourse on healthy living. I shall also briefly examine a fourth, that of medical certification, whose emphasis is slightly different. I shall consider the social context in which these discourses are located, and their implications for the meaning of chronic illness, both to those who are experiencing it and to those who are not.

These discourses and their implications will be considered in turn, as alternative ways of viewing health and disease. In practice, however, despite the fact that the discourses appear to be mutually incompatible in various respects, people often hold opinions about causes of and ways of combating disease which contain elements of more than one of them. This may be either because people are not consistent in their beliefs, or because they combine elements of the various discourses in such a way as to constitute a coherent view. None of these discourses is exclusively the preserve of any particular social group; in particular, medical discourses as discussed below refer to views of health and illness which are widespread in society, rather than to views which are necessarily held consistently by doctors, who may, for example, slip from a language of scientific power into one of patient responsibility when the solutions they offer prove to be inadequate (e.g. Williams 1989, p.150).

The discourse of medical progress: magic bullets and surgical miracles

I stated in the discussion of the sociology of chronic illness that the main feature situating its account of illness experience in the present is its acknowledgement of the importance of the institution of medicine, which not only provides care and relief, but also functions as a source of meanings and a system of knowledge and explanation (Bury 1982). I would contend, however, that the difference made by certain medical discourses to the experiences and beliefs about illness has not been fully explored in the sociological literature I have examined. In particular, the dramatic increase over the course of the 20th century in the number of previously intractable medical conditions which are now either treatable or expected to be treatable in the foreseeable future has brought with it expectations of progress according to which illness is seen as an unnecessary evil. This has radically affected the meaning of being ill.

Medical progress has received extensive and largely celebratory media coverage, which has tended to depict medicine as a soaring graph of progress (Anne Karpf, *Observer Magazine*, 15 August 1993). Despite the odd scare story, and the occasional critique of the overemphasis on medical technology at the expense of communication and primary care (e.g. *The Trouble with Medicine*, BBC2, 1993), stories about scientific breakthroughs which herald a new understanding of, and the prospect of a cure for, life-threatening diseases abound, as do reports of surgical 'firsts' involving, typically, multiple organ transplants. The euphoria apparent in some of the assessments of the prospective benefits of gene therapy also illustrates this mode of thought. According to this picture of medical success, all diseases can be eradicated given sufficient funds.

Medical discourses divide 'unwellness' into specific conditions which are capable of being diagnosed, treated or researched. The elimination, or at least alleviation, of any particular disease is perceived as always being possible. To be chronically ill, therefore (i.e. to suffer from a disease for which no remedy has yet been found) does not mean that one is undergoing a typically human, albeit highly unpleasant experience. Instead, it means, in a sense, to be an anachronism, to be caught in a mode of suffering for which science will have the answer tomorrow. Chronic illness is not only undesirable, it is anomalous.

The discourse of medical progress is reassuring to the healthy, because it presents illness as falling into finite, manageable categories which are actually or potentially under expert control. It has similar attractions for sick people, too. However, for the chronically sick, it constitutes ways of thinking about and acting on their situation which confirm their anomalous position and may limit their view of their political and personal options.

In order to benefit from medical science, it is first essential to fit into a medical category. People who feel ill, but who do not meet the criteria for any specific medically recognised disease or syndrome, may battle to have their symptoms acknowledged as forming a disease entity; the campaign for the recognition of myalgic encephalomyelitis (ME) is perhaps the best-known recent example of this process. (People who fail at this juncture also lose out economically and socially, as will be seen later.) The next logical step is to attempt to mobilise medical and public opinion, and to exert pressure for research funds; this is one function of patients' associations and self-help groups. If this is not done, people with a particular condition lose out on several fronts. First, they reduce the likelihood of a scientific advance that might restore them to health. Secondly, they forfeit the public sympathy which comes from having a complaint which doctors acknowledge as being serious and worthy of research. Thirdly, they may feel that they have been deemed unworthy of enjoying a human right. As will be seen later, health has come to be regarded as a precondition for self-realisation (Herzlich and Pierret 1984, p.286); to accept one's absence of health as inevitable may be seen as tantamount to accepting oneself as an inferior human being.

However, there are problems with this strategy. The level of expenditure necessary to 'crack the mystery of disease' is high, and funds are limited. Moreover, it has become increasingly clear that this situation of competition for resources is a permanent one, not just the result of the policy of a mean-spirited government in a period of recession. With the advance of medical technology and the rise in public expectations, potential expenditure on health is infinite (Harrison et al. 1990, p.41). Debate about whether the NHS is underfunded can mask the practical and moral issues arising from the fact that, even in a more prosperous and generous economic and political climate, some health needs will have to be given priority over others. If medical discourse prevails in defining the politics of health as the elimination of individual diseases, the following question inevitably arises. Whose disease gets the money?

The discourse of medical progress thus encourages groups of sick people to view each other as rivals, rather than forming links based on a common social disfranchisement (Zola 1983, p.212). It also constitutes the sick person as someone who waits for rescue by medical experts, and whose only aim is the restoration of health. These two aspects of medical discourse are inimical to programmes of political action with a non-medical slant, which would aim to make life more tolerable and less isolated for a wide range of sick and disabled people; such programmes might include the provision of better help in the home, better appliances, cheap and accessible transport, the creation of job opportunities, and a social security system suitable for people with limited or erratic capacity for work. Thought and action along these lines would entail the acknowledgement of chronic illness and bring about a demand for its integration into society, rather than its attempted elimination, which, in any case, is surely a mirage.

In the light of these considerations, it can be asked whether this type of medical discourse serves the interests of doctors – or at least of high-level medical pioneers and researchers – to the detriment of sick people, who are left with few other options for understanding their situation. Many doubts have been expressed about modern medical science. Its claims to have improved health on a large scale have been challenged, with the suggestion that the drop in mortality rates since the 19th century has had much more to do with the implementation of public health measures than with medical advances (Dubos 1960; McKeown 1976). Its more general value to society has also been questioned. The best-known critique is perhaps that of Illich (1976), who accuses modern medical practice not only of fostering expensive procedures which, even from a purely medical viewpoint, are ineffective or positively harmful, but also of depriving us of the social, cultural and personal resources which enable us to deal with pain and suffering. Illich advocates a reduction in medical dependency, claiming that medicine should revert to what he sees as its traditional sphere of enhancing natural healing processes (p.39).

However, these critiques of medicine must themselves be viewed critically. As far as effectiveness is concerned, for example, mortality rates do not tell the whole story. Whether or not medical science has saved large numbers of lives, procedures such as joint replacements may have made a huge difference to the quality of life (Klein 1989, p.166). Furthermore, expensive 'high-tech' procedures such as heart transplants, which were apparently counter-productive in their early days, are now far more successful in restoring patients to some kind of normality (John Illman, *Guardian*, 4 May 1993). While certain types of medical intervention have come under attack for the expense they involve or, as in the case of gene therapy, because they are perceived as potentially dangerous encroachments on natural processes, it must be remembered that they can bring results. In debunking the sometimes grandiose claims of advocates of medical advance, it is important to acknowledge the ravages that illness can cause. Illness ends lives, and disrupts and even wrecks lives that it does not end. And with all the sympathy and social support in the world, there are some people whose level of physical impairment is such that they cannot achieve a reasonable quality of life. The overwhelming majority of people, faced with the prospect of an early and painful death or with that of a prolonged and painful life, would like something done about their condition. In this context, social and medical compassion and understanding come a very poor second to physical relief. Everybody would choose cure over care.

For sick people to turn to medicine for a cure cannot therefore be seen as an instance of 'false consciousness', of people being lured by expertise which has no real advantages to offer them. There is, in any case, no way back to a pre-industrial age when we were supposedly in charge of our own health and able to handle pain (Illich 1976, p.134).[5.3] Awareness of the possibility of cure is now irrevocably part of the experience of illness. Thus incurably sick people have to cope with contradictory sets of needs and desires. Major illness, no doubt always experienced as an arbitrary disruption of a life in process, is now felt as all the more unfair because it is, in principle, preventable. Inevitably, there is anger at this disruption, and resentment at the fact that one's own disease has not been identified or 'solved' when others have. There is also inevitably hope that a medical breakthrough will eventually make possible a return to normality. (There may, too, be disbelief that medical science has nothing to offer, and a long and often fruitless search for a doctor who has the answer.) On the other hand, sick people also feel the need to be regarded – and to regard themselves – as people suffering a typically human fate, who need understanding and resources in order to enable them to participate in the social world to the extent that they are able to do so.

The discourse of medical certification

The discourse of medical progress, like the two discourses of individual responsibility which will be discussed shortly, is concerned with overcoming illness. Here I shall briefly consider an important type of medical discourse which constitutes the patient in quite a different way. The medical profession not only sets out to cure sick people; it also has the power and the duty to certify them as sick. On a formal level, this means that sick people rely on doctors to issue them with a certificate to enable them to take time off work, or to give them access to social security payments. However, a doctor's pronouncement to the effect that an illness is genuine and incapacitating is important in less formal contexts, too. It is often only in the light of a doctor's diagnosis that the patient's family and friends will accept that he or she is unable to perform accustomed tasks and carry out normal social commitments (Robinson 1988, p.23). To have symptoms which fit under a specific medical heading is therefore vital not only because it is a precondition for treatment, but also because it makes it economically and socially possible to rest.[5.4]

As was seen earlier, the categorising of sick people according to discrete disease entities results, within the discourse of medical progress, in a situation of rivalry between groups of patients. However, within this second discourse, which is concerned with the delimitation of sickness, the categorisation of people under distinct medical headings results in their being united in a single social category: those unfit for work. This is a characterisation which stresses and enforces the discontinuity between the sick and the healthy. Chronically sick people – at least those severely affected – may thus live in a state of permanent licensed dependency, but also in a state of social limbo. It has been claimed that the advent of waged labour forged a powerful link between occupational status and identity; thus the inactivity always associated with illness has now become intolerable, entailing as it does a kind of social death (Herzlich and Pierret 1984, p.222). This medical separation, while socially and economically necessary to the sick, confirms and compounds their isolation. If the discourse of medical progress presents chronic illness as an anomaly awaiting expert intervention, this discourse of separation renders it socially invisible.

The two medical discourses are thus distinct in the way in which they constitute the patient. What may link them, however, is the view of the medical profession which results from their combination, with the prestige that arises from the discourse or progress reinforcing the status which stems from the power to absolve patients from work, and vice versa.

Discourses of self-healing and self-care

I now turn to a consideration of discourses which present illness as being within the control of the sick individual. I shall discuss two different discourses which come under this heading, that on stress as the cause of illness, and that on healthy living and self-care. First, however, I wish to outline two possible reasons for the popular appeal of these discourses (Pollock 1988, p.381; Blaxter 1990, p.179).

The first lies in a reaction to the powerful discourse of medical progress. Within this discourse, the part played by the patient in the process of becoming ill and the process of cure is de-emphasised. Control over the body is assumed to be possible, but it is control by scientifically trained experts, not by sick or potentially sick people themselves. Moreover, the body over which this control is exerted is not a familiar one. Scientific analyses are couched in terms of cells, chromosomes and other entities which are invisible and inaccessible, whose nature and functions few people understand, and which appear to bear no relation to our own corporeal experience. It is therefore not surprising that this medical model of health may be regarded with a degree of ambivalence. On the one hand, it reassures, since disease can be conquered, but it also generates unease. Our bodies, so intimately part of us, are treated as alien to us, as objects whose functioning is mysterious, and which have nothing to do with who we are or, except perhaps in rare cases such as exposure to toxins, how we have lived our lives.

This unease is sometimes compounded by people's experiences at the hands of medical staff. The feeling patients often have of being treated as inert bodies with no need for reassurance, information or consultation about what is being done to them is well documented (e.g. Oakley 1980; Barber 1991). And while this objectification might be regarded as a price worth paying when medical treatment is successful, it is likely to become intolerable in cases where treatment fails, or none can be offered. Moreover, the physical reality of even effective therapy may be far removed from the 'cleanness' of the idea of technological progress; the miracles of modern surgery may be followed by prolonged pain and mess, by further, unforeseen operations, and by complicated and debilitating drug regimes. Thus both people's idea of medical science and their experience of medical care may incline them to wish to take a view of health and illness which minimises the importance of medical intervention.

A second reason for the appeal of ideas which place health and illness within individual control may lie in changing conceptions of the self. This is a complex and controversial area which can only be touched on here. Numerous commentators (e.g. Featherstone 1991; Giddens 1991; Friedman 1992) have pointed to the effect on self-identity of the decline of traditional, and in particular religious, values in giving meaning and direction to people's lives. There is now a plurality of authorities and of possible ways of life, and this multiplicity of options has enabled the self to become a project, something which can be worked on and reconstructed (Giddens 1991, p.5). Furthermore, care of the body has become an important component of the project of developing the self (Mellor and Shilling 1993, p.413). As already noted, in a culture which stresses the importance of self-fulfilment, a healthy body is a precondition of a worthwhile life. It is also to some extent a precondition of pleasures which are enjoyed through the body, particularly sexual pleasures. Moreover, the appearance of the body has taken on a new significance. Clothing, gesture, and bodily demeanour are now considered to be expressions of individuality rather than, as in the past, markers of social position (Featherstone 1991, p.189), and youth and beauty have become passports to the good things in life (p.185); this is, of course, particularly true in the case of women.

It is striking that the quest for a sleek, youthful appearance and the quest for health are often presented and understood as aspects of the same process. Health-enhancing activities are undertaken for their cosmetic effects (Featherstone 1991, p.183), and it is assumed that an aesthetic exterior indicates good health. 'Health and beauty' counters in chemist shops testify to the conflation of the two goals; indeed, a vast consumer industry has grown up around the maintenance cum beautification of the body. Appearance is something within our control, which can be endlessly reworked and 'improved' – at least in the short term. Thus, in so far as it is linked to appearance, health becomes not only a precondition for self-realisation, but part and parcel of it.

It may be questioned whether this new conception of the self exists throughout western society, or whether it is confined to people with a considerable degree of control over their lives, i.e. the better off. Nonetheless, in so far as the trend exists, it is consonant with a discourse which places individuals in charge of their own health.

The discourse on stress as the cause of disease

The discourse which links illness to stress might at first glance appear to be an unpromising means of conceptualising people as having control over their bodily processes. It has its origins in studies of the physiological reactions of rats to injury. These studies led scientists – perhaps most famously Hans Selye – to postulate the existence of a stereotyped response to a demand for adaptation (Selye 1975, p.36; Mackarness 1976). Whether stress actually causes an episode of disease is thought to depend on a number of factors. The chain of causality involved in any particular manifestation of illness is, as Selye concedes, complex and poorly understood (Pollock 1988, p.384); he maintains, however, that stress always plays some part in the genesis of disease (Selye 1975, p.47).

Selye's work has been immensely influential. He himself, writing in 1976, estimates that in the 40 years following his first publication, some 95 000 further publications had appeared on the subject of stress and disease (Pollock 1988, p.380). His work appears to have had resonances at the popular level as well; many laypeople, while vague about the physiological mechanisms involved, appear to believe that stress and disease are linked (Pollock 1988, p.382), while magazines commonly carry lists of life events, weighted according to stressfulness, inviting us to account for a past episode of ill health, or to predict the likelihood of a future one. The 'life event' approach is by no means confined to the popular press; within the social sciences, the Social Readjustment Rating Scale (SRRS), devised in 1967, and a subsequent refinement, the Psychiatric Epidemiology Research Interview (PERI) scale, list life-change events, each of which is given a standardised weight that is dependent on the amount of change it is deemed to entail (Holmes and Rahe 1967, quoted in Holmes and Masuda 1974, p.52; Young, 1980, p.140). It is notable that the life event approach ignores the subjectivity and agency of those who are allegedly placed under stress; the degree of change attributed to a specific life event, and the pathogenic effect of that change, are regarded as independent of the meaning which a particular person attaches to the event in question.

Not surprisingly – for it would seem to stand to reason that the way in which a person perceives a major life change must affect the stressfulness of that change – researchers in the field have questioned this assumption. It has been suggested that a number of factors, such as coping styles, personality traits and social support, mediate or modify the relationship between stressful events and disease (Maes et al. 1987, p.567). There is, therefore, a tension within the discourse on stress. On the one hand, there is an emphasis on physiological processes set off by specific quantifiable stressors. Since at least some of these stressors are beyond control (the most stressful life event in the SRRS scale, death of a spouse, cannot be avoided at will), the discourse on stress can take on a deterministic slant. This slant can also be found in those types of popular stress discourse which connect stress less narrowly to specific events, and attribute it to the effects of 'modern society' (Pollock 1988, p.388), in particular to the way in which modern society allegedly inhibits natural physiological 'fight or flight' responses (Coward 1989, p.83). Thus, while an explanation is offered for illness which reduces its randomness, the possibilities of averting it according to this schema may be limited. On the other hand, certain proponents of a link between stress and disease emphasise the perception of stressful events, thus opening the way to the idea that stress is best combated by a change of attitude or personality.

The idea that psychological traits mediate the effects of stressful events or conditions does not necessarily imply that illness is brought within people's control. After all, character traits such as inability to express anger (widely regarded as the main feature of the 'cancer personality' (Inglis 1981, p.87; Sontag 1991) might seem likely to be deeply ingrained; a psychoanalytic perspective, for instance, would certainly not view such characteristics as capable of easy change.[5.5] However, theorists who link personality type to disease seem, often unquestioningly, to assume that because illness is at least partly caused by mental factors, it can be eliminated by an effort of will (Coward 1989, p.86; Sontag 1991, p.58). Thus cancer and other major diseases are deemed to be conquerable by techniques such as visualisation (Inglis 1981, p.95) and positive thinking (Wilkinson 1988, p.92). Illness, although an expression of deepest fears or desires, can allegedly be overcome by a determined onslaught of the mind.

The prevalence of such beliefs about illness causation is hard to assess. Whilst they are not unknown within the medical profession (Inglis 1981; Jacobs 1990, p.169), it has been suggested (Coward 1989) that they are most common amongst alternative therapists and their clients (the latter presumably largely middle-class, since alternative therapies are rarely available on the NHS). However, these ideas also surface in a number of books on self-healing, and may thus reach a larger social range of people. One of the better known of these books (Hay 1988) takes the principle of linking the symptom to its alleged mental origin to the extreme; it devotes a chapter (pp.149–188) to an alphabetical list of disorders and their alleged causes, not only telling us that AIDS results from 'denial of the self, sexual guilt (and) a strong sense of not being "good enough"' (p.151), but also that ingrown toenails denote 'worry and guilt about your right to move forward' (p.171). Again, inadequacy, worry and guilt can be transcended; a recommended 'new thought pattern' accompanies each symptom.

The negative effects of this way of thinking about illness on those who are ill have occasionally been documented, and can easily be imagined. The belief that negative thoughts can reactivate or aggravate an illness is itself a source of stress (Smith 1985); whether or not one believes that stress is physically harmful, this can cause guilt and unhappiness. Patients who initially welcome the notion that they can cure themselves by changing their beliefs and attitudes may find themselves afflicted not only with disappointment, but also with anger and self-hatred if the strategy fails (Levine 1987, p.268); if illness expresses the self, inability to rid oneself of it must denote emotional as well as physical malfunction. A hierarchy of the sick arises, with those who have overcome serious disease designated as 'superstars' (Levine 1987, p.7), and recovery seen as a kind of heroism (Coward 1989, p.87). The chronically sick, according to these canons, could only be viewed – and view themselves – as people who lack moral fibre, who have failed to confront their true problems, and have opted out of life.

The attraction of these ideas for those who hold them is obvious. Illness is no longer feared as striking at random, irrelevantly intruding into our lives. Instead, it is supposedly related to who we are as people, and on some level to what we want; what happens to us is meant for us. Moreover, we no longer, according to this view, have to be reliant on the medical profession. While, to my knowledge, no proponent of these kinds of ideas would advocate dispensing with medical science altogether, the contention that illness and health reflect our inner selves and our desires, and that we can activate our own healing processes, clearly implies a downplaying of the possible contribution of medicine. Largely gone, therefore, are the concerns about the distribution of scarce financial resources as between diseases. Indeed, according to some commentators, the growth in medical expenditure is wasteful and counterproductive, and should be halted (Inglis 1981). Irrelevant, too, is our unease about the unfamiliar body presented to us by scientific research; if illness can by and large be accounted for by mental processes, the precise mechanisms whereby physical functioning becomes impaired are of academic interest only. Even environmental factors which, it may be admitted, play a role in the genesis of ill health, can be seen as having limited significance (Inglis 1981, p.320). This discourse, then, has attractions for both healthy and sick people. However, it tends to relegate the incurably ill to the status of moral inferiors who can only be despised for not helping themselves.

The discourse on stress and disease is harder to assess in one respect than that on medical progress, as well as that on healthy living (discussed below). However oppressive the effects of the last two may be in certain ways, it is clear that their claims are to some extent justified; medical procedures and/ or certain ways of living do improve health. It is far more difficult to make a judgement about the central claim of the stress discourse. Is there in fact evidence that stress – however defined – can, in certain circumstances, cause disease?

There appears to be little consensus on this issue amongst researchers in and reviewers of the field (Maes et al. 1987, p.569; compare with Mestrovic and Glassner 1983, p.1315 and Pollock 1988, p.385). Moreover, there is also widespread agreement, even amongst many of those inclined to believe that such a link exists, that the methodological problems of establishing it are legion (Mechanic 1974; Young 1980; Maes et al. 1987; Pollock 1988). Similar problems apply to attempts to establish links between personality types and disease; different studies, for example, may use different criteria for the assessment of a particular personality trait (Maes *et al.*, 1987, p.570).

Few people would deny that temporary stress can cause minor symptoms such as stomach pains or headache, for example. It does not appear implausible that more lasting and severe stress could cause more serious disease, and there seems to be a certain amount of consensus about the damaging effects of bereavement on health (Maes *et al.*, 1987, p.571). Even if the link exists, however, it does not follow that alleviating the stress would necessarily cure the disease; the initial physical damage may be irreparable. Neither does it follow that all illness is due to stress and nothing else. It is when this last claim is made, and stress is posited as a total or near-total explanation, rather than as one factor of variable significance in a complex set of determinants of health and disease, that this discourse becomes so oppressive of the chronically ill.

Healthy living and self-care

The idea that we can prevent disease, or, less commonly, mitigate the effect of those diseases we already have, by means of our lifestyle comes in various guises. Organisations such as the Health Education Authority publicise the link between particular types of behaviour and the risk of certain diseases (e.g. between smoking and lung cancer; between certain eating patterns and coronary heart disease and certain types of cancer). It is then considered to be the responsibility of the individual to choose to act rationally on the basis of this information. This responsibility for preserving one's health through rational choice extends to self-testing (e.g. for breast and testicular cancer) and to seeking medical help when appropriate (reporting well-known signs of early cancer as soon as possible, and making use of mass screening programmes). Less sober in tone and rather different in content, but resting on the same premise of individual moral responsibility, is the natural health movement, which enjoins the avoidance of products contaminated by artificial processes, and stresses the role of nutrition in abolishing disease (Coward 1989, p.123).

The belief that health depends to a large extent on behaviour and is in people's own hands is widespread within the population, even amongst the poorest (Blaxter 1990, p.162). About two-thirds of respondents questioned in the Health and Lifestyle Survey, conducted in the UK in 1984/85, claimed that people were 'guilty' of their own ill health, quoting smoking, poor diet, lack of exercise and other factors as reasons why this was so (Blaxter 1990, p.179). (Those who were themselves in bad health were, however, less likely to take the self-responsible view.) Thus the links frequently made in academic and political discourse between poverty and ill health do not seem to be taken on board by disadvantaged people themselves (Blaxter, 1990, p.162). One can only suppose that, as with the discourse on stress, people find an ethic of individual responsibility reassuring, allowing them as it does the impression of control over their bodies. They may be reluctant to confront the extent to which their health, so basic to their quality of life and possibilities of action, is affected by social inequalities which are, from their point of view, virtually immutable.

Adherents of the natural health movement also tend to stress individual responsibility and choice, while ignoring the wider context which constrains these choices. Individuals may opt for foods which have been grown organically or which are unprocessed – but the larger questions of how food production and marketing are organised are rarely addressed in a systematic way (Coward 1989, p.135). It is not in fact possible to buy one's way out of pollution risks; pollution is often invisible and lurks in the ordinary objects of daily life – including organic food. Information about how we are being harmed by pollution is virtually impossible to come by. Even where 'acceptable levels' for individual potential toxins have been determined and monitored, dangers remain. Not only are these levels arbitrary and subject to political dispute, scientific debate, and revision, but the effects of a combination of numerous substances on different individuals over time are rarely considered (Beck 1992, p.51). Denial of the magnitude of these problems and the belief that one can circumvent them by a strategy of wise consumer choice is an understandable reaction to fear and to bafflement as to how those responsible for pollution could possibly be brought under control.

An emphasis on healthy living also distracts attention from another kind of major fear, that of death itself. If we concentrate on particular causes of death and the possibility of being able to take action to avert each of these causes, the inescapable truth that everyone will in the end die of something does not have to be faced. One overwhelming worry is thus broken down into a series of minor worries, and each death becomes a matter of private responsibility, which caution could have averted (Bauman 1992a, 1992b).

It has been suggested that keeping oneself well is often regarded not only as personally desirable from a pragmatic point of view, but also as a duty (Herzlich and Pierret 1984, p.283). If this is so, to whom is this duty owed? Campaigns warning people of health hazards which they can avert by their own efforts are sometimes endorsed by the state, and in these cases it becomes obvious that the intention behind them concerns the saving of money as well as the saving of lives. Nonetheless, the duty of health seems not merely to be owed to others, in order to reduce the burden of health expenditure on society, but also to be something people owe to themselves, as a condition of a well-regulated life. The view of health as a duty to oneself contains mutually contradictory elements of puritanism and hedonism. On the one hand, it expresses a wish for constraint, a need to live in a disciplined and ordered way, while on the other hand, there is a desire to maximise health in order to make the most of oneself and one's life (Herzlich and Pierret 1984, p.286; Featherstone 1991, p.171). The problem is that if the need to live carefully is taken too seriously, self-fulfilment and enjoyment of life may be hard to achieve; the whole of life may fall under the shadow of death, with vigilance and defence of health having become a life-long labour

(Bauman 1992a, p.20). There is thus a fine line to be trodden here. The suspicion must be, however, according to the discourse of self-care, that the chronically sick have erred on the side of self-indulgence and feckless-ness, and are to be blamed for throwing away their health and hence their freedom.

Conclusions

The discourses I have outlined above constitute illness – particularly chronic illness – as something which can be averted. The problem of illness is, according to these discourses, to be resolved either by medical advance or by a change in people's mentality or behaviour. (The discourse of medical labelling, which acknowledges illness, does so only in order to remove the sick from the world of normal activity.) The implication is that a world without illness is possible.

These discourses create possibilities for thinking about and experiencing chronic illness. They are not exhaustive; in certain contexts, for instance, illness might be seen as the outcome of heredity, or as plain bad luck. I would argue, however, that the prevalence of discourses I have examined is increasing because they are related to important social trends. Both the development of technologies which affect health and the current dominance of vocabularies of individual responsibility and choice make it harder to think of ill health – or indeed of death (Bauman 1992a, 1992b) – as an aspect of human fate rather than as an avoidable affliction.

This construction of illness is detrimental not only to the sick but also, arguably, to the healthy. It is not surprising, given that illness is intrinsically undesirable, that healthy people should be eager to subscribe to the dis-courses outlined above, and to believe that they are immune from perma-nent illness provided that they seek expert help and/or adopt appropriate strategies of physical and mental self-care. However, this belief cannot really be sustained. Nobody can fail to be aware that bodies inevitably decay, some sooner rather than later. Moreover, virtually everyone has known their own body to let them down, albeit often in relatively unimportant and short-lived ways. Even the experience of short bouts of acute illness or of persistent minor symptoms may lead people to realise that illness does not always respond to their own or their doctors' efforts to cure it. These brief episodes of illness may also leave people with potentially frightening knowledge of how even minor physical disorders can disrupt their sense of their identity and of their boundaries, and their sense of security in the world. The incomprehension of the experience of chronic illness which healthy people tend to profess and to demonstrate may be based not on ignorance, but on denial of their knowledge, and this denial may in turn induce even greater fear. People who are under the sway of discourses which lead them to disclaim their own knowledge of corporeal frailty are left unable to confront the inevitable decline, either through illness or ageing, of their bodies.

These repressed fears afflicting the healthy compound the problems of the chronically sick. For people intent on self-actualisation which depends on control of the body, permanent illness may be as much of a scandal and an affront to reason as death; the chronically sick become an intolerable reminder of the frailty of the human body and of the precariousness of the lives we have constructed for ourselves, even under the most protected and favourable of circumstances. They are therefore shunned, and may be forced into complicated and sometimes unsustainable strategies of concealment in order to gain some limited access to and acceptance in the social world. At the level of social policy, too, discourses which constitute illness as invisible or anomalous operate to the disadvantage of the chronically ill, since they make it hard to challenge policies that deprive sick people of the structures and resources which would allow them some participation in social and economic life.

Demands for such participation seem utopian in the present political climate. At the time of writing, proposals have been made to tax benefits available to the sick, to impose more stringent medical tests[5.6] so as to weed out allegedly fraudulent claims, and to abolish, in all but a few cases, state compensation to employers whose workers are absent through illness. The last measure will make it harder for anyone with an ongoing medical problem to find employment; the first two measures will increase the isolation of those dependent on benefits. Both shortage of money and fear that capacity for any activity will be interpreted as fitness for work[5.7] confine and limit the sick; fear of failing to qualify for benefit also fixes them firmly in the patient role, since it is only by belonging to an accredited medical category that they can hope for a continuing income.

Government measures which impoverish and limit the sick make the spectre of illness still more frightening to the healthy, who become increasingly eager to maintain the barriers which divide them from those with chronic illness. Neither the sick nor the healthy are likely, under these conditions, even to attempt to challenge the discourses which so powerfully constitute chronic illness as separation from the social.

Endnotes

[5.1] The term 'discourse' is used here in the sense of a set of ideas, embedded in social practices, which people experience as external to them and as given. I am not assuming a Foucauldian relationship between discourse and power.

[5.2] In addition to the material cited here, the journals *Sociology of Health and Illness* and *Social Science and Medicine* are a good source of studies on chronic illness experience. *Social Science and Medicine*, Vol.30, No.11 (1990) is devoted to qualitative research on chronic illness.

[5.3] Critiques of medical technology may rely on deeply conservative assumptions about social arrangements. Illich's (1976) proposals for demedicalisation assume the existence of an unpaid army of caring women.

5.4 Some medical labels are more effective in this regard than others. Certain psychiatric labels, in particular, do not always exempt the patient from responsibility for his or her condition, or from the suspicion that an effort on the part of the patient would produce an improvement.

5.5 Classical psychoanalysis does not see emotional change as easy, or as achievable by an effort of will. However, this does not apply to various forms of popularised psychoanalysis which deny or underplay the importance of unconscious processes.

5.6 The extent of the power and autonomy of the medical professional has recently been called into question, in view of its unprecedented level of conflict with the state. Following accusations by government ministers that doctors have too readily certified patients as unfit for work, thus giving them access to social security benefits, a new type of medical test is to be introduced which will no longer rely on the judgement of the patient's GP, working as an independent professional, but on the capacity of the claimant, as assessed by a doctor employed by the state, to perform specified tasks. It remains to be seen to what extent the opinions and the diagnosis of the patient's own medical advisers will be taken into account when the new criteria are applied.

5.7 It is being reported that disabled charity volunteers are giving up their work for fear of being pronounced fit for paid employment by the DSS (*Observer*, 20 June 1993).

References

Anderson, R. and Bury, M. (eds.) 1988: Conclusion. In *Living with chronic illness: the experience of patients and their families*. London: Unwin Hyman, 245–257.

Armstrong, D. 1990: Use of the genealogical method in the exploration of chronic illness: a research note. *Social Science and Medicine* **30(11)**, 1225–1227.

Barber, P. 1991: Caring – the nature of a therapeutic relationship. In Perry, A. and Jolley, M. (eds), *Nursing: a knowledge base for practice*. London: Edward Arnold, 230–270.

Bauman, Z. 1992a: Survival as a social construct. *Theory, Culture and Society* **9(1)**, 1–36.

Bauman, Z. 1992b: *Mortality, immortality and other life strategies*. Cambridge: Polity Press.

Beck, U. 1992: *Risk society: towards a new modernity* (translated by Mark Ritter). London: Sage.

Blaxter, M. 1990: *Health and lifestyles*. London: Routledge.

Bury, M. 1982: Chronic illness as biographical disruption. *Sociology of Health and Illness*, **4(2)**, 167–182.

Bury, M. 1991: The sociology of chronic illness: a review of research and prospects. *Sociology of Health and Illness* **13(4)**, 451–468.

Bury, M.R. and Wood, P.H.N. 1979: Problems of communication in chronic illness. *International Rehabilitation Medicine* **1**, 130–134.

Charmaz, K. 1983: Loss of self: a fundamental form of suffering in the chronically ill. *Sociology of Health and Illness* **5(2)**, 168–195.

Charmaz, K. 1990: 'Discovering' chronic illness: using grounded theory. *Social Science and Medicine* **30(11)**, 1161–1172.

Conrad, P. 1990: Qualitative research on chronic illness: a commentary on method and conceptual development. *Social Science and Medicine* **30(11)**, 1257–1263.

Corbin, J. and Strauss, A. 1985: Managing chronic illness at home: three lines of work. *Qualitative Sociology* **8(3)**, 224–247.

Coward, R. 1989: *The whole truth: the myth of alternative medicine.* London: Faber & Faber.

Dubos, R. 1960: *Mirage of health: utopias, progress and biological change.* London: George Allen & Unwin.

Featherstone, M. 1991: The body in consumer culture. In Featherstone, M., Hepworth, M. and Turner, B. (eds), *The body: social process and cultural theory.* London: Sage, 170–196.

Freidson, E. 1988: *Profession of medicine: a study of the sociology of applied knowledge.* Chicago: University of Chicago Press.

Friedman, J. 1992: Narcissism, roots and postmodernity: the constitution of selfhood in the global crisis. In Lash, S. and Friedman, J. (eds), *Modernity and identity.* Oxford: Blackwell, 331–366.

Gerhardt, U. 1989: *Ideas about illness: an intellectual and political history of medical sociology.* Basingstoke: Macmillan.

Gerhardt, U. 1990: Qualitative research on chronic illness: the issue and the story. *Social Science and Medicine* **30(11)**, 1149–1159.

Giddens, A. 1991: *Modernity and self-identity: self and society in the late modern age.* Cambridge: Polity Press.

Glaser, B.G. and Strauss, A.L. 1968: *The discovery of grounded theory: strategies for qualitative research.* London: Weidenfeld & Nicholson.

Goffman, E. 1990: *Stigma: notes on the management of spoiled identity.* London: Penguin.

Harrison, S. et al. 1990: *The dynamics of British health policy.* London: Routledge.

Hay, L.L. 1988: *You can heal your life.* London: Eden Grove Editions.

Herzlich, C. and Pierret, J. 1984: Malades d'hier, malades d'aujourd'hui: de la mort collective au devoir de la guérison. Paris: Payot. Translated as *Illness and self in society.* (Baltimore and London: Johns Hopkins University Press, 1987: references here are to the French edition.)

Holmes, T.H. and Masuda, M. 1974: Life change and illness susceptibility. In Dohrenwend, B.S. and Dohrenwend, B.P. (eds), *Stressful life events: their nature and effects.* New York: John Wiley & Sons, 45–72.

Illich, I. 1976: *Limits to medicine.* London: Marion Boyars.

Inglis, B. 1981: *The diseases of civilisation.* London: Hodder & Stoughton.

Jacobs, G. 1990: *Candida albicans: yeast and your health.* London: Macdonald.

Jobling, R. 1977: Learning to live with it: an account of a career of chronic dermatological illness and patienthood. In Davis, A. and Horobin, G. (eds), *Medical encounters: the experience of illness and treatment.* London: Croom Helm, 72–86.

Jobling, R. 1988: The experience of psoriasis under treatment. In Anderson, R. and Bury, M. (eds), *Living with chronic illness: the experience of patients and their families.* London: Unwin Hyman, 225–244.

Klein, R. 1989: *The politics of the National Health Service,* 2nd edition. London: Longman.

Levine, S. 1987: *Healing into life and death.* Bath: Gateway Press.

Locker, D. 1991: Living with chronic illness. In Scambler, G. (ed.) *Sociology as applied to medicine*, 3rd edition. London: Bailliere Tindall, 81–92.

MacDonald, L. 1988: The experience of stigma: living with rectal cancer. In Anderson, R. and Bury, M. (eds), *Living with chronic illness: the experience of patients and their families*. London: Unwin Hyman, 177–202.

Mackarness, R. 1976: *Not all in the mind*. London: Pan Books.

McKeown, T. 1976: *The role of medicine: dream, mirage or nemesis?* London: Nuffield Provincial Hospitals Trust.

Maes, S., Vingerhoets, A. and Van Heck, G. 1987: The study of stress and disease: some developments and requirements. *Social Science and Medicine* **25(6)**, 567–578.

Mechanic, D. 1974: Discussion of research programs on relations between stressful life events and episodes of physical illness. In Dohrenwend, B.S. and Dohrenwend, B.P. (eds), *Stressful life events: their nature and effects*. New York: John Wiley & Sons, 87–97.

Mellor, P. and Shilling, C. 1993: Modernity, self-identity and the sequestration of death. *Sociology* **27(3)**, 411–431.

Mestrovic, S. and Glassner, B. 1983: A Durkheimian hypothesis on stress. *Social Science & Medicine* **17(18)**, 1315–1327.

Oakley, A. 1980: *Women confined: towards a sociology of childbirth*. Oxford: Martin Robertson.

Parsons, T. 1951: *The social system*. London: Routledge & Kegan Paul.

Pinder, R. 1988: Striking balances: living with Parkinson's disease. In Anderson, R. and Bury, M. (eds), *Living with chronic illness: the experience of patients and their families*. London: Unwin Hyman, 67–88.

Pollock, K. 1988: On the nature of social stress: production of a modern mythology. *Social Science and Medicine* **26(3)**, 381–392.

Riessman, C.W. 1990: Strategic uses of narrative in the presentation of self and illness: a research note. *Social Science and Medicine* **30(11)**, 1195–1200.

Robinson, I. 1988: *Multiple sclerosis*. London: Routledge.

Robinson, I. 1990: Personal narratives, social careers and medical courses: analysing life trajectories in autobiographies of people with multiple sclerosis. *Social Science and Medicine* **30(11)**, 1173–1186.

Scambler, G. 1991: Deviance, sick role and stigma. In Scambler, G. (ed.), *Sociology as applied to medicine*. London: Bailliere Tindall, 185–196.

Scambler, G. and Hopkins, A. 1988: Accommodating epilepsy in families. In Anderson, R. and Bury, M. (eds), *Living with chronic illness: the experience of patients and their families*. London: Unwin Hyman, 156–176.

Scambler, G. and Hopkins, A. 1990: Generating a model of epileptic stigma: the role of qualitative analysis. *Social Science and Medicine*, **30(11)**, 1187–1194.

Selye, H. 1975: *Stress without distress*. London: Hodder & Stoughton.

Silverman, D. 1985: *Qualitative method and sociology: describing the social world*. Aldershot: Gower.

Smith, C. 1985: Introduction to Lorde, A. In *The cancer journals*. London: Sheba Feminist Publishers, i–xi.

Sontag, S. 1991: *Illness as metaphor*. London: Penguin.

Strauss, A. 1990: Preface. *Social Science and Medicine*, **30(11)**, v–vi.

Turner, B.S. 1992: *Regulating bodies: essays in medical sociology*. London: Routledge.

Wiener, C.L. 1975: The burden of rheumatoid arthritis: tolerating the uncertainty. *Social Science and Medicine*, **9(2)**, 97–104.

Wilkinson, S. 1988: *M.E. and you: a survivor's guide to post-viral fatigue syndrome*. Wellingborough: Thorsons.

Williams, G. 1984: The genesis of chronic illness: narrative re-construction. *Sociology of Health and Illness* **6(2)**, 176–200.

Williams, G.H. 1989: Hope for the humblest? The role of self-help in chronic illness: the case of ankylosing spondylitis. *Sociology of Health and Illness* **11(2)**, 135–159.

Williams, G.H. and Wood, P.H.N. 1986: Common-sense beliefs about illness: a mediating role for the doctor. *The Lancet* **2**, 1435–1437.

Yoshida, K.K. 1993: Reshaping of self: a pendular reconstruction of self and identity among adults with traumatic spinal cord injury. *Sociology of Health and Illness* **15(2)**, 217–245.

Young, A. 1980: The discourse on stress and the reproduction of conventional knowledge. *Social Science and Medicine* **14B(3)**, 133–146.

Zola, I. K. 1983: Helping one another: a speculative history of the self-help movement. In *Socio-medical inquiries: recollections, reflections and reconsiderations*. Philadelphia: Temple University Press, 205–214.

Sociology of the NHS: when does the community decide?

June Greenwell

Introduction

The question that is central to this chapter concerns communities, both the possibility that they may be influential in determining their own health care, and the structures and processes involved in empowering or denying such a possibility.

For everyone in health care, 'community' is an exceedingly familiar adjective. Community care, community nursing and community medicine are terms used routinely. Patients are admitted from and discharged into 'the community', so describing the influence of the community in health care would seem to be a straightforward project. In practice this is far from being the case. An immediate difficulty is that the term community is frequently used in health care to indicate an activity that does not take place in hospital; community is effectively defined, not by what it *is*, but by what it *is not*. The hospital is positioned as the central institution and 'the community' is the amorphous locality that surrounds it. Before discussing whether or how a community can be influential, the nature of 'community' must be more clearly defined.

In recent years the concept of community has been discarded by sociologists as being largely meaningless. Previously, the emphasis had been on a simplistic division into two types of social groupings, described by the 19th century German sociologist Tönnies as *Gemeinschaft*, and translated as community, or *Gesellschaft*, indicating looser social links and translated as associations (Tönnies 1887). Gemeinschaft social groupings were considered to typify rural communities thought to have particular characteristics of kinship and cohesion, compared to the individualistic, competitive and divided groups found in urban society. When various studies found that these distinctions did not hold, and that there was no clear structural difference between social organisations in rural and urban settings, interest in the concept of community waned. An interest in the way that *place* produced social structures was overlaid by an emphasis on the *nation state* as the boundary within which such structures are generated.

The nature and influence of space and spatial distribution have become an increasingly important sociological concern (Giddens 1984). Empirical studies have demonstrated that social structures such as class, authority, and access to goods and services are negotiated differently in particular localities, so that an understanding of the influence of place is essential: 'place matters' (Gyford 1991). Arguments about whether or how hospital and health care services should be restructured or relocated, and about the potential impact of different patterns of distribution, are examples of a debate that is essentially about the spatial distribution of public goods. This is one of the central topics of this chapter.

An emphasis on *location* is not quite the same as a concern with community. Location indicates a position in space, while community refers variously to groupings of people, or to a particular kind of social group which may or may not be limited to a particular location. Confusingly, community is also used to indicate the territory served by public service providers, sometimes referred to as a public service community, or a community of collective consumption (Castells 1977, 1978). Health and local authority staff may also refer to their *district* in this way, as an alternative to talking of the residents or the population of the district.

At the same time, 'community' may be used to refer to a particular place, or to a social group within the district. This may be a community of place, such as a neighbourhood or a town, or a community of common identity, such as an ethnic or class-based group.

A further important and distinctive use of the term community is to refer to a grouping of people who display a warm and supportive mutuality, a community spirit, although there may be no grounds for supposing that socially supportive structures exist (Bell and Newby 1971). When hospital staff speak of discharging a patient into the community, the impression is given that the patient is going to a supportive environment, since one of the meanings of community is that of a social group whose members recognise and acknowledge each other. If staff referred to patients going to 'the district', or 'the locality', a very different image would be created. Constant reference to the community can be a way of ignoring the absence of supportive structures and minimising the isolation that can be experienced in 'the community'. If this is the situation, references to the community distort reality.

So far, four different concepts of local community have been discussed: public service communities determined by the boundaries of health or local authorities; historic communities such as villages, towns or cities; communities of identity, namely groups who see themselves as being the same sort of people; and mutually supportive groupings with a community spirit.

Some further points need to be made briefly. Communities of identity are 'imagined' communities (Anderson 1983). They exist only because the people involved see themselves as a community, one that is made up of 'people like us'. Imagined communities are therefore not essentially linked to a particular location, and can emerge and disappear. Nevertheless, imagined communities are powerful social constructions, which generate specific organisational structures to reflect the interests of the people who identify themselves as belonging. Nationality, race, religion, sexual orientation or lifestyle may be the basis for a community of identity.

Communities of interest, those which Tönnies identified as 'associations' or 'gesellschaften', are different. People can come together to defend or promote their interests without having a sense of being the same sort of people. However, in competing for scarce resources, whether control of land or access to public services, communities of common interest are particularly forceful when they represent groups who also see themselves as communities of identity. The possibility then exists for community activity to be centred around the exclusion of outsiders. Recently, in Tower Hamlets, competition for housing created some policy formulations designed to serve the interests of residents who had lived locally for more than one generation. These policies were thus serving an interest-based community (Burns *et al.* 1994). The fact that the long-stay residents were white and the incomers often non-white added to the intensity of the debate by drawing on images of identity; the community of interest in this situation was also a community of identity. The same authors noted a similar pattern with an association of affluent home owners in Los Angeles (Davis 1992, quoted by Burns *et al.* 1994). Such accounts of communities in action dispel the idealised depiction of community inherent in conceptions of gemeinschaft.

Communities that are the focus of social analysis vary widely; the particular community studied depends in part on the organisational level at which the study is situated, and in part on the purpose of the research. There is no entity called 'the community' that holds true in all discussion; what is meant by community depends on what is being discussed. However, there is a characteristic that must exist and which, if absent, means that there is no community: there has to be some element of reciprocity, of collective behaviour. This may be short-term and limited to the achievement of a specific goal, but if there is no collective element, there is no community. This is an additional reason why a focus on local districts is important, since it is at local level that collective behaviour is seen as most likely to re-emerge, to 'forego the temptations of private enrichment at the expense of public weal – in short to honour the "city" of which one is a member' (Bell, 1979, quoted by Marquand 1988, p.220). Community challenges individualism: the way that these two opposing principles influence health service provision is a topic to which I shall return.

In this chapter I shall address the possibility that health care services could be accountable downwards to users, rather than upwards to national level organisations or government. I shall also consider whether the values that encourage responsiveness to users have implications for the patient–professional relationship, and how local communities respond to proposed unwelcome change. Two communities are therefore of interest in the discussion: the communities of health service users, and the public service community of all of the residents of a local authority or health authority district, including health care staff. The discussion will make clear which community is being considered.

The main focus is therefore on the local district, but not in isolation from influences that shape and limit local service provision. The local district in the UK has limited power to determine the services that it provides, and the cross-cutting links between local and national structures are of particular interest.

Community involvement in local health services

To what extent can a local community influence patterns of service provision? What creates the momentum for change? How can such involvement be measured?

Health Authorities have for years consulted over plans for service change. Local authorities and professional organisations are among the consultees, and from 1974 there has been a system of statutory consultation with patients, as represented by Community Health Councils. Nevertheless, prior to 1991 and the introduction of an internal market, health service planning decisions were dominated by the views of hospital consultants. This was even more noticeable before the introduction of general management systems in 1985 (Strong and Robinson 1990). Since 1991, GPs have had significantly more influence in service planning, particularly since they have the option to exit from a reliance on the health authority, and become fundholders themselves. Apart from a system of formal consultation, health care planning has thus been largely detached from the views of users and other agencies in the local community. Two changes have occurred that have led to a wider pattern of community involvement in service planning: a greater focus on users' views, and the development of joint care systems for providing community care.

Joint care service provision

Policy directives since 1974 have urged collaboration between health authorities and local authorities for the provision of community care, but until 1991 the emphasis was largely on joint funding from the two agencies, rather than joint working to deliver services. Following the 1991 NHS and Community Care Act, the pressure for joint working increased.

Social service departments are part of local government, and are therefore controlled through a democratic structure of elected councillors; the NHS has a less democratic form of governance. Joint working required staff to work collaboratively, although they may be based in service areas with very different organisational cultures, forms of service delivery, and systems of financial control. A major review of the new arrangements reported health service frustrations with the slowness of social service decision-making. 'Managerial cultures . . . seem to have little time for the complexities of democratic representation and accountability' (Langan and Clarke 1994, p.88).

A democratic structure provides a mechanism for local accountability, but it is not a guarantee of responsiveness to community or user values or needs. An assessment of responsiveness to users is required to determine whether the community of service users is able to influence service provision and, if not, whether existing barriers are locally created, or relate to wider organisational cultures or structures.

User involvement in service planning

In 1992, health authorities were told that they should develop mechanisms for consulting users in planning and monitoring services, through a document entitled *Local Voices* (National Health Service Management Executive 1992). This was a top-down directive to health authorities to be responsive to users, but firmly within a service structure that had been imposed following the NHS reforms of 1991. A range of 'bottom-up' initiatives were developing at the same time (Dennis 1991; Joule 1992; National Consumer Council 1992). Together these marked a significant change in NHS culture, some drawing on management principles of 'closeness to the customer' although imposed by a central command, while others emerged from a base in the work of Community Health Councils (CHCs), the patient's 'watchdogs' in the NHS, or from the Patients' Association. They were aimed at patients as users of services, and eschewed the statutory model that had been used in 1974 to create the CHCs. CHCs continued to exist, interacting with the *Local Voices* initiatives in ways that varied between districts.

Local Voices challenged health authorities to become 'champions of the people' by involving service users through mechanisms such as focus groups, health forums, close working with Community Health Councils, public meetings and telephone hotlines. Responses to this initiative by health districts have been studied in one former health region (Lupton and Taylor 1995). A different study has looked at user involvement in the planning of community care services. Here the main focus was on the user's assessments of service provision, rather than on staff evaluations (Hoyes *et al.* 1994; Hoyes and Means 1994).

Before discussing the findings of these studies I want to look at two related systems for appraising the extent of citizen participation or empowerment. A description of community involvement in the form of a ladder of citizen participation was developed by Arnstein (1971). She suggested that there were eight 'rungs' to the ladder, extending from non-participation to citizen control. The rungs were as follows: manipulation of citizens; therapy; the provision of information; consultation; placation; partnership; delegated power; and citizen control.

It has subsequently been suggested that 12 distinct stages can be identified in relation to local government in the UK, and that these can be grouped into three categories: non-participation, citizen participation and citizen control (Burns *et al.* 1994). A simplified outline of this grid is given in Fig. 6.1. Readers with a particular interest in assessing user involvement are recommended to examine the original.

By using this scale it is possible to assess tentatively the findings of the two studies mentioned earlier. It provides an empirical base with which to start to answer an important question. One study looked at care services provided by Social Services as part of local government, while the other involved NHS staff who are not employed within a locally controlled, democratically accountable service. Does either model provide evidence of greater responsiveness to user values?

FIGURE 6.1 A LADDER OF CITIZEN EMPOWERMENT

12	Independent control	CITIZEN
11	Entrusted control	CONTROL
....		
10	Delegated control	
9	Partnership	
8	Limited decentralised decision-making	CITIZEN
7	Effective advisory bodies	PARTICIPATION
6	Genuine consultation	
5	High-quality information	
....		
4	Customer care	
3	Poor information	CITIZEN
2	Cynical consultation	NON-PARTICIPATION
1	Civic hype	

Source: Adapted from *The Politics of Decentralisation: Revitalising Local Democracy* by Burns et al. (1994, p.162).

The first point to note is that both studies reported considerable local variation between districts. Lupton and Taylor (1995) examined how District Health Authorities in the former Wessex Region were attempting to involve users in health service decision-making. They found that the form of involvement with users varied depending on the department that took the lead role. Public health departments encouraged community involvement in identifying health needs. Public relations departments were more likely to focus on media presentations and 'one-off' events. Quality assurance staff concentrated on feedback from service users to assist in service monitoring. The range of priorities identified indicates uncertainty of aim. This was confirmed by respondents, who welcomed public involvement in principle, but were uncertain about the purpose of the exercise.

The skills that staff felt were needed were only just beginning to develop, 2 years after the districts had begun to implement *Local Voices*. Key staff reported feeling isolated, and there were some reports of hostility from colleagues. There was frustration at the short-term nature of some of the processes being utilised. The involvement of users had a low priority where organisational change was creating uncertainty and upheaval. One of the more positive reports was of a general recognition that public involvement needed to become 'everybody's business'. While this was a cultural change apparently supportive of user involvement, it was leading to a situation where posts that carried specific responsibilities for encouraging user involvement were disappearing. If user involvement was everyone's responsibility, why have designated posts? While this was a rational approach, there was a risk that, if no individual was specifically responsible, user involvement would once again be marginalised.

An assessment of the published findings suggests that, on Burns' ladder of citizen participation, the health districts studied by Lupton and Taylor were at the bottom rungs of the scale, trying to engage in genuine consultation although unconfident as to their skills and objectives. There was some cynicism reported among staff who were not directly involved, which may produce non-participation if it emerged as a dominant attitude.

The study of user involvement in community care planning focused primarily on the views of users (Hoyes *et al.* 1994; Hoyes and Means 1994). Findings showed that almost all user and carer groups involved in planning for the 1992–93 plan had commented unfavourably on the nature of their involvement, but that there had been a 'less uniformly negative' set of reports from the 1993–94 exercise (Hoyes and Means 1994). Users expressed frustration that Social Services staff did not seem to know how they wanted to consult, or on what. Consultees' views were noted, but there was no involvement when strategic issues were discussed. The report spoke of the 'more professionalised' user and carer groups being involved in joint service planning. User involvement was at a locality (sub-district) purchasing level, within a macro framework created by key staff from a higher level of health and social services. The authors posed the question of whether this would be a strait-jacket or an empowering framework.

The impression given from the report of this study is of a move over a period of 1 year from poor quality information and token consultation to attempts at genuine consultation. Using Burns' schema (Fig. 6.1), users were seeing a move from non-participation to the lower rungs of participation.

Given that one of these studies was mainly of user views in social service planning, and the other was of staff views in health care purchasing, the findings are surprisingly similar. The answer to the question posed earlier is that the democratic structures that control social services do not appear to have produced a greater degree of user participation than the non-democratic form of governance in the NHS. In both reports, staff expressed misgivings about possible future trends that could leave user involvement as a marginal issue in service delivery.

Whether or not this happens will be at least partly determined by the nature of local service culture. If involvement of users only occurs in response to a directive from above, then the staff who are committed will be isolated within an unsupportive environment, and user involvement would cease if the directive changed. However, in some districts the move to involve users in service planning was compatible with local service values developed independently, and pre-empting the 1992 directive. For example, Rochdale had a strategic policy for involving users as part of a wider community development approach to service delivery, involving estate committees, community-based action committees, and community school councils (Burns et al. 1994). Developing user-led services requires a 'profound shift in the way services are planned and delivered' (Carpenter 1995, p.84). Carpenter (1995) reports on community care projects showing that user involvement often led to more cost-effective as well as to more user-sensitive service provision. A requirement that users chair the partnership groups in joint care planning was compatible with local service culture (Chapman et al. 1995). The weakness of studies of one aspect of user or community involvement is that, by focusing on one part of one service, the influence of wider aspects of local service culture may go unnoticed, or be outside the remit of the study.

The limits of responsiveness

One of the factors driving through the reforms of community care was a belief that professional values had been dominant in social service provision, at the cost of effective management, with a tendency routinely to ascribe inadequacies in service provision to cuts in government funding. Acceptance of a defined budget within a service culture that demands loyalty to the service, rather than to the service user, carries with it the risk of a different kind of failure, that of understating needs in order to meet budgetary requirements. The likelihood of this happening was made evident when a confidential circular was leaked in 1992 (Guardian, 30 December 1992). The Social Service Inspectorate's Chief Inspector warned councils not to let Social Service clients know of their entitlements unless there was funding available to meet identified needs. Social Services staff should record unmet need, but such information should be aggregated, so that while a Council could identify generalised unmet needs, no individual client could point to a written record suggesting that their own assessed needs had been ignored. Information about needs that could not be met should be filed in a way that makes it impossible for them to be ascribed to any individual client.

Public response to this leaked memo led to changed guidance, and since 1993 the Social Service Inspectorate has required an assessment of all assessed need be made and recorded. Even so, the point has been made that, unless informed staff encourage clients to express their needs, and unless there is as great a pressure on assessors to prove that they have completed an adequate assessment as there is to keep within budget, needs will be understated (Ellis 1993). Ellis (1993, p.3) concluded that assessors' 'preconceptions of policy, resources, and values precluded that dialogue with users and carers which should be the foundation of joint assessment'.

Patients as consumers or partners

So far, user involvement has been discussed mainly in relation to service planning, but this approach is inadequate. In health care, the most intense involvement of 'users' occurs when they are patients, and the key relationship for patients is with the professional staff who are providing care and treatment, not with service planners. Citizen empowerment in health care delivery is of limited value if it does not extend to the individual patient–professional relationship. Is this happening?

In a study of inter-professional relationships in hospital it was noted that staff not uncommonly referred to particular consultants as 'owning' the patient (Walby et al. 1994). It is a phrase redolent of the relationship between a passively dependent patient and a paternalistic professional, not inappropriate for a patient in intensive care, where the phrase was most frequently reported, but entirely inappropriate for the active collaboration between patient and professional required in all but the most acute health care situations. For some decades the relationship of patient to health professional has been evolving from a passive acceptance of treatment and care to something more like an active partnership (Greenwell 1995). The greater emphasis now being given to health promotion is one of the factors strengthening the trend toward partnership. A partnership relationship is further enhanced when someone who is a patient is also and at the same time a carer, and with an ageing population and a greater emphasis on providing care at home, this will be a common pattern. Carers can be accurately depicted as 'lay professionals', namely partners of health professionals in providing care.

However, the partnership model is only one way of conceptualising the patient–professional relationship. Another is to perceive the patient as a consumer who is able to claim a consumer's rights to good quality treatment and care. A third approach is to regard the patient or client as representing a collection of demands for treatment or care, which must be assessed in order to see whether these equate with needs as defined by the professional. These models of a patient's position carry strikingly different value assumptions.

Positioning patients as consumers in a market model of health care conveys an expectation that a patient's responsibilities are only towards their own needs. The language of rights is utilised, but within an individualistic framework. A 'consumer rights' approach finds some expression in the Patient's Charter, although this is perhaps better understood as part of a quality assurance system (Department of Health 1991). A consumer's role is to assess, select, demand and use services. Providers of services are required to respond to the demands of the consumers, but consumers do not have an obligation to help to sustain service delivery. There is no duty of active involvement laid on the consumer of health services, other than to obtain for themselves the best provision. Acknowledging the patient as an equal partner in health is a radically different notion; there is an implied responsibility given to the patient, and to the community of potential patients, to contribute to the partnership as a citizen willing to sustain adequate service provision.

The notion that individuals have duties as well as rights has been expounded by Etzioni (1993). His view is that it is both wrong and morally dangerous to emphasise rights without an equal stress on duties, a *communitaire* view of citizenship. There are criticisms to be made of his position, notably the lack of an equivalent stress on the duties of institutionalised power structures. However, Etzioni's notion of a citizen as someone who has duties as well as rights is central to the distinction between a perception of patients as consumers, and one that acknowledges them as partners in the provision of health care services.

A *communitaire* approach is implied in *Local Voices*, while a consumerist position is one of the elements informing the Patient's Charter. By using both of these models, the UK Government ensured that there was no clear direction capable of maximising support for improvements in health care. By stressing patients' rights, the UK Government could be seen as supporting service improvements without having to accept responsibility for funding the service at a level capable of meeting the standards, leaving local service providers to manage the process of reaching charter standards within ever tighter budgets. An emphasis on patients' duties alongside their rights was not made, and the one-sided nature of the patients' rights approach produced a vehement reaction at times (Brown 1991).

Health rationing and public participation

The inadequacy of a consumer model is further demonstrated when the issues relating to health service rationing are considered. Should users be involved in helping to determine service priorities, and sometimes in decisions not to supply some forms of treatment? Does the local community have any role in determining rationing in the UK? The state of Oregon (USA) has used the public to help determine a ranking list of health treatments available through publicly funded services, with some treatments unavailable except with private insurance (Klein 1992). Is there any equivalent response in the UK?

The UK health market has always been a market for rationed services, although it has usually been managed implicitly through waiting lists or clinical decisions (Aaron and Schwartz 1984). Transferring care or treatment from a free to a means-tested service provider is another way of rationing services, which will be discussed later. Rationing through explicit decisions began to be discussed openly in the early 1990s (Allen 1993). The appropriateness of involving users in making value judgements has been questioned (Freemantle 1994).

If users of services are primarily perceived as being consumers, and not citizens with responsibilities, it is difficult to see why it is appropriate for them to be involved in addressing such issues. Discussions of equity involve considerations of ethical values that do not fit within a consumerist approach to service delivery, but are consistent with the notion of users as citizens, and therefore as active partners in determining responses to ethical concerns in health care delivery (see Chapter 8).

The introduction of a market system in 1991 increased the need to address such issues (Harrison and Wistow 1992). While rationing had always existed, the use of written contracts within a market system of health care delivery, and the competition required to gain and retain service contracts, meant that rationing decisions became more transparent in the UK after 1991. The referral of patients for whom payment is not covered in advance through a contract is an example of the ethical dilemmas intrinsic to a market system. There is some evidence that health service providers have deliberately excluded particular services from unspecified block contracts, in order to price these higher under the extra-contractual referrals system, or within 'cost per case' arrangements (Johnstone 1994). This has direct implications for admission procedures.

Important rationing issues should surface as mainstream concerns in a parliamentary democracy, but in practice open discussion of health care rationing is uncommon within political parties. The management of political image leads political parties to dissociate themselves from unpopular issues (Beck 1992). The need to deal with image rather than open discussion was highlighted by reports that a junior health minister had cancelled a trip to investigate the system of rationing recently introduced in Oregon (USA). Apparently this was to avoid giving the impression that the Government supported health care rationing (*Sunday Telegraph*, 17 April 1994). Instead of addressing rationing decisions through central directives, these are devolved down to local providers and purchasers, and made explicit in the contracts required by the internal market.

A market system which compels rationing issues to be addressed without the need for directives has other advantages for governments. The market acts as a discipline, performing something of the same function that Foucault saw in Bentham's *Panopticon*; it provides continuous surveillance and internalises the values of the 'controller' (Foucault 1980). Blame for inadequate services is diffused and not forcefully directed at government. However, devolving blame also implies devolving responsibility, and the process of devolving responsibility points to public involvement, if only to legitimise difficult decisions.

As yet, this is only happening to a limited degree. *The Economist* magazine surveyed Health Authorities and found that only three had attempted to involve the public in making rationing decisions, although 12 out of 114 Health Authorities consulted reported that they would not pay for some specific treatments, mainly tattoo removal and infertility treatment. One Authority had set up an ethics committee of philosophers, lawyers and others to advise on medical priorities (*Economist*, 23 April 1994).

The change to a market system has sharpened the focus on ethical issues in health care. As these are confronted, further change will be generated, producing new concerns. Health care provides a quintessential example of the way in which reflexive change has become a characteristic feature of social structures (Walby *et al.* 1994; see also Chapter 2).

Community protest and health care services

So far the focus of the discussion has been on forms of involvement initiated by a 'top-down' approach to community involvement. This means that local concerns and values may be subordinated to central policy. Therefore what follows is a discussion of community involvement in health care service provision that is 'bottom-up', and sometimes confrontational, as distinct from user involvement encouraged from above, which must be contained within a centrally controlled agenda, or determined locally at an executive level.

How do such forms of community action emerge? How does the relationship between health authorities and local communities in any particular district become co-operative or conflictual? Why do some forms of hospital contraction proceed with public support, or at least acquiescence, while other closure programmes produce intense opposition? Why is local protest more evident at some times and in some locations than in others? And how does sociology inform these issues?

Opaque and transparent decisions

District level policies are largely determined centrally, whether for the NHS or for local authority services. However, there is a difference in the transparency of local council and local health authority decisions and actions. In local government, unpopular directives from central government are given publicity. In the NHS, chairs and members of health authorities are appointed centrally, and the model used for health authority and Trust boards resembles a commercial private limited company. Health Authority Members are specifically not appointed to represent local constituencies, and some see themselves as employees, with equivalent loyalty: 'As an employee of a public service having taken the Queen's shilling you have to temper your position to a certain point' (Watson 1994, p.78). CHCs have taken on the function of challenging local policy, but must do this in a manner that does not alienate them from health authority staff to the extent that they are unable to fulfil their important function of representing the interests of individual patients. Therefore usually the implementation of policy decisions in the NHS may not receive the same exposure to public opinion as local authority decisions, unless there is a proposed closure of a ward, clinic or hospital. It is around these issues that the nature of community protest or acquiescence will be examined. This includes acute and long-stay hospital changes, and changing patterns of long-stay nursing care for elderly patients.

Before looking at hospital closure in any detail, I shall summarise some of the approaches used in sociology to analyse community action.

Analysing community protest

One approach is to look at the agencies involved in producing a policy change. Pressure groups, parliament, the media, NHS Authorities, the consultative machinery, ministers and civil servants, industrial and commercial influence have all been listed in relation to health care in the UK (Ham 1992). The law and legal institutions need adding to the list, but the critical issue here is not whether all possible agencies have been mentioned, but how and where they become influential. Lists of agencies in themselves do not provide an analysis of the different structures that need to be present for any agencies to be influential, nor do they distinguish between those which operate at local and at national level, or in different ways at both levels. Rather than examining agencies, an analytical approach will be used in this discussion to try and determine the answers to such questions.

One theoretical position is that public protest is inevitable (Castells 1978). The nature of the state's response to protest is critical in determining the outcome (Pickvance 1985). Examination of how incidents come to command attention, claim legitimacy, and lead to change has also proved useful (Solesbury 1976). This is linked to what has been labelled 'the third dimension of power', the way in which a contentious issue may be kept out of public view in order to prevent the emergence of opposition (Lukes 1974). The way that knowledge is accessed or withheld, and the agencies involved in this process, are relevant concerns, as is the form of the law and the interrelationship of judicial and government authority (Beck 1992; Scheuerman 1994). A different analysis relies on an examination of the structures and resources that must be present before protest emerges (Bagguley 1991). None of these accounts can be examined in detail in this chapter, but all will be drawn on in discussion.

A Marxist analysis would suggest that conflict over the provision of important services is inevitable. Services are required to support workers so that their labour power can be constantly reproduced, but to create profit this will always be at a minimum level and will thus generate protest. A more sophisticated variation of this analysis recognises that, in modern society, most essential services are provided through public funds. The extent to which state-funded health care services can be provided is limited, so given that health care is a highly valued commodity, conflict will occur. Protest will be directed at the state through urban social movements that involve different class groups (Castells 1977, 1978). One of the criticisms of this analysis is that it ignores the capacity of the state to respond to protest (Pickvance 1985). The occupation of an accident and emergency department in Manchester in protest against a closure plan was an example of direct action that revealed a lack of effective contact with users, subsequently addressed by service providers (Emanuel 1993).

A different conflictual position emerges from a conceptualisation of the medical profession as a purveyor of sickness. Community-based health movements thus have to accept the inevitability of a challenge to medical domination of health care (Watt and Rodmell 1993). This is a very different approach to the 'urban movement' protest over the inadequate provision of health services.

The emphasis in this chapter is largely on the structures that determine whether services are provided, principally because this is a dominant issue in the mid-1990s. My stress is on the organisational and cultural factors associated with the implementation of plans, rather than the desirability or otherwise of any specific closure or rationalisation proposal. I will use these various analytical approaches to examine the changing pattern of support, acquiescence and protest that has been evident in relation to hospital contraction or closure in the UK since the early 1980s.

Changing hospitals: acute hospitals

Figures for hospital closures in England are difficult to obtain. Given the scale of information collection in the NHS since 1990, it is instructive that the Department of Health does not routinely attempt to collect this information. However, in 1995, House of Commons library staff were able to obtain information from all English regions almost equivalent in the time span covered to existing information for Scotland, Wales and Northern Ireland. The figures are listed in Table 6.1.

This pattern is consistent with a policy of attempting to concentrate acute hospital care that requires expensive equipment and specialist skills in around 24–40 sites, each servicing between 1–2 *million* people. Locally sited acute care facilities will concentrate on the diagnosis and treatment of less complex conditions, with fewer beds and buildings, and more flexible multi-disciplinary teams providing care and treatment in local centres. Local variation is anticipated (Institute of Health Service Management 1994a).

Table 6.1   Hospital closures

England	245 hospital closures since 1990
	85 psychiatric hospitals
	60 acute hospitals
	60 elderly care hospitals
	14 maternity hospitals
	14 specialist hospitals
	12 unclassified hospitals
Scotland	34 hospital closures since 1991
Wales	17 hospital closures since 1991
Northern Ireland	8 hospital closures since 1991

Source: House of Commons Library/*Guardian*, 1 May 1995.

This is in marked contrast to the policies laid down in the 1962 Hospital Plan for England and Wales (Ministry of Health 1962), or the equivalent Scottish and Northern Irish documents. These Plans proposed that a district general hospital should be provided for populations of around 125 000 people. Resultant hospital building developments took some time to be implemented, so that up to the early 1980s acute hospital closures were usually linked to the transfer of services to new larger hospitals. This pattern of acute hospital distribution is now being dismantled, or 're-configured'.

In the mid-1980s, budgetary pressure and the introduction of a centralised management structure led to a programme of hospital rationalisation (Flynn 1991, 1992). Figures for hospital closures are not available, but the numbers of beds declined, while at the same time turnover increased. There was overt local and media opposition, but with limited impact. The temporary closure of a children's ward in Birmingham produced an exceptional protest, but rather than halting the closure programme it led the then Prime Minister to announce a radical review of the NHS.

There are several reasons why there is a programme of hospital contraction in most western nations (Saltman and Von Otter 1992). Some pressures are from health-led concerns to devote more resources to the promotion of health rather than to the treatment of illness. Technological advances allow more treatment to be safely provided without an overnight stay in hospital, or with shorter stays, and specialist diagnostic skills can be provided at a distance. Time acceleration, and an ability to conduct social actions over large distances, have both been seen as characterising modernity (Giddens 1984). The policies that are being discussed for restructuring hospitals are linked to these features of society. A different emphasis comes from the concern to provide routine high-quality care by concentrating specialist services in a few centres where expertise can be enhanced by treating large numbers of patients. All of these point to a restructuring of hospitals, and the contraction of services on some sites (Ham and Appleby 1993).

The factors listed above can be described as being part of a *health-driven* agenda. Quite different trends produce a *finance-driven* agenda. But there is also a *political* agenda that has added to the health-based arguments for cost containment. The Executive Director of the Welsh Health Planning Forum has described the pressure for public sector spending restraint. The way in which his analysis relates the interests of leading European industrialists to the provision of NHS care is particularly interesting:

> ... the 1985 White Paper, Completing the Internal Market ... came into existence following the formation of a think-tank in the early 1980s of leading businessmen from large multi-national corporations, for example, Dekker from Philips and the Agnelli family from Fiat ... their objective was to be competitive in the global marketplace. But how was that competitiveness to be achieved? The answers lie in two directions: first ... through good management; and second, through decreased personal and corporate taxes. Within the UK, the Government have attempted to control public spending in all areas, health included, in order to reduce tax burdens in the hope of encouraging enterprise.
>
> (Warner 1992, p.129)

Warner's account illuminates the parameters that limit the effectiveness of local influence in health service provision. It requires a readjustment of familiar thinking to absorb the notion that the number of affordable hospital beds in an NHS district hospital relates to the influence of the owners of Fiat motors, but this is the nature of globalised economic processes. Local decision-making can only operate within policies determined by international structures operating globally.

There are therefore powerful pressures on service providers to restructure hospital provision, for reasons relating to treatment and health care as well as to finance and political policy. However, the arguments of service providers to support restructuring are matched by arguments for retaining existing hospitals that have an equally compelling force for the users of services.

Hospitals provide visible evidence of the existence of a caring function in the community. They embody by their existence a promise of available treatment when we are ill. To see a hospital close without a replacement being provided weakens the faith that has been placed in the NHS since 1948. The promise of community care is not a satisfactory alternative, partly because there is no visible presence in the shape of buildings, and partly because the experience of community care reforms suggests that care will not be free as it is in hospital.

Giddens (1984) has described late modernity as requiring trust to be based in disembedded systems, in contrast to the trust invested in kin, religion, and tradition in pre-modern societies. I suggest that the NHS has performed the function of being a trust-attracting institution, able to minimise anxiety by providing an assurance of treatment. Seeing a familiar hospital close can generate anxiety. A member of a Pensioner's Forum expressed these views to a policy think tank: 'Everyone I speak to is scared to death. It's wrong ... Ordinary people are afraid now that if they're ill they won't get treatment' (May 1994).

Certain factors have added to the mistrust that hospital closure generates in the 1990s. There is a sharper sense of financial insecurity, and thus an awareness of dependence on NHS provision. Fewer people are confident of being able to pay for private hospital care. There are more elderly people, and thus there is a greater need for hospital services. The growing public realisation that the NHS is ceasing to provide for long-term care adds perceptibly to anxiety, for if so significant a change could happen without public debate, then a commitment of trust in the service no longer seems reasonable. Protestations that acute care and treatment will remain freely available are questioned. Perhaps most influential is a widely held conviction that hospital closures are an unnecessary and politically directed change. The creation of NHS Trusts has weakened the sense of public ownership, ironically, since the presence of Hospital Trusts may emerge as one of the factors slowing down the hospital restructuring programme.

Hospitals contribute to self-identity; they are the places where the physical self was born, where children were born, and often where parents or siblings have been seriously ill or died. In that sense they have some of the functions of a monument; they are a point in space where significant personal events took place. NHS hospitals have also had another significance; they have conveyed a sense of ownership. It was quite possible for a politician in the mid-1980s to produce a book entitled *Our NHS* without any overtly cynical reaction (Owen 1988). The local NHS hospital is 'our' hospital. Given the emotional investment borne by hospitals, the transfer of acute hospital care from hospitals to an amorphous 'community' that lacks visibility in physical space is never going to be a popular move in so far as it involves hospital closure.

Nevertheless, it was noted some years ago that 'Britain has found it easier to close hospitals than have other countries . . .' (*Economist*, 19 November 1988). The reasoning behind this statement is that the NHS is untypical among western democracies in the extent to which hospital services are centrally controlled by government. Insurance-based or privately financed systems do not provide an opportunity to impose tight central control over funding and policy. Even in those countries that have a tax funded service, there is often an element of local control reinforced through local systems of tax distribution. Sweden is an example (Pollitt 1993). In the UK there is no local tax base to provide funds with which to challenge centrally controlled policies. In the Scandinavian countries, elected councillors can be put under democratic pressure to retain existing services by marginally increasing local taxation. The range of people critically involved in the decision, the nature of the pressures that can be placed on them, and the array of groups able to influence the decision would therefore be different to the position in the UK.

None of this has changed. If the lack of democratic or financial independence is the main reason why hospitals can be closed more easily in the UK than elsewhere, then patterns of closure should be consistent. The introduction of a market system into health care may have been expected to accelerate closure programmes, and this explanation was given when the hospital closures listed above were published. Yet in a quite remarkable way, and despite what might have been expected, public protest since 1993 has meant the abandonment of some provincial hospital closure plans, and the slowing down of the London hospital closure programme. This is an unexpected situation. It deserves a detailed analysis that is not yet possible, although some tentative explanations can be discussed.

Before 1992, there was a sense of inevitability in relation to hospital rationalisation and closure plans. In 1992, the Tomlinson Report on the reorganisation of the London hospital and GP services was published, arguing for a substantial reduction in the number of hospital beds in central London. This was based on extensive research by the King's Fund (King's Fund 1992; Tomlinson 1992). Initially there was a degree of public consensus supportive of the Tomlinson Committee findings (*Guardian* 16 October 1992). The press reaction was in general quite supportive, in marked contrast to the press reaction to the Birmingham ward closure in 1987 (see above). It seemed that public opinion had learnt to accommodate itself to massive structural change in the NHS.

One of the commentators who did not share in this consensus saw a hegemonic response developing that needed refuting:

> The reaction to Sir Bernard Tomlinson's report is a cause for wonder . . . there has been a general reaction of muted acquiescence. In the media, wise commentators have opined that everyone knows London has too many hospital beds. So authoritatively has this judgement been pronounced, it is now almost unchallengeable fact . . . Yet the assumption that London is awash with unneeded hospital beds is utterly and demonstrably wrong.
>
> (*Guardian*, 20 November 1992, p.6)

Immediate objection to the Tomlinson proposals was limited to opposition from some staff and user groups. Subsequently, opposition to the restructuring emerged, but surprisingly slowly. In April 1994, health service managers were noting that famous hospitals were set to close, yet the public response was still muted, and the British Medical Association's objections to closure were ineffective (Health Services Management 1994). In the following year this position changed abruptly: overwhelming opposition to hospital closure emerged. One local newspaper campaign was credited with success in slowing down the implementation of the programme (Butler 1995).

Similarly, community protests in provincial cities of the UK were reported as successfully blocking hospital and casualty department restructuring plans. A report by the Institute of Health Service Managers revealed that only one of several hospital restructuring proposals published by health authorities during the period 1993–94 had been successfully implemented. North West Surrey was unable to implement plans to transform an acute hospital into a community hospital, Birmingham Health Authority decided on bed reductions rather than hospital closure, and Bristol cancelled plans to close Accident and Emergency departments (Institute of Health Service Management 1994b).

The scale of the response to public pressure is in itself a remarkable change from the ineffectiveness of the protests that occurred during the period 1986–92. It is even more surprising in that it contradicts fears that were expressed when a market structure was imposed on the NHS in 1991. So what hypothesis can be put forward to explain this change? Why was it easier to implement hospital closure plans in the years 1985 and 1993, than was the case between 1993 and 1995?

As yet there is insufficient information to allow a definitive response to this question, although some tentative explanations can be provided. In a study that is relevant to this discussion, Bagguley examined why unemployment in the 1980s did not produce protest. He examines and rejects a range of explanations for this, and argues that protest is not inevitable, but requires the presence of particular structures and resources (Bagguley 1991). The section that follows examines several structural and cultural changes since 1993, which may have enabled public protest to achieve a far greater impact in the mid-1990s than was possible in the 1980s.

First, I want to return to the figures for acute hospital closure from 1990 (see above). The particular time span covered may mean that these figures are untypically high, because of structural changes in the NHS between 1985 and 1993.

In 1985, NHS management was restructured. The central features will be familiar to readers and will only be discussed briefly. The introduction of a system of general management at the level of the Health Authority and hospital was the feature that received most attention. A different aspect was the creation of a strong management link from the NHS Management Executive to the Districts, providing a pro-active style 'very different to the conventionally remote style in which civil servants had tended to work' (Levitt and Wall 1992, p.49). Together with the implementation of an array of management techniques, the effect was to alter the local/central balance of the NHS, tilting it towards a much greater degree of central control. Pressure on local managers to balance health authority budgets was much greater than had previously been the case. Hospital rationalisation schemes were planned in many districts (Flynn 1991; Walby et al. 1994). The time scale for implementing hospital closure plans was such that some instances contributed to the closure figures quoted earlier. In these cases, it is the implementation of general management, and not the introduction of the internal market, that will have been the pivotal factor. Unfortunately, without comparable figures for previous years no comparison is possible with the period 1985–90.

The introduction of the internal market will nevertheless have been influential in later closures. Applicants for Trust status had to show that they were capable of keeping within budget. It is difficult to believe that the obligation on Trust applicants to prove their financial competence did not create a greater motivation to close 'inefficient' hospitals. If so, this would become apparent in the figures for 1993. However, the structural and cultural changes that have taken place since then, as a result of the introduction of the purchaser-provider split and the formation of NHS Trusts, may emerge as one of the factors contributing to a different pattern of resistance to hospital closure since 1993. Far from accelerating hospital closure, the

1991 NHS reforms may have had the perverse consequence of introducing checks on restructuring that did not exist previously. This would indicate that the period 1985–1991 was an atypical time of strong centralised control that made it possible to enforce unpopular change, but which has since been transformed into a more fragmented structure with some degree of local autonomy.

A significant factor is the creation of NHS Trust hospitals, and the separation of 'purchasers' and 'providers' in health care. It is possible to move relatively quickly in making the decision to close or restructure a hospital that is directly managed by the Health Authority, as all hospitals were prior to 1991. The senior managers involved in managing change were in a line-management relationship with their Region, and required to implement policy directives. However, with the development of NHS Trust hospitals the pattern is different. The Trust Board can be expected to have an interest in its hospital's continued existence, and in maintaining a capacity to attract and retain contracts by retaining beds. It may want to stop providing some forms of care, but is unlikely to want drastic cutbacks in its bed provision. For a Trust, acute beds are part of the infrastructure needed to win contracts.

Furthermore, the Trust Executive has some independence from the Region, albeit less than was promised when Trusts were proposed (National Health Service Management Executive 1992). The Trust Executive has less reason to conform to the Health Authority restructuring proposals if these conflict with the Trust's aspirations. Where there is a conflict of interests, discussions between the Trust hospitals and the Health Authority will be more evident and protracted than was the case with the rationalisation of hospital facilities in the late 1980s. With lengthier negotiations there is time for opposition to be mobilised and become informed and knowledgeable.

Two aspects of protest may be crucial in determining whether protest leads to action: attracting attention and gaining legitimacy (Solesbury 1976; Ham 1992). The campaign by the London Evening Standard achieved the requirement of attracting attention (Butler 1995). However, alongside the publicity generated by the Standard, detailed professional and academic analysis showed that the statistics that were used to support the closure plans were deeply flawed (Jarman 1993; Raftery and Edwards 1995). The opposition to closure acquired legitimacy as well as attracting attention, but a swift implementation of the Tomlinson proposals would not have left time for the relevant information to be produced and disseminated, and to become influential.

A further causal factor was the changing popularity of the Government. The NHS reforms that were implemented in 1991 were deeply unpopular, but could be imposed by a government with a large Parliamentary majority. In the mid-1990s this was not the situation in the UK. Hospital closures were adding significantly to pressure on Ministers, particularly in relation to London. In response, guidelines on competition introduced to deal with hospital and health authority closures and mergers made it clear that non-economic reasons could be used in decisions relating to hospital changes. Consideration could be given to the implications of closing a unit which was popular with the public (National Health Service Executive 1994a). This marked a reversal of the kind of attitudes that forced through the 1991 reforms. However, it is a response to protest rather than a causal factor.

A different aspect of the post–1991 reforms may also have added to the resistance to closure. The initiative which required purchasers and providers to involve users in planning and monitoring led to the beginning of a cultural change in attitudes to user involvement, as discussed previously. Responsiveness to user opinion was accorded greater official importance in the 1990s than it was either in the profession-dominated service before 1985, or in the centralised management structure that held sway between 1985 and 1991.

Opposing the strongly expressed views of local people presents a greater cultural challenge to health authorities working closely with user groups than was the case for managers in the 1980s, who were not required to give undue credence to user opinion. Consequently, one of the likely features of confrontation over closure is that it will be successful in places where the Health Authority Board values user involvement. It may be unsuccessful where user opinion is dismissed as being of little importance. Local variations in outcome are likely.

Changing hospitals: long-stay hospitals

There is a different background pattern to the closure of long-stay psychiatric hospitals. Between 1965 and 1974 there was a succession of reports of ill-treatment of patients in long-stay hospitals in the UK (Martin 1984). These were vigorously contested at varying levels. They will be examined in more detail shortly. The point stressed here is that successive complaints and protests had to emerge in order to publicise what was happening, and to gain acceptance that the accounts given involved a legitimate protest.

In the process of investigating these incidents, traditional professional values were publicly questioned, an unusual event at that time. The alliances that emerged through the investigations were distinctly different from those that are evident in hospital closure protests in the 1990s. Patients' relatives, student and auxiliary nurses, the press, and some Government ministers backed investigations; senior medical and nursing staff were emphatic in declaring that 'lay people' could not assess their work, a view that was accepted by the members of several of the hospital management committees involved.

A notable feature was the interlinking of national and local protest. A series of local reports of disturbingly bad quality care began to emerge only after a national campaign had been instigated through the quintessential mechanism for establishment protest, a letter to *The Times* (10 November 1965) (Lord Strabolgi *et al.* 1965; Robb 1967). This achieved Solesbury's first condition for successful protest. It attracted attention, but the complaints were dismissed after an internal enquiry; the protest did not acquire legitimacy. Back-bench Labour MPs were particularly hostile to criticism of NHS care (Martin

1984). However, the report that was published helped to create a cultural change that encouraged some staff in long-stay institutions to be critical of standards of care. Equally, relatives' complaints were taken more seriously.

Professional resistance to 'lay' criticism was strong. Professional autonomy was held to be absolute, although the quality of care was shown in some incidents to be poor. The result was to create a climate where there was a favourable response to a planned programme of transferring care away from long-stay hospitals. The 1970 proposals for a feasibility study in favour of a move to a more community-based psychiatric service was based around a development implemented by psychiatric service staff at Worcester's Powick hospital; it was a professionally led change (Department of Health and Social Security 1970; Hall and Brockington 1991). Psychiatric hospital closure was generally perceived to be a progressive move aimed at improving the quality of health care provision. The development of a range of appropriate drugs was a critical aspect of the change.

By the mid-1990s, attitudes to community psychiatric provision were changing. A complex mix of service provision had evolved, with different claims on an inadequate budget. The Mental Health Act Commission carried out over 1000 visits to districts, and reported that rapid throughput and premature discharge of detained patients were creating a crisis in the inner cities (Mental Health Act Commission 1993). This kind of report is a classic example of the interaction of local and national structures, able to draw on the experiential knowledge held at the local level, while acting as a conduit to Ministers. Shortly after its publication, a patient suffering from schizophrenia, and inadequately supervised in the community, murdered a passing stranger. This event highlighted the inadequacies of community psychiatric supervision, and made this a high profile issue.

The danger for those users who have gained from an unpopular service change is that their concerns and interests become marginalised. Pressure groups representing users have to ensure that their views are collected and published. A competitive scrabbling for resources for preferred forms of treatment is generated by inadequate finance, or finance that cannot be made available (Audit Commission 1994). Currently unfashionable forms of treatment have to be given overt support using claims that are recognised to have legitimacy. West Birmingham's home treatment services for patients with psychiatric illness featured in a publication that stressed user support for a community-based service in a multi-ethnic area (Cobb 1995). The development of the service required funding that could only come from the closure of hospital facilities, a policy aspiration usually characterised as working against the interests of inner city patients, but here shown to be *empowering* them.

Long-stay care beds for elderly patients

In the 1980s, long-stay beds for elderly patients were closed in a number of health authority districts, although not in others. This local variation is in itself of interest, but a further dimension is the length of time it took for any public debate to emerge (Age Concern 1991). One of the reasons is that the hospital statistics which were collected at the time did not distinguish between beds for the rehabilitation of elderly patients, and beds for long-stay patients; that is, for the rest of the patients' lives. Because information was not collected and made available, the running down of long-stay provision proceeded without any national level democratic debate. This is Lukes' (1974) 'third dimension of power' in operation, namely the power to prevent an issue becoming known. In order to evoke change, local knowledge had to be obtained by national pressure groups that were able to get the issue discussed, but it required financial pressure through the quasi-legal structure of the Health Ombudsman to compel a response.

However, before looking at the way in which this situation has been dealt with, I want to examine the mechanisms through which local decisions were made either to retain or to close down long-stay NHS beds. This leads to a very basic question. Why have some districts retained some long-stay services for NHS patients, while others have shelved responsibility for providing such care?

A key factor is that NHS care is 'free at the point of use', but residential and nursing-home care is means tested. Elderly people given long-term nursing care in an NHS ward do not pay for their care; the cost is borne by the Health Authority who either (prior to the formation of Trusts) ran the hospital, or (after their formation) purchased the care. Thus all health districts retaining long-stay beds are adding significantly to their financial responsibilities. In deciding whether or not to keep long-stay beds, the same formal mechanism for consultation is applicable to all districts. It is difficult to conceive that the closure of a free service would gain popular support in any health district, so how was it that, in some districts, the consultative process allowed all continual-care NHS beds to disappear, while in other districts they were retained?

Box 6.1 shows a local process of consultation which led to the retention of more NHS continuing-care beds than had been initially proposed.

An important factor may have been that managers presented the views of the consultant geriatricians to the Health Authority. Members were therefore aware that these senior medical staff did not support the reduction in bed numbers. Comparative studies of other similar consultations would have to be made in order to confirm the hypothesis that medical opinion is a key factor in influencing the decisions of Health Authority or Trust Board members. If confirmed it would show the continued domination of medical opinion, but not why this has led to marked variations in NHS long-stay bed provision.

A different issue is the relative visibility of medical and nursing staff in the consultation process, and this is exemplified in the above account. The views of nursing staff had to be provided through their union, since nursing staff were employees and therefore not people who could be directly consulted about the decisions of their employer. Geriatricians were able to respond directly because they were not employed by the Health Authority, but by the

---

BOX 6.1 USER INVOLVEMENT IN THE NHS; A 1991 EXAMPLE

Lancaster Health Authority; Proposed Relocation of Services for Elderly People requiring Long-term Care

Lancaster Health Authority submitted proposals for a reduction in the number of long-stay beds for elderly patients in the summer of 1991. There was no plan to close all such beds as had happened elsewhere, but a reduction from 100 long-term care beds to 48 beds was proposed. This would involve the closure of four wards in an old building where it was impossible to provide a high degree of privacy. Improved support from NHS paramedical staff was proposed for private nursing homes. A revenue saving of £98 000 was anticipated. Nursing care on the wards was accepted as being of a high standard.

At that time there was a statutory obligation on Health Authorities to consult formally locally before agreeing a ward closure. A summary of responses from 10 agencies was provided at the monthly public meeting of the Health Authority, including the views of the consultant geriatricians and nursing unions. Responses from health professionals either expressed serious concern or stated that they could not support the application. The local Community Health Council had discussed the proposals with relatives of patients, and in their public meetings. They opposed the plan and submitted alternative proposals. The Board accepted a revised proposal from managers to reduce bed numbers by 14 rather than by 52 beds.

Source: Lancaster Health Authority Meeting, 2 October 1991, Agenda Item 5a.

Regional Health Authority. Public debate was thus informed by open debate among different groups of health service staff. Such openness has been seen as a necessary feature of environmental risk assessment (Beck 1992). I suggest that it is equally critical in allowing users to assess the value of different patterns of service provision.

With the formation of Trusts, medical staff are no longer as free to comment publicly on controversial service decisions, and contact between health authority purchasers and Trust-employed consultants may also be actively discouraged. Mumford argues that 'Keeping them apart is a recipe for disaster' (1993, p.5). A slightly different claim would be that staff should be actively encouraged to collaborate, while retaining sufficient independence to ensure that contested decisions are publicly and adequately debated.

The differences between districts point to the importance of local service culture in determining patterns of service provision. Before the 1980s, local NHS service variations existed within a national framework of patient entitlements to NHS care, but for the continuing care of elderly patients this is no longer the case. One particular incident was pivotal in clarifying the issues involved. A patient who had suffered a severe stroke was discharged from an NHS hospital in Leeds in 1991. He was sent to a private nursing home where his family were compelled to make up the shortfall in costs of over £6000 per year. The Health Service Commissioner – often referred to as the Health Ombudsman – responded to a complaint, and ordered the District Health Authority to meet the costs and reimburse the family (Health Service Commissioner 1991). For some Health Authorities this ruling had serious financial implications.

In August 1994, the Secretary of State for Health announced new 'Guidelines' purporting to set out NHS responsibilities for meeting long-term health care needs (National Health Service Executive 1994b). These stated that a patient does not 'have the right to occupy indefinitely an NHS bed', but he or she does have the right to refuse to be discharged from an NHS bed into a nursing or residential home. The confusion inherent in these rulings is evident. It is an example of a process of devolving unpopular rationing decisions downwards from the centre to local districts, and means that local variations in service provision are inevitable.

The involvement of the quasi-judicial agency of the Health Ombudsman was the key element in compelling the Government to produce guidelines. The Parliamentary system of checks on government had failed to achieve this, although the publications of the House of Commons Social Services Committee ensured that the issue was well understood. The legal system had to be utilised to compel action in the face of the failure of the democratic process. The use of judicial review to compel government to address unpopular issues has been described in relation to environmental issues in Germany, where the legal system is used to put government '. . . on the defendant's bench more and more frequently' (Beck 1992, p.196). The changes to long-term care in the UK show that a transference of trust from the democratic to the legal system is also occurring in relation to service provision.

NHS law is 'de-formalised' law. It does not set out a precise duty to provide a service, but a discretionary duty. An NHS Chief Executive made it clear that there was 'no general duty on a health authority to provide in-patient medical or nursing care to every patient who needs it' (*Health Service Journal* 1994, p.17). The duty of the NHS is constitutionally determined by the Secretary of State, who is responsible for providing services '*to such extent as he considers necessary to meet all reasonable requirements*' (Dimond 1994). This contrasts with the specific ruling that charges cannot be levied for NHS care, unless there is a clear statutory law, as there is with prescription charges.

It has been argued that deformalised law is necessary to allow welfare service provision to be responsive and flexible (Habermas 1976). I would suggest that this assumes that governments are committed to the maintenance of the welfare state. Without a commitment to welfare provision, the existence of deformalised law enables governments to abandon welfare service responsibilities without the need to do this through the democratic system of parliamentary debate. There is empirical evidence from the USA that formal law is more effective in safeguarding welfare entitlements than deformalised law (Scheuerman 1994). The evidence of long-term care service provision in the NHS over the last decade and a half is that deformalised law has not provided an adequate protection to service users.

Conclusions

This chapter began by questioning whether it was possible for local communities to influence the nature of health service provision in their district. The limitations of local power have been made evident. Policies and funding levels are centrally determined and districts have to operate within them. Democratic structures are capable of publicising the limitations within which local policies have to operate, but cannot alter these limits. Neither social services nor the health service have routinely extended citizen empowerment in relation to health and social care beyond the level of genuine consultation, and in some districts user involvement in service planning may be vulnerable if central support for this policy is to be withdrawn.

The changing nature of the patient–professional relationship in health care is based on either a consumerist, a needs-led, or a participative partnership model. I have argued that only the last of these is capable of producing a community commitment to sustain health service provision and respond to difficult issues relating to health care rationing.

The issue over which community protest most frequently emerged was the contraction or restructuring of hospitals. The reasons for persistent opposition to hospital closure are related to the security engendered by the visible presence of hospitals, and their implicit promise that treatment will be available when it is needed. Trust in the NHS has been weakened by the intensity of change, and in particular by the transfer of long-stay elderly care services from the NHS.

The pressures that have led to a policy of restructuring hospitals arise from fundamental shifts in the way that health can be delivered; they will not disappear. Imposing change is possible, but alienates both local communities and the wider public, and could lead to a withdrawal of support for public health care services. The restructuring of psychiatric hospital provision has shown that it is possible to win support for change, but for this to happen there has to be trust that such change is inspired by a concern to improve levels of health care provision. In a publicly funded health service, community involvement is an inescapable element in developing such trust.

References

Aaron H.J. and Schwartz, W.B. 1984: *The painful prescription: rationing hospital care.* Washington: Brookings Institute.

Age Concern 1991: *Under sentence: continuing care units for older people within the National Health Service.* London: Age Concern.

Allen, I. 1993: *Rationing of health and social care.* London: Policy Services Institute.

Anderson, B. 1983: *Imagined communities: reflections on the origins of nationalism.* London: Verso.

Arnstein, S.R. 1971: A ladder of participation in the U.S.A. *Journal of the Royal Town Planning Institute* **April 1971,** 176–182.

Audit Commission 1994: *Finding a place: a review of mental health services for adults.* London: HMSO.

Bagguley, P. 1991: *From protest to acquiescence: political movements of the unemployed.* London: Macmillan.

Beck, U. 1992: *Risk society.* London: Sage.

Bell, C. and Newby, H. 1971: *Community studies: an introduction to the sociology of the local community.* London: Allen and Unwin.

Bell, D. 1979: *The cultural contradictions of capitalism.* London: Heinemann.

Brown, C. 1991: Do as you would be done by. *Health Service Journal* **101,(5)**, 26–28.

Burns, D., Hambleton, R. and Hoggett, P. 1994: *The politics of decentralisation: revitalising local democracy.* London: Macmillan.

Butler, P. 1995: The standard bearer. *Health Service Journal* March 1995, 12–13.

Carpenter, J. 1995: Implementing community care. In Soothill, K., Mackay, L. and Webb, C. (eds), *Interprofessional relations in health care.* London: Edward Arnold, 75–87.

Castells, M. 1977: *The urban question: a Marxist approach.* London: Edward Arnold.

Castells, M. 1978: *Class, city, and power.* London: Macmillan.

Chapman, T., Hugman, R. and Williams, A. 1995: Effectiveness of interprofessional relations. In Soothill, K., Mackay, L. and Webb, C. (eds), *Interprofessional relations in health care.* London: Edward Arnold, 46–61.

Cobb, A. 1995: Crisis? What crisis? *Health Service Journal* **January 1995**, 22–23.

Davis, M. 1992: *City of quartz: excavating the future in Los Angeles.* London: Verso.

Dennis, N. 1991: *Ask the patient: new approaches to consumer feedback in general practice.* London: College of Health.

Department of Health 1991: *The patient's charter: raising the standard.* London: HMSO.

Department of Health and Social Security 1970: *Worcester development project: feasibility study for a model reorganisation of mental illness services.* MO(M1)56. London: HMSO.

Dimond, B. 1994: How far can you go? *Health Service Journal* **April 1994**, 24–25.

Ellis, K. 1993: *Squaring the circle: user and carer participation in needs assessment.* York: Joseph Rowntree Foundation.

Emanuel, J. 1993: When people won't take 'closed' for an answer. *Health Matters* **16**, 6–7.

Etzioni, A. 1993: *The spirit of community: rights, responsibilities, and the communitarian agenda.* New York: Crown.

Flynn, R. 1991: Coping with cutbacks and managing retrenchment in health. *Journal of Social Policy* **20(2)**, 215–236.

Flynn, R. 1992: *Structures of control in health management.* London: Routledge.

Foucault, M. 1980: *Power/knowledge: selected interviews and other writings 1972–1977*, Gordon, C. (ed.), New York: Pantheon.

Freemantle, N. 1994: The public and professional face of rationing. In Harrison, S. and Freemantle, N. (eds), *Working for patients: early research findings.* Leeds: Nuffield Institute for Health.

Giddens, A. 1984: *The constitution of society: outline of the theory of structuration.* Berkeley: University of California Press.

Greenwell, J. 1995: Patients and professionals. In Soothill, K., Mackay, L. and Webb, C. (eds), *Interprofessional relations in health care.* London: Routledge, 313–331.

Gyford, J. 1991: *Does place matter? Locality and local government.* Belgrave Paper No.3. Luton: Local Government Management Board.

Habermas, J. 1976: *Legitimation crisis.* Boston: Beacon.

Hall, P. and Brockington, I. 1991: *The closure of mental hospitals.* London: Royal College of Psychiatrists.

Ham, C. 1992: *Health policy in Britain,* 3rd edition. London: Macmillan.

Ham, C. and Appleby, J. 1993: *The future direction of the NHS.* Birmingham: National Association of Health Authorities and Trusts.

Harrison, S. and Wistow, G. 1992: The purchaser-provider split in English health care: towards explicit rationing. *Policy and Politics* **20,** 123–130.

Health Service Commissioner 1991: *Annual Report 1990–91.* London: HMSO.

Health Service Journal 1994: Opinion: a financial time-bomb set to explode. *Health Service Journal* **August 1994,** 17.

Health Services Management (HSM) 1994: Is public opinion really public? Health Services Management Journal **90(4),** 3.

Hoyes, L. and Means, R. 1994: Open plan. *Health Service Journal* **August** 1994, 23.

Hoyes, L., Lart, R., Means, R. and Taylor, M. 1994: *Community care in transition.* York: Joseph Rowntree Foundation.

Institute of Health Service Management (IHSM) 1994a: *Policy Consultation Documents.* London: Institute of Health Service Management Policy Unit.

Institute of Health Service Management (IHSM) 1994b: *Reconfiguring acute services.* London: Institute of Health Service Management Policy Unit.

Jarman B. 1993: Is London overbedded? *British Medical Journal* **306** 970–982.

Johnstone, J. 1994: Extra-contractual referrals: squaring the circle. In Harrison, S. and Freemantle, N. (eds), *Working for patients: early research findings.* Leeds: Nuffield Institute for Health.

Joule, N. 1992: *User involvement in medical audit: a spoke in the wheel or link in the chain?* London: Greater London Association of Community Health Councils.

King's Fund 1992: *London Health Care 2010: changing the future of health care in the capital: King's Fund Commission on the future of acute health services in London.* London: King's Fund Institute.

Klein, R. 1992: Warning signals from Oregon. *British Medical Journal* **304,** 1457–1458.

Langan, M. and Clarke, J. 1994: Managing in the mixed economy of care. In Clarke, J., Cochrane, A. and McLaughlin, E. (eds), *Managing social policy.* London: Sage.

Levitt, R. and Wall, A. 1992: *The reorganised national health service,* 4th edition. London: Chapman and Hall.

Lukes, S. 1974: *Power: a radical view.* London: Macmillan.

Lupton, C. and Taylor, P. 1995: Coming in from the cold. *Health Service Journal* **March 1995,** 22–24.

Marquand, D. 1988: *The unprincipled society: new demands and old politics.* London: Fontana Press.

Martin, J. 1984: *Hospitals in trouble.* Oxford: Blackwell.

May, A. 1994: Equity in the balance. *Health Service Journal* **September 1994,** 14.

Mental Health Act Commission 1993: *Fifth biennial report, 1991–1993.* London: HMSO.

Ministry of Health 1962: *A hospital plan for England and Wales.* London: HMSO.

Mumford, P. 1993: The future of the acute hospital; managing staff in hospitals. *King's Fund Newsletter* **16(4),** 4–5. London: King's Fund Institute.

National Consumer Council 1992: *Involving the community: guide-lines for health service managers.* London: National Consumer Council.

National Health Service Executive 1994a: *The Operation of the Internal Market: local freedoms, national responsibilities.* Leeds: NHS Executive.

National Health Service Executive 1994b: *Responsibilities for meeting continual care needs*. Leeds: NHS Executive, Community Care Unit.

National Health Service Management Executive 1992: *Local voices*. London: HMSO.

Owen, D. 1988: *Our NHS*. London: Pan Books.

Pickvance, C. 1985: The rise and fall of urban movements and the role of comparative analysis. *Environment and Planning: Society and Space* **3**, 31–53.

Pollitt, C. 1993: Running hospitals. In Maidment, R. and Thompson, G. (eds), *Managing the United Kingdom*. London, Sage.

Raftery, J. and Edwards, N. 1995: *Beds and bed usage in London*. London: London Health Economics Consortium, London School of Hygiene and Tropical Medicine.

Robb, B. (ed.) 1967: *Sans everything: a case to answer*. Edinburgh: Thomas Nelson.

Saltman, R.B. and Von Otter, C. 1992: *Planned markets and public competition: strategic reform in northern European health systems*. Buckingham: Open University Press.

Scheuermann, W. 1994: The rule of law and the welfare state: toward a new synthesis. *Politics and Society* **22(2)**, 195–213.

Solesbury, W. 1976: The environmental agenda. *Public Administration* **winter issue**, 379–397.

Strong, P. and Robinson, J. 1990: *The NHS – under new management*. Milton Keynes: Open University Press.

Tomlinson, B. 1992: *Report of the inquiry into London's health service, medical education, and research*. London: HMSO.

Tönnies, F. [1887]1995: *Community and association: gemeinschaft und gesellschaft*. London: Routledge & Kegan Paul.

Walby, S., Greenwell, J., Mackay, L. and Soothill, K. 1994: *Medicine and nursing; professions in a changing health service*. London: Sage.

Warner, M. 1992: Health strategy for the 1990s: five Areas for substitution. In Harrison, A. and Bruscini, S. (eds), *Health care UK*. London: King's Fund Institute.

Watson, P. 1994: Public health medicine and D.H.A. members: a crucial interface in medicine. In Harrison, S. and Freemantle, N. (eds), *Working for patients: early research findings*. Leeds: Nuffield Institute for Health.

Watt, A. and Rodmell, S. 1993: Community involvement in health promotion: progress or panacea? In Beattie, A., Gott, M., Jones, L. and Sidell, M. (eds), *Health and wellbeing: a reader*. London: Macmillan, 6–13.

7

Views of the body, stigma and the cancer patient experience

Carolyn Featherstone

Introduction

Although it is a fact which we would all like to ignore, one in three of us will develop cancer. We have then, at the very least, a personal vested interest in understanding the cancer patient experience. The word cancer has frightening connotations, and cancer patients suffer not only from physical pain but also from a very fundamental impairment of self-image which accompanies damage to the body, both visible and unseen. While one might believe that this would be a secondary concern in the desire to survive, people with breast cancer, for example, are very much affected by their changed body.

In today's society the body has become an object of obsession. We are surrounded by messages that bodies matter and judgements are made not only about the raw material with which we are supplied, but also about how much we 'achieve' with it. Bodies in late western societies have become 'projects'.

To understand the full impact of serious illness in general, and the cancer experience in particular, we need first to look at two related issues in social attitudes to the body and the stigma of cancer. Secondly, we shall review the patient experience in 'high technology' treatments, particularly radiotherapy and chemotherapy. The doctor–patient relationship in cancer treatments is very problematic, requiring exceptional skills on the part of cancer specialists. Sadly, for many reasons these skills are so thin on the ground that, as Sherwin Nuland argues, there may be a need for a redefinition of the notion of 'hope' (Nuland 1993).

Views of the body

Sociologists have only recently begun to recognise the importance of the body and our perceptions of it in all social action. While there are a variety of models, the 'socially constructed' and 'body-as-project' theorists would seem to have most to contribute to an understanding of the body experience in cancer sufferers, and the perceptions of this disease in our culture. A major objective of these theorists is their critique of 'naturalistic theories'. The naturalistic perspective will be considered first to provide a context for social constructionism and phenomenological views (see Chapters 3, 4 and 5).

Naturalistic theories

The most prominent theorists are the sociobiologists. Sociobiology is an extremely controversial approach, because of the social and political implications of its views. Naturalistic theorists argue that the capabilities and limitations of bodies are the determining factor in producing particular relationships between people. Furthermore, these relationships are not seen as changeable; inequalities between genders, races and classes are seen as 'natural' and, therefore, legitimate.

In the late 19th century, for example, the exclusion of women from British universities was justified on the basis of 'natural inferiorities' (Gunew 1990). Gould (1981, p.104) reports that Gustave le Bon measured 13 skulls in 1879 and from this deduced that women were an inferior form of life, 'closer to children and savages than adult civilised man'. Unfortunately, these views were not only widespread at that time, but continued to be promulgated in the 20th century.

Opponents of demands for equal participation in the labour force utilised the theories of writers such as Wilson (1978) and Dawkins (1978). They attempt to establish genetic differences between men and women as a basis for particular social practices, e.g. family structures and childrearing norms. The basic unit of explanation in sociobiology is the gene, which is seen as being responsible for *all* human behaviour, including socio-psychological mores and morality. Examples of behaviour claimed to be determined genetically include incest taboo, parent–child conflict, war, ethnocentrism, and homosexuality (Hawkins 1994).

The purpose of human life, according to Dawkins (1978), is to serve as a 'survival machine' for genes. Survival machines are unaware of their real purpose. Present-day society is seen as the *successful* outcome of competition and aggression – natural and inevitable. Any attempt at reformist societal change to overcome inequalities between genders, races and classes will necessarily fail.

The sociobiologists present their views as 'scientific and non-ideological'. They have, however, been the focus of widespread criticism, even outrage. These criticisms can be divided into three groups: first, on the grounds of their reductionism; second, on account of their poor science; and third for the socio-political implications of their work. According to Midgeley, in *The Ethical Primate*, Wilson appears to believe that 'because we need our limbic systems in order to think about standards, we shall therefore find the right standards (or morality) by investigating the limbic system' (Midgeley 1994, p.74).

The second group of criticisms focuses on the poor scientific status of sociobiology. Shilling argues that 'while sociobiology makes assumptions about the relationship between the body and society, it is unable to provide any mechanisms which would account for the collective structuring of human life and social institutions, or the likely direction of social change' (Shilling 1993, p.52).

The most widespread criticism has come from those who are horrified by the ready use made of these ideas to 'justify' social inequalities. Sociobiologists have often disowned any adherence to a political or ideological position. They deny an association with Social Darwinism, since it was used to legitimate Hitler's activities concerning racial purity.

However, as Hawkins (1994) points out, what they explicitly deny is beside the point. Social Darwinism, he argues, is not in itself a fully fledged social or political theory: rather, it is a world view. As such, it is embodied in a wide range of theories and ideologies – including capitalism and socialism, partriarchy and feminism, militarism and pacificism.

According to Hawkins, the assumptions of Social Darwinism are seen to be as follows.

1 Biological laws discovered by science are applicable to the whole of organic nature, including human beings.

2 The pressure of population growth on resources generates a struggle for existence between organisms and their environment, between species of organism, and between organisms of the same species (the latter is the most intense struggle).

3 Biological traits conferring an advantage on their possessors would enable them to survive and reproduce, thus ensuring that such traits would, through inheritance, be passed on to descendants and would spread throughout the population.

4 This process would, over time, account for the emergence of one species and the extinction of others.

5 Natural selection would ensure the evolution of a range of social and

socially relevant psychic features (e.g. the emotions, reason, altruism, the institutions of kinship, religion, warfare, gender relations).

Hawkins contends that sociobiology *does* meet these criteria, despite its protests, while Wilson is confident that the progress of biological science will point the way to a biologically based ethics. Hawkins argues that they

> . . . are confident that they know what it is to be human and that the answer to current social problems is to be found, not in social change and political reform but in engineering deviant versions of human nature so as to bring them into line with current social reality.
>
> (Hawkins 1994)

It is clear that we must look carefully and critically at the assumptions of sociobiologists. At a less extreme level, there is a temptation to use naturalistic medical models of 'appropriate behaviour' which are different for men and women (Shilling 1993, p.54). For example, aggression is seen as healthy for men, but not for women.

Social constructionists

Social constructionists' accounts of the body are exemplified in the work of Foucault (1979a) and Goffman (1959). While the emphasis of these two writers is clearly different, they share a view of the body as fundamental to the lives of embodied subjects, while also maintaining that the significance of the body is ultimately determined by social structures which exist beyond the reach of individuals (Shilling 1993, p.70).

We will briefly consider the work of these theorists. Goffman's (1959) work, *The Presentation of Self in Everyday Life*, is centrally concerned with issues of body management. The body, for Goffman, is one of the resources utilised to present a particular view of the self. People need the support of significant others in successful presentation and identity management. There are limits to the possible 'selves' which those around us will find acceptable, and we assess ourselves by the response of others. If those whom we care about do not confirm our view of ourselves, then it is difficult for us to sustain this. We are left with the choice of modifying our self-image or seeking alternative sources of support in a different group.

Goffman's views of the self and stigma are very pertinent to the diseased body, and particularly those with cancer. Management of a diseased body poses particular problems. Goffman defines stigma as a 'special discrepancy between "virtual" and "actual" social identity – that is the difference between the characteristics we expect an individual to have and those he is proved to possess' (Goffman 1968, p.12).

One type of stigma is classified as 'abominations of the body'. These may occur when a body is difficult to manage (as in colostomy) and interactions are likely to embarrass 'normals' – or perhaps where the disfigurement is such as to arrest everyday interaction responses: 'normals tend to find disfigurement difficult to look at and the eye contact necessary for sustained social interaction is absent' (Goffman 1968, p.25).

Many stigma sufferers have so internalised the standards and expectations of 'normals' in the socialisation process that they see themselves as others do, inevitably causing themselves, if only for moments, to agree that they do fall short of what they really ought to be. Depending on a number of factors – visibility, 'known-about-ness', obtrusiveness and perceived focus – the stigmatised person will be treated differently. So illnesses such as diabetes may cause no problems in face-to-face social contact, but the sufferer may be seen as a 'non-person' in employment contexts (Goffman 1968).

Consequently, there is a high level of motivation for those whose stigma is less visible to attempt to 'pass' as normal, but there is a constant worry about being 'found out'. Clearly, this tension has as much to do with consequent loss of trust as with the recognition of 'differentness' if discovery occurs. A clear example of this is a woman who wears a prosthesis after mastectomy, or a man who is infertile following chemotherapy. Such people are forced to present themselves falsely in almost all situations, having to conceal their unconventional secrets because of everyone having to conceal the conventional ones. Goffman (1968, p.95) clearly believes that everyone accepts their stigmatised relationships. Does he overstate the reactions of others as a source of self-identity? After all, many groups of disabled people have begun to question these social categorisations.

Mike Featherstone *et al.* (1991) and several other writers have criticised Goffman for his failure to recognise that we resist others' definitions, particularly in the process of ageing when a youthful self is experienced as trapped within a declining and decaying body. Research reports people feeling that they have the same self as when they were young, despite being treated as middle-aged or old. Similarly, groups of disabled people have made great efforts to confound societal perceptions of restricted ability by, for example, participation in Olympics and marathons. There have also been politically active individuals who have opposed campaigns for better provisions for people with disabilities, on the grounds that they fundamentally dispute the oppositional categories of 'able-bodied' and 'disabled'.

Foucault (1980), while sharing Goffman's position on social constructionism, differs substantially in the direction of his interests. It is difficult to talk about Foucault's ideas in general terms – they are complex, change over time, and his language is obscure. Foucault's interests include three significant areas: (1) how bodies are constructed by 'discourse'; (2) how bodies are *controlled* by those in power; and (3) how sexuality is socially constructed.

'Discourse' is a key concept in Foucault's writings. According to Dreyfus and Rabinow (1982), 'discourse' is concerned with expert statements of powerful groups, i.e. statements which are taken seriously by a community of experts. Foucault is particularly interested in medical discourse. According to Busfield (1986, p.129), 'Foucault sees ideas and meanings forming holistic structures, rather like the paradigms described by Kuhn (1970), which constitute social reality and define what counts as knowledge'. So we are talking about a mental model of reality, as used by expert groups. It will include the language, concepts and criteria of evaluation which are seen as legitimate for discussion of, for example, medical issues (see Chapter 10).

For Foucault (1980), knowledge and power are inextricably linked. The power of the medical profession is located in its discourse or ideas. Much of our thought about our bodies, then, is constrained by medical ideas which change over time.

In his work on the history of sexuality, Foucault (1979a) considers that the interest in sexuality in the Middle Ages was oriented to the after-life. In the 18th and 19th centuries, this changed to 'a concern with governmentally approved forms of sexuality which would produce life'. Furthermore, the 20th century has seen a partial development of this trend as sexuality has become harnessed to expressions of self-identity and life style (Shilling 1993, p.77).

Other key concepts are his ideas on bio-power and the docile body, in his account of how governments seek to control populations. Capitalism requires 'docile bodies'. According to Foucault (1979b), the spread of capitalism was accompanied by 'a parallel increase in usefulness and docility'. In the 20th century, the human and social sciences are seen to be heavily involved in the refinement of disciplinary technologies – in prisons, schools and social welfare agencies.

In late capitalism the body is largely 'self-controlled'. Foucault argues that the power of the state is subtle, that the control exercised over everyday existence, is, to a large extent, unrecognised. These ideas are an implicit critique of naturalistic theories, on the grounds that bodies are not limited by their biology. Bodies are seen as, to a great extent, responsive to discourse, to interpretation. The assignation of gender roles is equally flexible. This view has led his work to be taken up by many feminist writers.

Shilling, however, is strongly critical of Foucault.

> His writings on the body are somewhat disembodied. The body is present as object of discussion, but absent as a focus of investigation. He is deeply concerned with disciplinary systems and sexuality . . . but the body tends to become lost . . . as a real, material object of analysis.
>
> (Shilling 1993, p.80)

Foucault's analysis contrasts very strongly with the discussion of Goffman which describes graphically what it is like to be and act as a human body. Turner makes a similar point: 'My authority, possession and occupation of a personalised body are minimised in favour of an emphasis on the regulatory controls which are exercised from the outside' (Turner 1984, p.245). This may be a fundamental weakness of his work.

The body as project

More recent contributions to the body in sociology have built on social constructionism, but have focused on an important issue, that the body is 'unfinished' at birth, and goes through constant change and manipulation.

Many of these changes are part of the maturation process, but we also have considerable control and a substantial role in determining what we do with our bodies. The organic physical body itself clearly both constrains and enables this process. 'It is all very well saying that the body is socially constructed, but this tends to tell us little about the specific character of the body' (Shilling 1993, p.10).

A version of this perspective addresses the particular case of the body in the late 20th century. The body in consumer culture is seen as a 'project'. As a result of developments in all areas of technology, biological reproduction, genetic engineering, plastic surgery and sports science, the body is increasingly becoming a phenomenon of options and choices. Furthermore:

> Consumer culture latches on to the prevalent self-preservationist conception of the body, which encourages the individual to adopt instrumental strategies to combat deterioration and decay (applauded too by state bureaucracies who seek to reduce health costs by educating the public against bodily neglect) and combines it with the notion that the body is a vehicle of pleasure and self-expression.
>
> (Featherstone 1993, p.170)

People are persuaded that with (constant) work they can achieve a desirable body, so they are, therefore, responsible for how they look. Losing control of the body (e.g. as a result of smoking, poor diet, etc.) is seen as a *moral* weakness (see Chapter 5).

We have not, however, conquered death. No matter how much control is exerted over bodies, death is 'the great extrinsic factor to human existence' (Giddens 1991, p.162). We deal with a problem by ignoring it. As Aries (1976) argues, death in the late 20th century is seen as a failure, isolated and under professional supervision. We are unable to confront it, and are relieved that it is routinised and confined. Serious illness is seen as a brush with death. When we encounter it in someone we know, it reminds us of our own mortality. For this reason, cancer has a particularly problematic status in our society, and is in fact stigmatised. The reasons for this will be considered later.

Medical professionals and the body

Freund and McGuire (1991, p.6) argue that the professional medical role relies upon a particular view of the body. The first component of this is 'mind-body dualism', the assumption that physical diseases are problems of the body and can be treated in isolation from other aspects of the person. The body is seen as a 'machine', a complex system of parts, which can be treated for piecemeal repair of the system (see Chapter 3). Illness is located in the individual: it is not perceived as a property of communities. The individual is seen as at least partly responsible for his or her own health in terms of lifestyle. While individuals are held at least partly responsible for their own disease, medical successes are, on the other hand, seen as the outcome of the technological search and production of 'magic bullets' (Dubos 1968).

The many negative consequences which follow from this have been rehearsed many times. There is, for example, a failure to recognise the interaction of mind and body, a disregard for environmental factors in health, and a refusal to acknowledge alternative medical treatment as having any validity. In addition, there is a widespread tendency to disregard the 'whole person' (i.e. socio-psychological factors) in the definition of successful practice. There is an unwillingness to recognise fears about body image and the impact of high technology treatments as a legitimate concern of the patient. In many cases, women with breast cancer who have questioned the need for mastectomy have been made to feel that their distress is 'trivial' or 'cosmetic'. In the pursuit of the 'safest' treatment option, the specialist will often pursue the most radical path. The fundamental concern in our society with the complete and undamaged body, and the significance placed on the breast in particular, with regard to both female self-image and sexual attraction, does not appear to be acknowledged by medical professionals. Their narrow focus of concern often results in the communication of a diagnosis and proposed treatment which is brutal. One patient was told, without preamble, 'You've got cancer, you'll have to lose the breast'. The professional perception of the body, then, tends to be mechanistic and apparently unconcerned with the cultural values with which bodies are endowed. For the cancer patient, the medical profession is likely to argue for high-technology treatments. The outcome of these is very doubtful in term of prolonging life, and the 'quality of life' tends not to be seen as a relevant concern.

At this point it is worth quoting an American specialist at length. He admits that:

> Too often physicians misunderstand the ingredients of hope, thinking it refers only to cure or remission. They think it necessary to transmit . . . the erroneous message that it is still possible to attain months or even years of symptom-free life. When an otherwise totally honest . . . physician is asked why he does this, his answer is likely to be . . . 'Because I didn't want to take away his only hope . . .'
>
> (Nuland 1993)

Nuland believes that it is really in order to maintain his own hope that the doctor deludes himself into a course of action whose odds of success seem to be small.

> Rather than seeking ways to help his patient face the reality that life must soon come to an end, he indulges a very sick person and himself . . . This is one of the ways in which his profession manifests . . . society's current refusal to admit death's power.
>
> (Nuland 1993)

The death of the body, then, is associated with medical failure. There is a cultural unwillingness in advanced western societies to recognise that life has a beginning, middle and end. This, together with the confrontation with serious illness (evidence of ultimate lack of control), accounts for some of the fear and stigma associated with cancer. This problem will now be explored further.

The stigma of cancer

The fantasies inspired by TB in the last century, and by cancer now, are responses to a disease thought to be intractable – and capricious . . . a disease not understood, in an era in which medicine's central premise is that all diseases can be cured.

(Sontag 1989, p. 6)

While the causes of cancer are not yet known, research has identified factors such as the environment, lifestyle and sometimes genes as likely to be implicated in a complex interaction. As Sontag (1989, p.6) notes, many people with cancer 'find themselves being shunned by relatives and friends and are the object of practices of decontamination by members of their household'. Sontag was herself a cancer patient.

The medical profession is well aware of the power of the cancer label. It has been suggested that many people labelled as terminally ill – and this is how cancer is seen – will lose the will to fight the disease and may well die earlier. This is often used as a justification for *not* telling the truth to patients. The solution, Sontag proposes, is 'not to stop telling cancer patients the truth, but to rectify the conception of the disease' (Sontag 1989, p.6). She states that

as long as a particular disease is treated as an invincible predator, *and not just as a disease*, most people with cancer will indeed be demoralised by learning what disease they have. The solution is *hardly to stop telling cancer patients the truth* but to rectify the conception of the disease, to *demythicize it*.

(Sontag 1989, p.7; my italics)

While there is indeed plenty to fear rationally about cancer and its treatment, this is often augmented by non-rational perceptions. This view is supported by research by Stahly (1988), who found that seriously ill heart-disease patients are less stigmatised than cancer patients. It seems that heart disease is more easily accepted as the consequence of an unhealthy lifestyle. Heart disease is therefore, to some extent, 'avoidable', while cancer seems to have a more random causation in public perception.

Thus one component of the stigmatisation seems to be the enigma of its causation and occurrence, and particularly the perceived technical failure of medicine to deal with it. It is also seen as beyond the control of the individual; having done the right 'body work' is no guarantee of immunity. An additional component of the fear is the corruption of the body:

Malignant tumours continue to be viewed as repugnant sources of self loathing and decay, a humiliating abomination to be concealed behind

euphemisms and lies . . . The residual heritage of its odious connections is the one most difficult for our generation to expunge.

(Nuland 1993, p.215)

The stigma of cancer is not just a product of its danger to life; it is seen as
corruption of the body leading to likely mutilation. In a culture where the
acceptable self is associated with a healthy, whole, aesthetically pleasing
body, these aspects of the disease become even more problematic (Hammick
1992). Cancer is associated with a painful death. It is also associated with
painful treatment. It is hardly surprising that the illness is feared, but given
the fact that some cancers are curable (e.g. about 60% of breast cancer, many
paediatric tumours, testicular cancer), the fear goes beyond the actuality of
the case:

Cancer was, as TB has been, a condition to which a superstitious dread
adhered, as well as a rational and understandable fear – to talk about it
was to invoke it, to speak briefly or in a lowered voice was to leave it
sleeping.

(Blaxter 1983, p.41)

Cancer is seen as unselective, general, indiscriminate in its 'victims'.
Contact with serious illness, any illness, forces people to consider their
own mortality. On a day-to-day basis health is a state that is taken for
granted. Encountering serious illness forces us to face fundamental questions: 'Can I allow myself to recognise the suffering of the other? Can I accept
what other bodily contingencies have imposed on it as being possibilities
also for my own body?' To emphathise is difficult, because the ill body
'threatens my healthy image of myself and my fundamental need to trust
this health as a "natural" condition' (Featherstone et al. 1991, p.93).

We have a general problem, then, of engaging with the seriously ill. The
nature of cancer adds an additional repulsion – it is associated with bodily
corruption, decay and pollution. While the disease is ostensibly random,
people are often seen as 'responsible', either directly, in terms of smoking
or diet, or more generally. This has been reflected in the widespread
research into what has been called the 'cancer personality'. The 'C' type
behaviour proposed by Morris (1980) is characterised by abnormal inhibi-
tion of aggressive responses and emotions, conformism, a tendency to
avoid conflicts in personal relationships, submission and patience. 'C'-
type personalitites have been claimed to have particular problems in dealing with stress. Cooper and Watson (1991, p.48) report some 18 studies
supporting a correlation between this behaviour pattern and the occurrence
of cancer.

However, the role of stress in carcinogenesis has been disputed. There is a
general problem with regard to such psychosocial factors in the unreliability of
measuring techniques. There are all kinds of reasons why stressful events may
be under-reported (Guex 1994, p.9). Equally, in the search to make sense of the
disease in terms of the 'narrative' of their lives, cancer patients may look for
factors to which they can assign a causal significance. They are looking to make

sense of the illness. There is a more concrete consequence of this cultural fear of cancer: it may lead to late presentation for treatment (Stahly 1988).

We must remember that there are now cures for some cancers. People who have had cancer treatment are alive, well, and performing their economic roles in a manner no different from everyone else. There is, however, evidence that employers and life insurance companies discriminate against cancer patients. Hammick (1992) concludes her discussion with a plea for the 'normalisation of cancer'.

While many medical professionals refuse to engage with these problems by hiding the truth from their patients, it will be difficult to achieve that end. There is evidence that social support is a great aid in coping with cancer, but many people keep their hospital visits secret. This all adds to the burden of dealing with serious illness. The high-technology solutions currently available, and the implications for the patient experience, will now be considered in detail.

High-technology solutions: the problems of evaluating cancer research and treatment

Biologists now have considerable understanding of how cellular growth is controlled in our bodies. In the course of our lives, cells divide 10^{16} times. The control of this complex process can sometimes go wrong, producing cells which do not obey the rules for normal cell growth and which can multiply indefinitely. This local growth causes primary tumours, but primary tumours 'can usually be cured by surgery or radiotherapy, even when enormous'. It is generally the spread of cancerous cells by metastasis away from the original site which causes clinical problems (Sikora and Halnan 1990, p.3).

However, 'cancer' is not just one disease; it is a number of diseases grouped under the same name. Some of these are curable. Great advances have been made in the treatment of, for example, testicular cancer, leukaemia, lymphoma and choriocarcinoma. Cure has been achieved even when the disease has spread. This is the good news, but it has to be said that these are very rare cancers. While lung cancer is the most common tumour worldwide, it has remained resistant to treatment; there has been little change in mortality rates (Sikora and Halnan 1990, p.4).

It is difficult to establish exact mortality rates since, given the major advances made in diagnostic techniques over the last 50 years, epidemiologists cannot be sure that misdiagnosis did not occur during the early years of cancer treatment. Mortality is usually expressed in relation to the 'stage' of the cancer, which depends on the size of the primary tumour, its presence in the appropriate lymph nodes, and whether there is evidence of metastasis. There is now quite significant standardisation of staging criteria, but people have been using a number of different systems over the last 40 years, and there is a problem of compatibility over time. There is a further problem in comparing outcomes in different geographical centres; factors other than the cancer treatment alone may intervene, e.g. referral patterns.

Radiotherapeutic developments

There are a number of changes in radiographic and radiotherapeutic tech-niques which have contributed to more effective treatment. Radiotherapy works by delivering an accurately aimed dose of ionising radiation which damages cancer cells. The objective is to kill the tumour cells. The damage, however, may be sub-lethal, and there seems to be a significant ability of the cancer to repair the damage. The extent of the effectiveness of treatment depends on a number of factors.

Some tumour types are inherently more sensitive than others. The degree of oxygenation of these cells is also important; well-oxygenated cells are more radiosensitive. The degree of damage also depends on the type of beam used, that is, the kind of energy source employed. The treatment protocols take account of these differences in both level of dose and frequency of treatment.

The use of heavy-particle radiation with high linear energy of transfer, which is considered to have greater accuracy and effectiveness, is likely to improve cure rates of primary tumours. However, Sikora and Halnan (1990, p.13) argue that the effectiveness of radiotherapy is likely to improve for two more significant reasons. The first of these is the widespread use of more precise tumour demarcation methods linked to computerised radiotherapy planning. Most interestingly, they suggest that increased skill dissemination, better training and the installation of modern equipment at those centres involved in radical radiotherapy will have the greatest impact on outcomes. It seems that the treatment offered and received depends on geographical location in the country and whether there is a major specialist centre nearby.

Chemotherapy

As far as chemotherapy is concerned, dramatic progress has been made over the last 30 years in curing Hodgkin's disease, leukaemia and testicular cancer. However, it is argued by leading specialists that a 'plateau' may have been reached. 'It is not likely that existing drugs in new combinations will have any significant effect on mortality' (Sikora and Halnan 1990, p.13). Research is now focusing on understanding drug resistance, and on attempt-ing to improve the acceptability of the treatment experience, which is both harrowing and has serious side-effects. The patient experience of cancer treatments will now be discussed in detail.

The patient experience of radiotherapy

Of all the cancer treatments, radiotherapy is perhaps the one about which prospective patients are most ignorant and fearful (Guex 1994, p.87). There is, amongst the lay public, a generalised fear of radioactivity, which is associated with burning and carcinogenesis. It is counter intuitive to this general perception that radioactivity should heal. Furthermore, its invisibility is disturbing. 'It's easier to believe in an operation that takes it all away, rather than a treatment you can't see' (Henegan 1993, p.33).

At best, it is described by Guex (1994) as 'treating evil by evil'. The treatment and the disease may be viewed with equal horror. The thought of undergoing an 'invisible' treatment, without noise, and alone in a room frightens the patient in an altogether understandable way. The fears are not alleviated by the fact that 'explanations given by specialists are not always clear and go beyond people's capacity to understand' (Holland and Rowland 1990).

Very rarely do radiotherapy patients receive the full story about the treatment procedure. The treatment itself should be painless, but the equipment, which is taken for granted by the professionals, can be alarming for the patient, and fear of an unknown technology is high:

> What if the machine breaks down and burns a hole right through me?
>
> (Henegan 1993, p.27)

These fears are not entirely irrational. Radiotherapeutic accident and failure to inform patients of clinical trials on radiotherapy have hit the mass media. A pressure group has been formed by those who believe themselves to have suffered long-term damage from radiotherapy, which they attribute to a large extent to a lack of honesty and information from medical professionals. The group is called RAGE (Radiotherapy Action Group Exposure).

There are more specific fears of infertility, loss of sexual function, burning and disfigurement. The *likely* actual side-effects are nausea, vomiting, fatigue, alimentary problems and skin sensitivity. Patients should be advised to take less fibre and high levels of protein in their diet. This is frequently not discussed by the doctor; such omission may be defended on grounds of lack of time, and/or the possibility that patients, if told about side-effects, are more likely to get them; furthermore, it is suggested that too much information may be confusing.

It is often assumed that radiotherapists will deal with this problem. The best cancer centres provide booklets for their patients. However, Henegan found that patients were unprepared for the severity of side-effects. The patients mentioned 'absolute total exhaustion', and 'losing mauve skin everywhere'. One (out of 30 patients) had lost movement in her arm. However, none of these women indicated that they would have refused treatment if the side-effects had been explained more fully. Many did not understand that radiotherapy is cumulative in its effect and therefore the strongest reaction will occur after treatment ends (Henegan 1993, p.30ff).

There are aspects of the treatment planning process which patients also find difficult. For precision, to ensure accurate positioning in the treatment of head and neck cancers in particular, the patient must be kept absolutely immobile. This is obviously a practical problem over a long treatment period, and to achieve such immobility, perspex head shells are made to fit each individual patient. These are then fixed to the treatment couch. Making these can involve totally covering the head with a moulding material. Anxious patients are likely to find this experience claustrophobic. On other parts of the body, the location of the treatment focus is marked on the body itself, as a tattoo. The patient has to make sure that these marks are not removed, in order to ensure adequate reproduction of each treatment (Souhami and Tobias 1986, p.75).

In the initial stages of treatment, patients are often apparently so anxious that their muscles are tensed and the marking for treatment has to be re-done when their body is in a more relaxed state. Radiotherapeutic treatments of testicular cancer involve procedures which patients find very embarrassing. In addition, older patients in particular find the necessity to be naked very difficult to deal with, as do members of some religious groups, including Muslims and Hindus.

None of this is painful, but it can be appreciated that it adds to the patient's experience of not being in control, and of alienation from their body. It is seen as just one more process to be endured. The more patients are told about the process, the more prepared they are to deal with it. Patients need to be told about the accuracy of modern equipment, about the small risk to healthy tissue, and if possible to be shown equipment and the procedures outlined before they start treatment (Guex 1994, p.88). This has been shown to increase tolerance considerably (Holland and Rowland 1990, p.138). It is hardly surprising that reactions to 'sham' radiotherapy were severe for 75% of the groups. This indicates genuine fear of the *process*, and also that this fear is likely to be underestimated by professionals.

Chemotherapy – the patient experience

A great deal of research is done on making chemotherapy more acceptable to patients. Once having experienced the nausea and vomiting caused by the cytotoxic drugs themselves, the prospect of treatment causes anticipatory nausea and vomiting in 60 per cent of patients (Holland and Rowland 1990, p.423). While in France and Switzerland the use of psychological desensitisation techniques is widespread (Guex 1994, p.89), in the UK clinical psychologists are employed at only a few leading centres. It is argued that Progressive Muscle Relaxation (PMR) training, while normally undertaken by clinical psychologists, could be performed by specifically trained nursing staff (Watson 1991).

A more serious side-effect of chemotherapy is, of course, hair loss. This is frequently seen as an attack on the whole identity, and does not seem to be any more tolerable for older patients (Guex 1994, p.89). While in British society young people may choose to shave their heads as a fashion, baldness associated with stigmatised illness will be seen as an alienating mark, drawing attention to one's diseased state. For many women, sexual attractiveness is closely linked with their hair; perceptions of beauty in western society put a high value on both quantity and quality of hair. When people see themselves in the mirror it is a continuing shock, a constant confrontation with a 'strange' image.

However, the most serious fear is that of sterility, which is clearly very problematic for young patients. Sperm banking can be offered, as long as the cancer has not already affected the sperm. Sterility is not inevitable, but since this is a possibility, it is a source of great fear for patients. Fertility is not only a concern in the more obvious context of potential childlessness, but is also strongly associated with symbolic perceptions of youthful identity. In many cultures fertility is strongly linked to 'machismo' as a definition of 'maleness'.

Chemotherapy is an extremely stressful experience which continues over many months. Cancer specialists admit that patients may find the reality of this treatment even worse than they imagined. This may lead the patient to wish to give up the treatment. Where there is a potential cure (e.g. Hodgkins disease, testicular cancer, lymphoblastic leukaemia) it is argued that the specialist and GP should do all that they can to support the patient through to completion of treatment. Unfortunately 'For many cancers of adult life, the benefits of chemotherapy are much less clear . . . the worst outcome is that a patient is made to feel wretched by the treatment and guilty at stopping' (Souhami and Tobias 1986, p.114).

Variations in treatments and outcomes

Not only is there variation in the knowledge of treatments of different types of cancer, but also there is evidence that a problem exists in disseminating state-of-the-art cancer knowledge to GPs and non-specialist hospitals (Calman 1994). I propose to look at the case of breast cancer, which is one of the most common cancers and one about which there is considerable current concern.

In the UK women have a one in 12 chance of developing breast cancer in the course of their lives. It is the most common cause of death in women aged 35–55 years (Houlston *et al*. 1992, p.691). Women between the ages of 50 and 64 years are currently routinely screened by mammography. This service has been offered since 1986. One-tenth of those screened are recalled for further investigation, and one-tenth of those recalled are found to be symptomatic.

The treatment offered varies considerably, but most commonly surgery is undertaken, with or without radiotherapy. Until relatively recently mastectomy was regarded as a 'standard' response. Now it is recognised that, for many women, lumpectomy is adequate. Surveys have indicated that the more patients that are seen by a particular specialist, the *less* radical the treatment undertaken. In other words, those specialists with more experience are much less likely to 'over-treat' (Williams 1992, p.437).

There has been wide variation in the treatment people have been offered, and also what information they have been given regarding alternatives. In some provincial general hospitals the appropriate experience, to offer women the 'best' choice, appears to be lacking. This concern is the focus of the proposals made by the government's Chief Medical Officer for standardisation of patient care and protocols (Calman 1994, p.13). These proposals will be outlined later.

In a state of shock following diagnosis, many women have granted 'open-ended' permission to surgeons to use their judgement as to what is necessary to deal with the cancer. Granted this permission, it is perhaps not surprising that they opt for mastectomy for 'safety'. It is, however, within the patient's right to specify agreement to a more limited procedure, with the recognition that, if more radical treatment is proved to be necessary, a second operation could be undertaken. This is not a popular option amongst hard-pressed surgeons, and it is not highly publicised. In fact, patients have experienced pressure against this choice.

Radiotherapy combined with surgery is not considered to improve survival, but it is used to prevent local recurrence and as a palliative treatment. Again there is variation in treatment, but common practice in London teaching hospitals is 25 daily treatments over a period of 5 weeks. Sometimes this is boosted with additional treatments, if required. Thus a course of treatment could last for up to 7 weeks (Henegan 1993, p.8).

While cytotoxic drug therapy is now not considered to improve survival, hormone treatments (e.g. Tamoxifen) have been found to be beneficial for 50 per cent of patients whose bodies 'accept' the hormone treatments. There is currently a great debate about the possibility of using Tamoxifen as a preventative therapy for those who are at high risk of breast cancer. Negative side-effects are relatively low, about 6 patients in 10 000 per year, but this is an expensive treatment and the estimates are that preventative use would improve mortality rates by only a few per cent.

While less radical treatment is obviously desirable, there is a substantial change of body image even with lumpectomy, where the breasts are likely to be asymmetrical after surgery (Fallowfield 1990, p.555). There is a widespread view that doctors grossly underestimate the importance of the breast in both self-image and patients' attitudes to sexual activity.

Guex (1994, p.86) reports that research on emotional distress following breast surgery is inconclusive. Some researchers have found no difference in emotional distress in the months immediately following surgery, between mastectomy and lumpectomy – lumpectomy patients are equally displeased with the results (Fallowfield 1990). Others have noted that the immediate response to mastectomy was greater distress than the response to lumpectomy (Guex 1994, p.86).

An explanation may be that *any* significant change to the breast will cause a very fundamental change to the self-image of most women. However, it may be that surveys should have been conducted at a greater time distance from the operation, which in itself is a major shock. Many women take years to come to terms with this; some find it affects their image of self for ever.

Reconstructive surgery is often requested to deal with this. Wellisch *et al.* (1985) studied two groups of women; one group was given immediate reconstruction (in the same operation as the mastectomy), while the other group had reconstruction delayed for a year. There was no difference in aesthetic evaluation – 85% of women found this satisfactory. However, the emotional response of the two groups was very different with regard to the entire breast loss experience. Those who waited suffered stress and depression, while the group who had immediate reconstruction did not suffer loss of attractiveness, femininity or impaired sexual relationships. They were also less fearful of cancer in general.

In summary, there is a need for standardisation of treatment, greater honesty about options, and a greater recognition of the fears and losses of breast cancer patients. HM Chief Medical Officer has argued that cancer care should be restructured in order to ensure that 'all patients should have access to a uniform quality of care wherever they may live to ensure the maximum possible cure rates and best quality of life'. In order to do this there needs to be 'public and professional education to help early recognition of symptoms', and 'patients, families and carers should be given clear information and assistance in a form they can understand about treatment options' (Calman 1994, p.2).

To achieve this, the Expert Advisory Group on Cancer (Calman 1994) advocates setting up three levels of provisions.

1   Primary Care – there must be detailed discussion between primary care teams, cancer units and centres in order to clarify patterns of referral.

2   Designated Cancer Units – to be created in many district hospitals. These should be large enough to house teams with sufficient facilities and expertise to deal with the commoner cancers.

3   Designated Cancer Centres – providing expertise in the management of all cancers, including common and rarer cancers. They will provide specialists, and diagnostic and therapeutic techniques, including radiotherapy.

There will need to be strong links between cancer centres and cancer units. They argue for the necessity for common personnel, common treatment policies, audit arrangements and participation in clinical trials. It is hoped that implementation of these proposals would go a long way towards improving the cancer patient experience, but little has been done so far.

Problems in the doctor–patient relationship

Research indicates that doctors generally have great difficulty in dealing with medical uncertainty. There is evidence that clinical training still educates them to see death as technological failure rather than an inevitable end (Freund and McGuire 1991, p.233). While there is a prospect of patient death, or medical error in disputed treatments, doctors may deal with this uncertainty by limiting the information given to patients and their families (Millman 1976), often in order to minimise the possibility of 'blame' at a later stage.

In the 1950s in the USA, 90 per cent of physicians studied by Oken (1961) stated that they did not reveal the diagnosis of cancer to the patients. This survey was repeated by Novack *et al.* (1979), and 95 per cent of respondents claimed that all the necessary information was disclosed to patients. USA legislation on patient rights may well be responsible for this change. However, there is still a belief that what the doctor includes in his perception of all that is relevant may well not meet the expectations of the patient. 'Many patients are dissatisfied with both the *amount* and *quality* of the information they receive' (Freund and McGuire 1991, p.233). This issue was the subject of extensive complaint by Henegan's (1993) interviewees. One saw herself as 'an intelligent, educated woman' and as such expected to 'get it from the hip'. These findings support earlier studies which concluded that doctors 'consistently underestimated their patients' level of comprehension'. Freund and McGuire argue that doctors stereotype patients in order to 'justify information control'.

Keeping patients ignorant of their condition allows the doctor to avoid dealing with emotional response which physicians find disruptive or unpleasant. One of the problems is that doctors are not trained to deal with this. 'They sure never had a course on this part of medicine when I went to school, but let me tell you, I sure could use it now' (Taylor 1988).

'Normalisation' of cancer cannot occur when doctors are anything less than honest. Lack of honesty about a medical condition which is already stigmatised underlines and confirms the stigma. It also undermines the patient's confidence in the doctor's competence and judgement, when the truth finally becomes apparent. For the patient then, the doctor needs to be seen to be a professional who disregards the stigma, who is not frightened by the word 'cancer'.

A good doctor for the cancer patient is one who gives all the information he or she has available, presenting the picture in the most optimistic way possible, and who is prepared to support the patients in their emotional reactions. The doctor must be prepared to do this on several occasions, since the patient is unlikely to absorb the information at one meeting. This must include *detailed* discussion of *all* treatment options, *all* the uncomfortable and embarrassing procedures, and *all* the known consequences.

Henegan's (1993) study and that of Guex (1994) indicate that patients will be unlikely to reject the treatment on the grounds of greater knowledge, but will rather have a realistic view of what is required of them. At the moment it is likely that patients will receive a generalised account of procedures and some side-effects. Patients prepare themselves mentally for distressing treatments, but may find that the reality is worse than they anticipated. People may feel in consequence that they have 'not coped', that they are failing. Patients need a clear, honest account. Honesty and clarity are supported by Souhami and Tobias:

> In explaining the diagnosis, 'cancer' is the only word which unequivocally conveys the nature of the complaint. Many physicians use the words 'malignancy', 'tumour' or 'growth' with the best of intentions, but this carries the risk that the patient will fail to realise the true nature

of the disease (indeed, this is often what is intended).

(Souhami and Tobias 1986, p.110)

Some specialists have argued that the emotional support for patients should be carried out by another professional.

In some units, part of the work of talking to patients is taken over by psychiatrists, psychologists, social workers and other counsellors. Invaluable though help from these persons may be, we do not think it desirable that doctors should see themselves as technical experts and when human feeling intrudes into the medical situation, the patient should be sent to talk to someone else. . . .

(Souhami and Tobias 1986, p.110)

All of this takes time. Lack of time is often cited as a reason for telling patients only part of the story. Time management has become a primary goal.

A study by Byrne and Long (1976) quotes the following GP:

The doctor's primary task is to manage time. If he allows patients to rabbit on about their conditions then the doctor will lose control of time and will spend all his time sitting in a surgery.

There is no evidence that recent NHS changes have done anything to undermine this perception of professional efficiency. However,

It is to be regretted that some doctors and most health administrators regard heavily booked clinics as a sign of efficiency. A 5-minute consultation with a cancer patient is nearly always bad medicine. These are conditions which may be forced upon doctors but should never be accepted by them.

(Souhami and Tobias 1986, p.110)

Paradoxically, the Patient's Charter includes the standard that patients should not be kept waiting for over half an hour. This is having the negative consequence of leading cancer centres being put under pressure to *reduce* the amount of time spent with patients by doctors. Good cancer practice has prided itself in recent years on giving patients the opportunity to ask questions:

The manner in which the explanation is given is critical. The doctor should be unhurried . . . look at the patient's face while speaking and show that he is not frightened or discomfited by the diagnosis. There is a limit to the number of facts a patient can assimilate . . . particularly under stressful circumstances . . . not infrequently the patient may seem to understand, but in fact be too anxious to take in anything . . . When a patient is able to ask questions . . . he or she has understood at least part of the explanation.

(Souhami and Tobias 1986, p.111)

This is a very good objective which, however, can only be met if doctors treating cancer are not held to artificial time limits. The failure among conventional practitioners to appreciate what is important for cancer patients has been one of the reasons why such patients consult complementary practitioners.

Who uses complementary practitioners?

While some 35 per cent of the population of the UK has consulted some form of complementary medicine (Sharma 1991), statistical data are not available to indicate how many of these are cancer patients. Studies indicate, however, that while 90 per cent of patients in French-speaking Switzerland use complementary therapies, 25 to 45 per cent of cancer patients do so (Guex, 1984, p.93). The reasons for people using alternative medicine, in general, derive from three main causes (Sharma 1991).

1 Technical failure of conventional medicine, whereby bio-medicine has been unable to provide a cure or management of chronic illness; in such circumstances, people seek symptom relief from complementary therapists.

2 Failure of the doctor–patient relationship on an interpersonal level. Many patients, particularly women, believe that their symptoms are not taken seriously by their doctors (Roberts 1985), or that they have been dealt with in an unsympathetic or patronising way. Symptoms may have been discussed as 'psychosomatic'. This is often the case in patients with conditions such as Myalgic encephalitis (ME) or allergies, who are essentially seeking confirmation of their personal illness experience. They may well be labelled 'problem' patients or hypochondriacs by NHS doctors (Featherstone 1993).

3 Ideological commitment to holism, which involves a belief in seeking positive health and well-being, rather than just avoidance of illness. Patients usually have some kind of background belief system or world view, such that consulting a complementary practitioner is seen as being consistent with that set of values.

What needs are cancer patients, in particular, expressing? They are not necessarily seeking a cure for cancer; in fact this is rare. Instead, they are seeking certainty in terms of some kind of symptom control. They also require treatment for the side-effects of conventional treatments, and most patients will be using complementary therapy as an adjunct rather than a replacement for such treatment (Guex 1994, p.93).

Patients also need psycho-social support and confirmation of self-identity. As we have seen, many conventional doctors refuse to discuss the outcome of death. There is a willingness to talk about this reality among complementary therapists, so that the person can make realistic choices, and has control over what may be the final months of his or her life (Guex 1994, p.96).

What these therapists are offering, it seems, is empowerment – returning choice and control to a situation where events have left the cancer sufferer feeling out of control of his or her life. The positive power of talking about the illness is well documented. People need support on three levels – instrumental, informational and emotional. There is evidence that having a family is a significant factor in promoting cancer survival (Cooper and Watson 1991, p.112). There is also evidence that friends are quite likely to withdraw support for the cancer patient because of the stigmatised status of the disease (Cooper and Watson 1991, p.114). Friends of cancer patients report that they do not know what to say or how to help. The role of complementary practitioners is also to promote the self-esteem of their patients. They are non-judgemental. Each patient is seen as worthy of support; each body, however damaged, is seen as worthy of care.

Which treatments are most often used in the UK? *Acupuncture* is quite widely used for pain control and as an anti-emetic (Guex 1994, p.98). There are some doctors in the NHS who are already offering this. *Aromatherapy* has been shown to ease tensions and anxiety. It increases circulation, helps to break down scar tissue, and also stimulates the lymphatic system (Guex 1994, p.98). Aromatherapy is widely available in hospices and cancer hospitals. *Spiritual healing* is sought by a number of people, usually those in the most extreme stages of the illness. *Nutritional therapies* are some of the most widely used approaches. While strict adherence used to be demanded, cancer centres and Moerman and Gerson therapists are now more flexible. These therapies are seen to aid in improving prognosis and in reducing side-effects (Guex 1994, p.102). It has been noted that this is an area where patients can feel in control again. If diets are experienced as 'depressing' then it is recognised that they are likely to be counterproductive (Thompson 1989, p.23). *Reflexology* is a popular treatment, widely available in European hospitals and becoming increasingly so in the UK. As Guex points out, this is a treatment which, because it deals entirely with the feet, is quite easy for the patient to use. This is particularly effective in easing stress and insomnia (Hall 1991).

While there has been a hostility to complementary therapies in the UK, there is much to be gained from taking a positive attitude. Improvement is needed in the interpersonal dimension of our consultations (Guex 1994, p.97). It is important to respect the patient's autonomy and to encourage his or her desire to explore therapies which make him or her feel better, even if there is little impact on the prognosis. If we condemn complementary therapies, the patient will simply have recourse to them without informing clinical staff (Guex 1994, p.98).

Conclusions

We have seen that western attitudes to the body in modern society are a strong contributory cause of the stigma surrounding cancer. We are seen as being responsible for our bodies; we feel an obligation to do the best possible job, and engage in all kinds of 'body work' to achieve this. Not to do the best possible job is seen to be almost immoral. 'She has let herself go' is not simply a descriptive statement, but a judgement on inadequate 'body work'. When people's bodies change in the course of a serious illness, the general public is repelled. It is frightened by the randomness of cancer, because not even good 'body work' can guarantee protection against it. Death and serious illness remain out of our control.

There are three negative consequences of this stigma in particular which seem to impinge on the doctor–patient relationship in cancer treatments.

1   There is likely to be late presentation for treatment because patients may deny symptoms.

2   The stereotyped views which some doctors hold imply that patients lack the ability to understand their disease, treatment and outcomes. Many doctors underestimate the seriousness of the disease outcome to patients, justifying this by the notion of maintaining hope. Some do not believe that honesty will give back control to the patient, and that even if the patient chooses not to have treatment, it is the doctor's professional duty to support that choice.

While some cancer sufferers may not choose to talk about their imminent death, doctors should be prepared to communicate frankly and sympathetically with those who do. One of the reasons for consulting complementary practitioners is that these specialists recognise the positive psychological effect on patients if they are able to discuss their condition.

3   There has been a tendency in the past for doctors to persuade their patients to embark on radical treatment (e.g. mastectomy for breast cancer). This stems in part from a fear of being seen 'not to do enough'. However, it reveals an insensitivity to the very severe psychological consequence of losing a breast. Again, this is a particular problem in a society which values the complete and perfect body so highly. Even women with long-standing marital relationships have not allowed themselves to be seen naked at home after surgery.

What can be done to 'de-stigmatise' cancer? There need to be two levels of 'attitude change' in the wider society. Such an illness should be 'normalised', without underestimating its seriousness. Employers, insurers and the wider public should be aware of the successes of cancer treatments: patients *do not* all die (Hammick 1992).

In addition, the medical profession should be aware of the advantages to the patient of less invasive treatments. The *full range* of treatment options should be discussed. Clinicians should be trained to be more sensitive to the impact of the body in social identity and relationships. Patients are rational beings, who should be told the truth about serious illness. At the moment, minimal time is being devoted to this in medical education. To quote Sontag

(1989, p.7) again, 'The solution is hardly to stop telling cancer patients the truth, but to rectify the conception of the disease, to de-mythicise it!'

References

Aries, P. 1976: *Western attitudes to death from the Middle Ages to the present.* London: Boyars.

Blaxter, M. 1983: The causes of disease: women talking. *Social Science and Medicine* **17(2)**, 59–69.

Busfield, J. 1986: *Managing madness.* London: Unwin.

Byrne, P.S. and Long, B.E. 1976: *Doctors talking to patients.* London: HMSO.

Calman, K. 1994: *Consultative document: a policy framework for commissioning cancer services.* London: Department of Health.

Cooper, G. and Watson, M. 1991: *Cancer and stress: psychological, biological and coping studies.* Chichester: John Wiley and Sons.

Dawkins, R. 1978: *The selfish gene.* London: Paladin.

Dreyfus, H.L. and Rabinow, P. 1982: *Michel Foucault – beyond structuralism and hermeneutics.* Brighton: Harvester Press.

Dubos, R. 1968: *Man, medicine and environment.* London: Pall Mall.

Fallowfield, L. 1990: *The quality of life: the missing measurement in health care.* London: Souvenir.

Featherstone, C. 1993: *The use of alternative therapies in the management of ME (myalgic encephalitis).* Paper presented to the Medical Sociology Group Annual Conference, University of York, September 1993.

Featherstone, M., Hepworth, M. and Turner, B.S. (eds) 1991: *The body: social process and cultural theory.* London: Sage.

Foucault, M. 1979a: *The history of sexuality. 1: an introduction.* London: Penguin Books.

Foucault, M. 1979b: *Discipline and punish. The birth of the prison.* Harmondsworth: Penguin.

Foucault, M. 1980: Body/power. In Gordon, C. (ed.), *Power/Knowledge: selected interviews and other writings 1972–1977* by Michel Foucault. Brighton: Harvester Press, 55–62.

Freund, P.E.S. and McGuire, M.B. 1991: *Health, illness and the social body.* Englewood-cliffs, NJ: Prentice-Hall.

Giddens, A. 1991: *Modernity and self-identity: self and society in the late modern age.* Cambridge: Polity Press.

Goffman, E. 1959: *The presentation of self in everyday life.* New York: Anchor Books.

Goffman, E. 1968: *Stigma: notes on the management of a spoiled identity.* Harmondsworth: Penguin.

Gould, S.J. 1981: *The mismeasure of man.* London: Penguin.

Guex, P. 1994: *An introduction to psycho-oncology* (translated by Goodare, H.). London: Routledge.

Gunew, S. 1990: *Feminist knowledge: critique and construct.* London: Routledge.

Hall, N. M. 1991: *Reflexology.* Bath: Gateway.

Hammick, M. 1992: The stigma of cancer. *Radiograph Today* **58**, 467–470.

Hawkins, M. 1994: *Social Darwinism in modern social thought: the case of socio-biology.* Paper presented to the European Research Centre Seminar, Kingston University, October 1994.

Henegan, E. 1993: 'Exploration of the experience of radiotherapy in women with cancer of the breast.' Unpublished PhD thesis, University of Kingston, UK.

Holland, J.C. and Rowland, J. 1990: *Handbook of psycho-oncology.* Milton Keynes: Open University Press.

Houlston, R.S., Lemoine, L., McCarter, E. *et al.* 1992: Screening and genetic counselling for relatives of patients with breast cancer in a family cancer clinic. *Journal of Medical Genetics* **29**, 691–694.

Kuhn, T. 1970: *The structure of scientific revolutions.* Chicago: University of Chicago Press.

Midgeley, M. 1994: *The ethical primate.* London: Routledge.

Millman, M. 1976: *The unkindest cut: life in the backrooms of medicine.* New York: William Morrow.

Morris, T. 1980: A 'type' for cancer? Low trait anxiety in the pathogenesis of breast cancer. *Cancer Detection and Prevention* **3**, 102.

Novack, D.H., Plumer, R., Smith, R.L. *et al.* 1979: Changes in physician's attitudes toward telling the cancer patient. *Journal of the American Medical Association* **241**, 897–900.

Nuland, S.B. 1993: *How we die.* London: Chatto and Windus.

Oken, D. 1961: What to tell cancer patients: a study of medical attitudes. *Journal of the American Medical Association* **175**, 1120–1128.

Sharma, U. 1991: *Complementary medicine today: practitioners and patients.* London: Tavistock/Routledge.

Shilling, C. 1993: *The body and social theory.* London: Sage.

Sikora, K. and Halnan, K. (eds) 1990: *The treatment of cancer,* 2nd edition. London: Chapman and Hall Medical.

Sontag, S. 1989: *Illness as metaphor.* London: Penguin.

Souhami, R. and Tobias, J. 1986: *Cancer and its management.* Oxford: Blackwell Scientific Publications.

Stahly, G.B. 1988: Psychosocial aspects of the stigma of cancer: an overview. *Journal of Psychosocial Medicine* **6**, 3–4.

Taylor, K. 1988: Telling bad news: physicians and the disclosure of undesirable information. *Sociology of Health and Illness* **10(2)**, 109–132.

Thompson, R. 1989: *Loving medicine: patient's experience of personal transformation through holistic treatment of cancer.* Bath: Gateway.

Turner, B. 1984: *The body and society.* Oxford: Basil Blackwell.

Watson, M. 1991: *Psychologically-based nausea and emesis: assessment and treatment.* Paper presented to a Workshop on Psychiatric and Psychological Treatments for Cancer Patients, Royal Marsden Hospital, September 1991.

Wellisch, D.K., Schain, W.S., Barrett Noone, R. *et al.* 1985: Psychosocial correlates of immediate versus delayed reconstruction of the breast. *Plastic and Reconstructive Surgery* **76**, 713.

Williams, C.J. (ed.) 1992: *Introducing new treatments for cancer: practical, ethical and legal problems.* Chichester: John Wiley & Sons.

Wilson, E. 1978: *On human nature.* London: Tavistock.

8

Medical therapeutic research: ethical and legal issues in randomised controlled trials

Christopher Hibbert

Introduction

Put simply, a randomised controlled trial is a piece of research which enables two medical procedures or types of treatment to be compared in a systematic manner. There is, or course, nothing particularly new about the idea of making progress in medicine through the observation and comparison of different practices. Back in 1857, a Hungarian doctor noticed that puerperal fever was more prevalent in women who had been examined by medical students than among those who had been examined by midwives. Further observation revealed that the medical students had been dissecting corpses prior to examining the women, but when they were made to wash their hands in disinfectant before proceeding with the examination, the number of deaths from the fever dropped significantly (Faulder 1985). However, it was not until the streptomycin trial in 1946 that the observation of patients became more systematic by making use of randomisation. What happened was that patients suffering from tuberculosis were randomly allocated to either a treatment group or a control group, those in the treatment group being given streptomycin, which was withheld from the control group (Burkhardt and Kienle 1983).

A controlled trial featuring randomisation is now considered to be the most scientific way of generating information about the effectiveness of new treatments, because it places a strong emphasis on systematic observation and removes human bias from the point where a decision is made about which treatment to allocate to a patient. Over the years, the randomised controlled trial (RCT) has been further developed to test a whole range of medical interventions including surgery, radiotherapy, screening procedures and new drugs. Nevertheless, although RCTs are in widespread use, and a substantial number of patients may be taking part in them at any given time, they are not without controversy. Testing and research are activities about which people rarely feel completely neutral, and no patient wants to think that he or she has been recruited as an unwitting subject of an experiment. On the other hand, no patient wishes to receive a treatment which has not been properly tested. Given that there is a need for properly tested treatments, there remain certain ethical questions concerning the way in which a trial is carried out.

This chapter will focus on two issues of what might be called procedural ethics. The first of these is the question of whether a patient should be informed that he or she is taking part in a trial and the fact that the treatment will be allocated randomly. Clearly, consent rests at the very nub of the doctor–patient relationship, and it will be necessary to consider how much information needs to be imparted to the patient for consent to be effective. The second matter to be considered will be the ethical requirement of equipoise, which means that it will be morally justifiable for a patient to be entered into a trial only in cases where the doctor has no clinical preference for either of the treatments on offer. Although the structure of the chapter keeps separate the notions of consent and equipoise, it must be stressed that the two issues are closely interrelated, with informed consent playing an important part in how equipoise itself might be analysed. Having prepared a foundation with the ethical issues, the chapter will examine just how far the ethical requirements of a properly conducted randomised controlled trial are reflected by law.

Informed consent: what is the ethical requirement?

As already noted, medicine is heavily dependent on research in order to test new treatments and to monitor the continuing effectiveness of existing ones. While in many cases the subjects of the research will be patients who perhaps stand to benefit from the therapy being tested, in other cases the research subjects will be recruited from among healthy volunteers. In the case of healthy volunteers becoming the subjects of research, it is clear that the individuals concerned are out to gain little if any benefit from the research, while on the other hand medical science and generations of future patients stand to benefit a great deal. In order to ensure that volunteers will continue to come forward, it is important that their altruism is not met with abuse. One way to achieve this is by stringent requirements in relation to consent.

On this footing the Declaration of Helsinki (1975) makes a number of recommendations regarding experimentation on human subjects:

> each potential subject must be adequately informed of the aims, methods, anticipated benefits and potential hazards of the study . . . The doctor should then obtain the subject's freely given informed consent, preferably in writing.
>
> (extract from Basic Principles, paragraph 9)

It must be noted, however, that the Declaration makes a distinction between therapeutic and non-therapeutic research, and that the above recommendation is directed at the latter category.[8.1] Where therapeutic research (referred to in the Declaration as 'Medical Research Combined with Professional Care') is concerned, the requirements for consent are not as stringent. In fact, the Declaration recognises that there may be situations where a 'doctor considers it essential not to obtain informed consent . . .'(paragraph 5). It is well to remember that the Declaration of Helsinki cannot be enforced in the same way that a law can, but rather it amounts to what society believes to be ethically good practice in the conduct of research. As a code of practice it puts pressure on doctors to abide by its recommendations, but it is clear from the wording that it leaves the doctor with considerable freedom to decide whether informed consent should be sought in the context of a clinical trial. For example, let us imagine that a doctor is treating a patient and that the appropriate treatment, such as drugs or surgery, is only available as part of a randomised controlled trial. Should the doctor inform the patient of the existence of the trial? Furthermore, should the doctor inform the patient that there are in effect two competing therapies, but instead of choosing between them the patient will be allocated to one of them on a strictly random basis? What are the arguments in favour of not informing the patient about these aspects of the treatment?

The case for non-disclosure

One objection to providing full information is the burden it would place on the doctor in having to explain such matters as the nature of the patient's condition, the uncertainty surrounding the effectiveness of different treatments, and the need for randomisation. It is true that there is often not enough time to enter into long explanations with patients about the circumstances of their illness, and furthermore many patients may lack the technical understanding of medical matters needed for them to be able to converse meaningfully with their doctor. Besides, some patients may have no wish to know all the medical details, but have simply come to the doctor for a cure. To this part of the argument there is no single response except to say that a doctor endeavours to be sensitive to the information needs of each individual patient. If, however, there is a problem in making the information understandable to the patient, this may perhaps be more to do with the skill and commitment of the doctor in communicating than with the ability of the patient to grasp such medical information.

What about the uncertainty of the different treatments? It might be argued that the case for non-disclosure gains strength here, because the doctor may wish to protect the patient from the uncertainty. The patient has come to the doctor and relies on him or her to use medical expertise to effect a remedy. It is almost as though the doctor and patient then become partners in a common enterprise, with the patient happy in the knowledge that the doctor knows what he or she is doing. If the patient were now to be told that the proposed remedy may or may not be as good as another, that would have the effect of eroding the patient's confidence in the doctor, and the resulting anxiety might in fact slow down the effectiveness of the treatment. In other words, the treatment works best when both doctor and patient are convinced of its effectiveness.

The same type of argument might be applied to the decision not to disclose the fact of randomisation. As stated earlier, randomisation is used in order to prevent any bias from creeping in when patients are allocated to one or other of the trial treatments. Furthermore, it allows statistical tests to be carried out, so that any differences between the two treatments at the end of the trial cannot be attributed to the trial subjects themselves. This is because any one of the patients could have received either of the treatments in the trial. So why should this information be troublesome for a patient? Once again it would bring home to them the uncertainty inherent in the treatment, but there is another way in which anxiety might be kindled. The patient might be unhappy about the idea of missing out on a new and possibly more effective therapy simply because he or she has been randomly allocated to the standard treatment. In the eyes of the patient this might appear like the future being determined by the luck of the dice, particularly if the patient is in the throes of a serious illness and has a particular treatment preference.

What the above arguments have in common is that they are based on the doctor's wish to protect the patient from information which at best will carry little benefit, and at worst will cause distress. This concern for the patient's welfare accords with the doctor's duty of beneficence, an ethical principle which ensures that the doctor always acts with the best interests of the patient foremost. This does of course raise questions about what the 'best interests' of the patient are and who determines them, but for the time being the gist of the argument is that acting in accordance with beneficence means shielding the patient from potentially troublesome information.

Another type of argument against disclosure suggests that giving the patient full information about the trial will often lead to their refusal to participate, and that on a much wider scale this will lead to trials failing to take place due to the difficulty of recruiting subjects. Is this argument sound? With regard to the criteria that clinical trials should satisfy, David Sackett (1980) states that every trial must be valid in the sense that its results are true, the results themselves must be generalisable in the sense of being widely applicable, and the trial itself must be affordable and still leave resources available for other patient care. The first requirement – validity – is non-negotiable because it means not drawing a false conclusion that a treatment is effective. A trial needs a sample of the right size in order to be valid. Too few subjects will jeopardise the trial because it will be difficult to determine trends in the treatment.

However, is it realistic to suggest that patients will be discouraged from taking part in trials once they know of their existence? Michael Baum (1990) recounts what happened with the Cancer Research Campaign (1983) breast conservation trial. At the time there was a division in med-ical opinion about how to treat a woman diagnosed with breast cancer. Some surgeons favoured lumpectomy followed by radiotherapy, while other surgeons were quite convinced that removal of the whole breast (mastectomy) was the best treatment. The debate as to which was the best treatment eventually led to the setting up of a clinical trial in which women who did not have a stated preference for either lumpectomy or mastectomy would be randomised to receive either treatment. After 3 years the trial had to be abandoned because it had 'frightened off' most of the surgeons and most of the patients.

Michael Baum's account does not specify what it was about the trial that 'frightened off' the surgeons and the patients. Perhaps it was the uncertainty of the two treatments with which the patients found themselves confronted. Perhaps it was the fact of randomisation that the patients found to be unpalatable. What the account does illustrate, however, is a trial that set out to achieve a high level of morality through full disclosure, but which foundered for that very reason. The irony was that even without the trial both treatments were being given randomly, because it was largely a matter of chance which surgeon's preference a patient with breast cancer would encounter (see Chapter 7).

So far two main arguments against seeking fully informed consent have emerged from the discussion. The first is placed in the setting of the doctor's duty of beneficence, while the latter is concerned more with the long-term difficulties of recruiting patients for trials in the future. The approach in the latter argument bears the hallmark of utilitarianism, a theory of morality which asserts that the most moral course of action in any situation is that which maximises happiness or minimises suffering.[8.2] Although a doctor must attend to the particular needs of the patient and treat each patient as an individual, he or she cannot help but look at treatment from a broader perspective as a result of treating a large number of patients. Since society would be horrified at the idea of patients receiving untested treatments, it then becomes imperative that clinical trials continue to be carried out. A preliminary response to this line of argument comes from within the utilitar-ian approach itself, namely that once patients become aware that they are being recruited into trials without their consent they may in turn lose faith in the medical profession and become less ready to seek medical intervention. This is just one response to the utilitarian argument. Perhaps it is now timely to look at some of the arguments in favour of seeking fully informed consent before entering a patient into a trial.

The case for informed consent

Fully informing a patient about a proposed treatment by reference to its method, benefits, likely risks and possible alternatives allows the patient to make a choice on the basis of the information given, and thus to exercise the right to self-determination. The patient's right to self-determination corresponds to the ethical principle of respect for autonomy which, like the ethical principle of beneficence mentioned earlier, circumscribes the doctor's duty to the patient. Autonomy literally means 'self-ruling', and in the context of the doctor–patient relationship it means that any treatment proposed by the doctor must take into account the fact that the patient is a rational being with individual desires and preferences and who is capable of choosing between the available options. In relation to the clinical trial this would mean informing the patient of all the relevant matters, including the fact of randomisation, and thereby allowing him or her to decide whether to be entered.

What becomes apparent at this point is that there is a conflict between the principle of beneficence and the need to respect the patient's autonomy. The version of beneficence discussed above was that the patient needs to be protected from information and decision-making that he or she would find difficult to cope with, whereas respect for autonomy requires all the cards to be placed on the table. However, the conflict can to some extent be resolved by arguing that the doctor's duty of beneficence includes a duty to respect and promote the patient's autonomy. In this way, the concept of beneficence or 'best interests' is given a broader meaning, which enables the patient's wishes to be brought within the analysis.

So far so good, but there is still a challenge to the main argument which needs some discussion. A doctor who favours keeping the patient in the dark about the trial may suggest that, while autonomy is an important considera-tion, this is an occasion when autonomy takes second place to beneficence. Furthermore, a utilitarian in this situation would simply see considerations of autonomy as a complete obstacle to getting a clinical trial under way. So how can these arguments be countered?

First, autonomy is often expressed as the right to self-determination, which means that once we begin speaking about the right of a patient to make choices we are placing him or her at the forefront of the analysis. The patient's right to self-determination thus engenders the doctor's duty to respect the patient's autonomy. The important thing is the order: the right comes before the duty. Those who argue in favour of a morality where autonomy is the starting point in the analysis are unlikely to accept an argument which places the doctor's duty of beneficence above the patient's right to choose. After all, the whole point of having a right is that it serves as a check against well-intentioned but unwarranted medical decision-making and, in response to the utilitarian approach, it serves to protect the individual from the sharp edges of what society as a whole would consider to be desirable goals.

A second and further response to the utilitarian approach comes from Kant's theory of morality.[8.3] Kant asserted that the ability to reason is what gives people their capacity to be moral. By virtue of their ability to reason, people are able to recognise in themselves the capacity to make choices and are likewise able to recognise this capacity in others. All human beings are entitled to equal respect and therefore it is wrong to treat others in a way that we would not wish to be treated ourselves. The fact that people have their own individual expectations and desires makes them 'ends in themselves' who ought to be respected as such and never used merely as a means to achieving someone else's plans and desires. In the case of the doctor–patient relationship it is necessary for the doctor to take into account both the individual desires of the patient, and the fact that to override these by entering the patient into a random trial would be morally wrong because it would amount to using the patient as a means to an end for gaining further knowledge.

Perhaps this is overstating the case. After all, if the trial was about to test a therapy unrelated to the patient's condition, then it would be quite easy to make a case that the patient was being treated simply as a means to an end. That is why healthy volunteers need to be fully informed about non-therapeutic research before they agree to take part in it. However, in the case in question, the trial is being conducted as an integral part of the treatment and the patient stands to benefit from it if allocated to what turns out to be the arm of the trial with the more effective therapy. In situations where the treatment is not part of a trial, the patient is unlikely to expect lengthy explanations from the doctor, and indeed the doctor would be surprised if he or she had to go into detail about routine therapy. So why should the additional fact of the trial make a difference to the amount of information usually given?

This point is taken up by Raanan Gillon (1989), who observes that in the doctor–patient relationship the patient will often dispense with requests for information about the treatment, and simply rely on the doctor to make the best choice. In the absence of explanations given to the patient, consent will be inferred because the relationship is based on trust. So where does the trust spring from? It would seem that it is based on two assumptions. The first of these is that any medical treatment proposed is intended to benefit the patient rather than others, and the second is that a treatment will only be proposed once the doctor has formed the opinion that it carries a net benefit over harm for the patient. Clearly, a clinical trial fails to meet the criteria of the first assumption because one of its aims is to benefit patients in general. The point then is that a failure to inform the patient about the trial would damage the trust at the basis of the relationship, and by implication would weaken the consent which would otherwise be implied.

Placebos – can the deception be morally justified?

While on the subject of trust as the basis of consent in therapy, it is worth spending a little time considering the use of placebos in clinical trials, because placebos bring with them their own ethical problems. Let us imagine that a trial has been set up to test the efficacy of a new drug. One group of patients is randomised to receive the new drug, while the other group is randomised to receive a placebo. The placebo is actually a dummy drug which may look exactly like the drug being tested but is really no more than a concoction of lactose, starch or herb extracts. Furthermore, the trial is run 'double blind', which means that both doctor and patient are unaware of whether the patient is receiving the drug or the placebo. The way in which the placebo functions is therefore as a form of deception, but can such deception be morally justified?

The answer from a utilitarian point of view is not difficult to anticipate. If patients are told that they will possibly receive a placebo instead of the new drug, they are likely to withdraw from the trial, but as generations of future patients depend on the systematic testing of new therapies, there is much to be gained for the price of a small, perhaps even trivial, deception. So how is this argument to be countered?

As seen above, utilitarianism works rather like a pair of scales. It puts all the likely benefits of the trial on one side of the balance and sees whether they outweigh the regrettable aspects, such as the deception of the patients participating in the trial. This type of calculation is attractive to the medical researcher, but its reasoning is flawed because, as Beth Simmons (1978) points out, 'it is the subject alone who is in the unique position to make such a judgement: he alone knows the relative value he places on risks, benefits, and deception'. Doctors and other investigators may have vested interests in carrying out the trial, these interests being the cause of science or perhaps the advancement of their own careers. This is not to say that doctors are behaving cynically towards their patients or adopting a mercenary approach to the way in which they offer treatment. What is being argued is that the pressure to carry out research may gradually bring down the value of truthfulness, so that it no longer holds the same value for the physician-investigator as it does for the patient. Thus, the utilitarian argument is weakened by the attempt to set up an objective calculation of benefits and burdens, when in reality different individuals place different values on the factors in the balance.

A further objection to deception within the utilitarian framework, which has perhaps already been hinted at, is the long-term consequences. Margaret Mead (quoted by Simmons 1978) suggests that the doctor who makes use of deception as part of research risks becoming accustomed to manipulating other human beings, and that when this takes place on a wider scale it simply encourages 'styles of deceptive research'. For the utilitarian, the message is clear. If deception goes unchecked it will ultimately sour patients towards research, with a consequent loss of confidence in the medical profession.

This in turn gives rise to the question of whether forms of deception such as placebos are only unethical due to their likely consequences. Is recourse to utilitarianism the only satisfactory way of answering this question? It may in fact be a flimsy argument to suggest that deception is necessarily wrong because of its consequences, for there may be occasions when lying promotes the overall good. An example of this might be a case where a doctor refrains from telling the truth to a patient in a critical state in order not to jeopardise the patient's recovery.

An alternative analysis would be to suggest that deception in itself is morally wrong, regardless of its consequences, although in order to sustain this position it would be necessary to assert that the doctor and the patient have a duty of fidelity to each other. A duty of fidelity is no less than a duty to deal honestly, which would mean not telling lies and, as far as the doctor is concerned, not misrepresenting the nature of the treatment by allowing the patient to receive a placebo. It is a Kantian notion that telling a lie violates a principle of right, even though the lie may not bring about untoward consequences. This is similar to the notion of not treating others merely as a means to an end, for to do so would be wrong even if the person so treated actually benefited as a result. To summarise, then, acting deceitfully breaks an implicit promise to behave honestly towards others. This is particularly significant within the treatment context, due to the degree of trust which the patient invests in the doctor.

A further challenge to the practice of deception would be the manifest way in which it undermines the patient's autonomy. In what way? It has already been argued that a patient has a right to self-determination, but that this right can only be exercised effectively if the patient is provided with sufficient information to be able to make an informed choice. Lying to a patient has the effect of supplying that individual with a false premise for making decisions. Thus it might be argued that, although a deceived patient can still act rationally on the basis of information given, the state of misinformation which arises from the deception will serve to limit the scope for autonomous decision-making.

Does this mean that the use of placebos can never be morally justified? Alternatively, if placebos are to be used, what requirements of informed consent would render their use ethical? Beth Simmons (1978) suggests a research design involving three groups of patients. Group 1 are told that they will receive the active experimental drug and it is administered to them accordingly. Groups 2 and 3 are told that they will receive either the experimental drug or the placebo, but one group receives the experimental drug while the other receives the placebo. What this in effect means is that patients in Groups 2 and 3 are aware of the deception and agree to be deceived for the purpose of this particular treatment. Since they have consented to the deception as well as to the treatment, their autonomy has not been compromised. (This does, of course, raise the rather interesting question of whether deception exists once consent has been given. A preferable alternative formulation might be that once consent has been given, the patient is simply in a state of uncertainty as to the precise nature of the treatment received.) The attraction of this research design, however, is that it allows a systematic comparison to be made between the trial groups, but still manages to satisfy the requirements of a fully informed consent.

As an endnote to her discussion of placebos, Beth Simmons presents an imagined scenario where an experimental drug has a potentially life-saving effect, but can only be tested in a trial where the patient subjects are kept in the dark about the placebo. To inform the patients would be to jeopardise the trial. Can such a trial ever be ethical? The author suggests that a prerequisite for such a trial would be to interview a very large number of potential volunteers and ascertain whether they would consider the deception to be extremely trivial in the light of the benefits to be gained. If the overwhelming response from the potential volunteers was that they would not mind such a deception, it would be possible to infer from the response that a reasonable person considers the deception in this situation to be morally acceptable and, as such, not compromising to the patient's autonomy.

What this line of argument attempts to achieve is to square the deception with the duty of fidelity by arguing that the duty to tell the truth is not absolute when there is much good to be gained as a result, and where the promise itself is trivial. Furthermore, where a large number of people have no moral objection to the deception, it still manages to accord with respect for autonomy. Where the argument falls down, however, is in trying to harness the priorities of truth-telling and autonomy with the trappings of utilitarianism. The fact that 99 out of 100 patients have no objection to deception does not make whole-scale deception morally acceptable. The point is that respect for autonomy means respecting the choices of the individual, and any standard of the 'reasonable person' is completely irrelevant to the analysis. Surely the essence of autonomy is being able to make the very choices that others might consider wholly unreasonable.

Consent and randomisation

Having dealt with the issue of placebos, it would now be useful to give some further thought to the question of randomisation. As discussed earlier, randomisation is held to be of paramount importance in obtaining valid scientific results, because it removes any bias from the way in which patients are allocated to the treatment groups in the trial. Nevertheless persuading a patient to consent to receive randomised treatment is still a major hurdle in getting a trial under way. The traditional method is to seek consent before randomisation, but a variant on this, developed by Marvin Zelen (1979), is to randomise all the patients prior to obtaining consent. The patients who are randomised to the control group receive the standard therapy but are given no information about the existence of the trial. However, the patients randomised to the experimental treatment are fully informed and their consent is sought, but if they refuse consent they are allocated the standard therapy.

On the face of it, the Zelen method offers an attractive compromise in seeking informed consent, but what are the justifications for withholding information from the control group? The reasoning behind the Zelen method is that patients assigned to the control group will receive the best standard therapy already in existence, and because they would expect to receive this anyway as part of their treatment there is no need to inform them of the trial. Furthermore, information about the trial would only prejudice patients against it and prevent it from running. So what are the objections?

A first objection is that the method undermines the autonomy of patients in the control group by not informing them that there is an alternative treatment. Unless patients are clearly informed about the possible alternatives to the treatment proposed, they are unable to exercise their right to self-determination by choosing between the treatments on offer. This leads on to the second objection, which questions whether there is such a thing as a 'best' standard therapy once the patient's preferences have been taken into account. This is an issue which will feature more fully in the later discussion on equipoise. Finally, to offer the standard treatment as part of a trial without the patient's knowledge is to undermine the implicit trust that any treatment offered is intended to benefit the patient and that patient only. Any undisclosed intention to benefit other patients has echoes of using the patient merely as a means to an end which, as the earlier discussion suggested, violates a principle of right.

A more recent suggestion made by Zelen, perhaps in response to some of the above objections, is to randomise as before but then to seek the consent of patients in both the control and the experimental groups. What this means is that every patient is fully informed as to which treatment group they have been randomised to, and then asked whether they will agree to take part in the trial. This method certainly meets the requirements of consent, but there is a lingering fear that, depending on how the information is put across, compliance with (what appears to be) the doctor's choice of treatment will seem to be the most appropriate course of action for the patient.

The ethics of equipoise

In addition to the need for fully informed consent, there is also the requirement of 'equipoise' for a clinical trial to be ethical. Equipoise means that there is genuine uncertainty as to which of the two therapies in the trial is the more effective. In other words, the doctor is poised between the two treatments, with the relative advantages and disadvantages of the two weighing equally on both sides. Equipoise is required because the doctor has a duty to act in the best interests of the patient (the principle of beneficence), so if the doctor formed the view that one of the treatment options offered a better chance of success for the patient, he or she would be ethically required to withdraw the patient from the trial. However, there may be occasions when the requirements of equipoise are difficult to meet. The discussion which follows looks at situations where either the patient's or the doctor's preference can tip the balance, and then goes on to explore the ethical dilemma raised by an early trend in the course of the treatment. First, the question of a patient preference will be considered.

Situations where the patient has a treatment preference

An interesting question to raise at the outset is why a patient's preference should be relevant when neither treatment in the trial has a proven superiority. There might be some strength in this assertion if the two treatments were similar in all important respects, but where the treatments differ in terms of their inconvenience and side-effects it is likely that the patient will wish to be the one who makes the choice. A good example of this would be a case where a woman with breast cancer is asked to participate in a trial which is designed to compare the success of mastectomy with that of lumpectomy. In terms of mortality, neither treatment has yet proved to be superior, yet for many women the loss of a breast would have such profound consequences for their sexuality and psychological well-being that they would prefer to keep the breast at all costs.

What is beginning to emerge here is a rather more extended meaning of the duty of beneficence, or acting in the patient's best interests. In the context of the trial, acting in the best interests of the patient means more than making sure that neither treatment is disadvantageous – it means allowing the patient to decide what weight to attach to the likely benefits and burdens. Thus, in the eyes of the patient, the 'best' treatment is not necessarily the one that turns out to be the most medically efficacious, but the one that best accommodates the priorities and values of the patient. In other words, the 'best' treatment is the one which gives fullest expression to the patient's autonomy. An argument along these lines is adopted by Schafer (1982), who suggests that when a doctor favours one treatment over another equipoise is disturbed, but once the patient makes the ultimate choice equipoise is restored, even though the patient's choice may not correspond to the doctor's. However, this suggestion does not find favour with Freedman (1987), who doubts the ethics of giving a patient an inferior treatment. Nevertheless, this does seem to beg the question of what is meant by an 'inferior' treatment. If Freedman means by this 'less efficiacous', then that surely is what the trial is seeking to determine and hence cannot be known at the outset.

Situations where the doctor has a treatment preference

Just as problematical for the requirement of equipoise is a case where the doctor has a treatment preference. This can arise in a number of ways. For example, the two treatments in the trial may have no proven advantage in terms of medical efficacy, but one of them has diminished quality-of-life factors which cannot be overlooked. This might be the case in a trial for chemotherapy, where the doctor is aware of the fact that the unpleasant side-effects can be particularly demoralising to a patient who is already very ill. A further treatment preference on the part of the doctor might be a case where the doctor simply has a hazy notion that one of the treatments is better. This notion might derive from the preliminary results of an uncontrolled study that took place in advance of the full-scale clinical trial. If the results from the preliminary study look particularly promising, this might jolt the doctor out of equipoise and into recommending the new experimental treatment. However, Sacks, Kupfer and Chalmer (cited in Schafer 1982) suggest that there is a danger in publishing the results of a study which has not been subjected to the utmost scientific rigour, because it misleads doctors into believing the treatment is more effective than it really is. On the other hand, Hollenberg, Dzau and Williams (cited in Schafer 1982) are quick to point out that unless there is some early evidence, albeit from an uncontrolled study, in support of the new therapy, it may be difficult to recruit patients for the full-scale trial.

Another way of expressing the idea of the doctor having a hazy notion is to say that he or she simply has a hunch or an intuition that one of the treatments is better. The nature of a hunch, however, is that it inhabits a region just outside the boundary of reasoned argument, and the doctor who pays attention to it could be accused of substituting irrationality for cool scientific logic. In defence of the doctor, what the hunch could mean is that, during the course of interaction between the doctor and patient, the doctor picks up a nuance (not always open to empirical observation) that for this particular patient one of the treatments is more advantageous than the other.

What is needed now is to locate these often hazy preferences within a framework for analysis, because the picture which is beginning to emerge is one in which equipoise is rarely achieved, and in the absence of equipoise the morality of the trial is seriously called into question. To aid ethical analysis, the preferences mentioned above are explained by means of a device known as theoretical equipoise. Theoretical equipoise refers to a situation where the individual doctor has a balanced uncertainty about the relative merits of the trial therapies. This balanced uncertainty will derive

> from a variety of sources, including data from the literature, uncontrolled experience, considerations of basic science and fundamental physiologic processes, and perhaps a 'gut feeling' or 'instinct' resulting from . . . other considerations.
>
> (Freedman 1987)

The problem with theoretical equipoise is that it is fragile, and it does not take much for a doctor to favour one of the treatments. As has already been seen, once the doctor believes that there is a difference in the therapies, perhaps on the basis of anecdotal evidence or the results of an earlier study, equipoise is disturbed regardless of whether the perceived difference actually exists. It is almost as though the doctor's uncertainty, in the words of Freedman, is 'balanced on a knife's edge', so that even a hunch will topple it. So what is the alternative?

The alternative is to employ the concept of clinical equipoise, which takes a broader view and looks at the opinions of doctors collectively. Clinical equipoise exists when there is a division of opinion in the clinical community over the relative merits of the treatments. After all, the whole point of the clinical trial and indeed what makes it ethical is that there is collective uncertainty as to which of the treatments is better. Each treatment will have its own supporters, but with each side conceding that the evidence for the other treatment is just as convincing. As far as the running of the trial is concerned, clinical equipoise will have implications for the requirements of consent, because the patient needs to be informed of the honest disagreement among the experts as to which treatment is better. Put like this it may go some way toward alleviating the fears of the doctor who believes that expressing uncertainty about the effectiveness of the treatment will simply undermine patient confidence.

But what about cases where the doctor does have a preference? If the preference is more than just a hunch, disclosing it would accord with the duty of beneficence, for it would provide the patient with the benefit of the doctor's opinion, but the doctor would need to let the patient know that this is not a preference shared by all doctors. It is then up to the patient to decide. The argument against disclosing the hunch would be that a hunch is no more than an irrationality, and the doctor has no duty to promote irrational decision-making in the patient. On the other hand, respect for autonomy may require the disclosure of any piece of information that a patient would consider relevant to making a choice about treatment.

The essence of the argument then is that individual doctors can justifiably ignore their treatment preferences when these are placed in the broader context of doctors' uncertainty generally. Collective uncertainty is ethically more important than the uncertainty of individual doctors. However, the objection that might be raised to this is that it entails a move away from patient-centred therapy, while the expectations of the patient are that any treatment offered will be specifically tailored to individual needs. This type of objection is met by Fried (cited in Freedman 1987), who argues that ethical medicine is social rather than individual in nature, in the sense that progress relies on consensus within the medical community. Ethical medicine is that which is practised by individuals with an understanding of the need for scientifically validated knowledge, and not by those who are skilled in guessing. To believe otherwise would make it largely a matter of chance which particular doctor and hence which doctor's preference the patient encounters. Furthermore, the law (which will be considered in more detail later) looks to the standard of the medical community, rather than the individual doctor, when determining whether an appropriate standard of care has been provided.

Given that clinical equipoise refers to the collective uncertainty of doctors in general, an interesting question to ask is just how much uncertainty there must be. Must there be an equal division of opinion with, say, 50 per cent of doctors favouring treatment A and the other 50 per cent preferring treatment B? Is there equipoise when the supporters of treatment A far exceed those of treatment B? An attempt to answer this question involved performing an experiment in which laypeople were presented with a number of trial scenarios, and for each one were asked to indicate what they considered to be an acceptable level of doubt for voting in favour of the trial at an ethics committee (Johnson *et al*. 1991). The reason for choosing laypeople rather than doctors or patients was to neutralise as far as possible any bias the participants might otherwise have, enabling the subjects to think of themselves as future patients in need of protection, but at the same time being able to view the different sides of the debate objectively. The experiment revealed that when collective opinion was split more than 70:30, more than half of the subjects considered the trial to be unethical, and when the ratio changed to 80:20 the trial found favour with less than 3 per cent of the subjects.

This experiment provides interesting data, but the question still remains as to whether clinical equipoise is accessible to this kind of measurement. Furthermore, it proceeds on the basis that each individual doctor's preference carries the same value, whereas in reality it would be necessary to take into account the strength of the preference and not just the number of doctors expressing it. What the experiment does indicate, which the authors point out, is that where complete equipoise does not exist (and in most cases it does not), patients are prepared to make some trade-off from their own individual good for that of future patients who are likely to benefit from the results of the trial. Until now the discussion of equipoise has centred around the ethical implications of either the patient or the doctor having a treatment preference. Both issues are relevant to the decision as to whether the patient should be entered into the trial. Once the patient is in the trial, however, there is another matter to consider. The remainder of the discussion will examine the question of early trends appearing during treatment. What happens, for example, when one of the treatments begins to show signs of being superior to the other?

Early trends in the treatment

A doctor is under a continuing duty to act in the best interests of the patient during the course of the trial, which means that when early results show the patient to be receiving the less favourable treatment, the doctor is faced with a dilemma. Beneficence requires that the doctor withdraw the patient from the trial in cases where the patient stands to receive no benefit from it and may even be harmed, but withdrawing the patient may jeopardise the trial itself, with the consequent loss of benefit to patients generally. This amounts to a conflict of priority between the individual patient and the statistical group (Burkhardt and Kienle 1983). While the statistical group is important, it should not be overlooked that the treatment itself is administered to individuals. Indeed, the Medical Research Council is quite clear about where the doctor's duty lies:

it is axiomatic that no two patients are alike and that the medical attendant must be at liberty to vary his procedures according to his judgement of what is in his patient's best interests.

(cited in Burkhardt and Kienle 1983)

A line of argument developed by Vere (1983) is that, while withdrawing a patient from the trial appears to overcome the ethical objection that the patient is not receiving the best treatment, this should be done only in cases where the patient is suffering as a result. To withdraw the patient because the early results of the other treatment are promising is a decision arising from no more than a belief about the relative merits of the two treatments. What Vere is arguing, then, is that a treatment preference springing from an early trend is equivalent to a subjective belief that is still a long way from being verified by the statistical group. As such, the statistical group takes priority over the individual patient, because until statistical significance is reached the best treatment for individual patients is still speculative.

Even if the doctor feels happy about keeping the patient in the trial until statistical significance is achieved, should the patient be told about the early trend in the other treatment? If the patient is not told, this might amount to vitiating the ongoing consent, because arguably it is a piece of information that would be relevant to the patient's decision whether to remain in the trial. So what is the answer? Schafer suggests that the patient should be informed right from the outset that a clinical trial requires the doctor not to act on any trends in the data that might emerge at an early stage. This would then be a factor for the patient to take into account in deciding whether to be entered in the trial.

Legal aspects of informed consent and equipoise

The law works in such a way that when a conflict arises and the case is brought to court, the issue is decided by referring to earlier cases which have features sufficiently similar to be relevant to the present dispute. Once a final decision has been reached, possibly after one or more appeals, that case in turn becomes a source of guidance or a precedent for later ones, and thus a body of case law develops. Where the difficulty arises, however, is that at the moment there is no law in the form of either case law or legislation that deals specifically with clinical trials. As such, the discussion which follows can only speculate on what the law might be, reasoning by analogy with what the law has already established in relation to treatment which is not part of a trial. The law in any case ought to reflect sound ethical reasoning, and it will be interesting to explore just how far the law would give force to the ethical requirements of informed consent and equipoise so far discussed.

It was seen earlier that informed consent is a prerequisite for autonomy, because unless a patient is presented with all the information needed to make a realistic choice about treatment, there is an obstacle to exercising fully the right to self-determination. From the point of view of ethics, a patient who is about to be entered into a trial would need to be more fully informed than a patient who was simply being given routine treatment. This is because a trial has the additional aim of gaining knowledge to help other patients. So what information should a patient be given? Good ethics demand that the patient be told of the existence of the trial, that the treatment will be randomised and what this means. The patient would need to have information about material risks in the treatment as well as any additional burdens that the treatment might incur, such as having to remain in hospital for longer, or a change in daily routine. The patient would also need to be informed of the treatment alternatives, the fact that there is freedom to withdraw from the trial at any time and still be entitled to the best standard treatment, and that any treatment preferences which the doctor may have now or during the trial cannot be taken into account. From a legal standpoint, Kennedy (1988) suggests that the law would begin with the presumption that all this information will be provided unless there is a compelling reason for withholding it. Moreover, the 'compelling' reason would need to be more than something along the lines that full disclosure would inconvenience the trial. To give the patient less than full information could render the doctor liable for battery or negligence.

Battery

What exactly is battery? Perhaps it might help to imagine the following situation. An individual awakens from a gentle slumber in a deck-chair in a park only to discover that while he was sleeping a passing hairdresser had noticed his dishevelled appearance and, caught up in a sudden rush of beneficence, set about giving him a complete new hairstyle. The result is stunning – everyone says how much better the sleeper now looks – but what makes the hairdresser's action fundamentally unlawful is that the haircut was carried out without the individual's consent. The essence of an action in battery, therefore, is to give force to the right of an individual not to be touched without his or her consent, and in the context of treatment it means that a patient is legally protected from receiving a therapy which he or she has not agreed to.[8.4] Given that agreement is a prerequisite for treatment to commence, how much information is required by law for the agreement to be recognised as a valid consent? The requirements of consent for avoiding a claim in battery are discussed in the case of *Chatterton v Gerson* [1981 3 WLR 1003], where a patient claimed that her doctor had failed to provide her with enough information about an operation which, although carried out competently, led to the patient suffering from an unpleasant side-effect of which the doctor failed to warn her. In dismissing her claim in battery, Bristow J (the judge) said 'once the patient is informed in broad terms of the nature of the procedure which is intended, and gives her consent, that consent is real'. This means that in order for consent to be valid the patient must be told in broad terms what is going to be done and why.

Applying this to the trial, the patient would need to be informed of the trial itself, the fact that treatment will be randomised and that the patient will be treated as a member of a group. These facts go right to the nature of the procedure, because the purpose of the trial is not simply to treat that particular individual. Thus a doctor who does not disclose this dual intention could be liable in battery for providing a treatment which the patient would not ordinarily agree to receive. However, this still leaves the question of whether the risks of the treatment must be disclosed, because the trial may allocate the patient to a treatment which has no proven benefit, and possible harmful side-effects. Could it be argued that the risks are inextricably bound up with the nature of the treatment itself, that not to disclose them would wipe out the patient's consent? A case which tried to bring non-disclosure of risks within the scope of battery was *Hills* v *Potter* [1984 1 WLR 641], where a patient had undergone an operation for a neck deformity and consequently suffered paralysis, a side-effect which she had not been warned about. However, the judge rejected the patient's claim on the basis that it was more appropriate to an action in negligence. Furthermore, the Court of Appeal in *Sidaway* v *Bethlem Royal Hospital Governors* [1984 2 WLR 778, 790] took the view that consent will only be invalid if it is 'obtained by fraud or misrepresentation of the nature of what is to be done', a view later endorsed by the House of Lords when the case went to appeal. The prevailing view, then, is that failure to provide information about the nature and purpose of a particular treatment comes within the province of battery, while failure to provide information about risks or side-effects belong to an action in negligence. So how might an action in negligence arise?

Negligence – what is the duty to inform?

The requirements for a successful action in negligence were discussed by the Law Lords in the case of *Sidaway* [1985 2 WLR 480], which involved a patient who had undergone an operation on her neck vertebrae. Although the operation was carried out with all due skill, the patient still suffered damage to her spinal cord, a risk which she claimed the surgeon had not warned her of, and so had been negligent. When the case came to trial, expert testimony revealed a difference of opinion among neurosurgeons as to whether it was appropriate to warn a patient in this situation of the risk of damage to the spinal cord. The case eventually reached the House of Lords, who dismissed the patient's appeal by reaching a decision which can be summarised as follows.

The doctor has a duty of care to the patient, and this includes a duty to inform the patient about any treatment proposed. In the light of the doctor's skill and experience, however, there may be times when the doctor decides not to disclose a piece of information, and this course of action will be lawful as long as it is in the patient's best interests and other doctors in the same situation would adopt a similar approach. Nevertheless, a doctor must respond truthfully to questions asked, and even in a situation where no questions are asked but information is simply volunteered, the courts reserve the right to review a decision not to inform if it is thought that

> disclosure of a particular risk was so obviously necessary to an informed choice on the part of the patient that no reasonably prudent medical man would fail to make it.
>
> (Lord Bridge in Sidaway)

What this means, then, is that subject to a limited right of intervention by the courts, the standard of disclosure is determined by doctors themselves. It is an extension of the principle in *Bolam* v *Friern Hospital Management Committee* [1957 1 WLR 582], where the judge described medical negligence as the failure by a doctor to act

> in accordance with a practice of competent respected professional opinion . . . A doctor is not negligent, if he is acting in accordance with such a practice, merely because there is a body of opinion who would take a contrary view.

By extending this principle from treatment to information about treatment, the court in *Sidaway* is in effect saying that doctors decide what the patient ought to know. This raises the question of whether such a standard of disclosure applies to clinical trials. If it does, then a patient need not be warned of the risks of the trial where a respected body of medical opinion takes the view that disclosure is not called for.

From the point of view of ethics, *Sidaway* does not give full weight to patient autonomy, as it restricts what a patient might need to know in order to make a fully informed choice about a proposed treatment. In order for the law to give due regard to the right to self-determination in the context of trials, it will be necessary to argue that there is some feature of clinical trials that makes them sufficiently different from standard therapy for the legal principle in *Sidaway* not to apply. One possibility would be to argue that *Sidaway* is concerned solely with treatment, whereas clinical trials are only partly concerned with treatment, their other aim being to furnish knowledge to benefit patients in general. Therefore, to the extent that the treatment in the trial is different from that which the patient would ordinarily receive, the patient needs to be informed accordingly. Furthermore, a higher standard of disclosure is required not only because of the different treatment but also because the treatment has no proven benefit and may even have harmful side-effects.

The gist of the argument so far, then, is that the standard laid down in *Sidaway* applies to treatment, but is too restrictive for trials. In other words, where the procedure is not simply treatment but treatment plus something else, a higher standard of disclosure is required. But is there any case law to support this? One case of relevance to this issue is *Gold* v *Haringey Health Authority* [1987 3 WLR 649], where the plaintiff agreed to undergo sterilisation but was not warned of the risk of the sterilisation reversing itself, nor was she warned that the alternative, male vasectomy, carried a lower risk of reversal. In her action for negligence following the birth of a child, the trial judge allowed her claim on the basis that *Sidaway* need not be followed because it applied only to therapeutic interventions. The plaintiff's operation was non-therapeutic because it was carried out for contraceptive purposes rather than for treatment of a medical condition. As such, the plaintiff was entitled to a higher standard of disclosure, and ought to have been given all the information a sensible and reasonable patient would wish to recieve. When the case went to the Court of Appeal, however, the decision of the trial judge was reversed and the court ruled out any distinction between treatment and non-therapy in the doctor's duty to disclose. In other words, both were subject to the principle in *Bolam*. According to Lord Justice Lloyd in *Gold*, to differentiate between therapeutic and non-therapeutic 'would be to go against the whole thrust of the decision of the majority of the House of Lords in [*Sidaway*]'.

The Court of Appeal's decision in *Gold* appears to give little if any support to the notion that a clinical trial requires more information to be given because it is situated somewhere along the continuum between treatment and a non-therapeutic procedure. Perhaps in many cases a clear distinction between therapy and non-therapy is more real than imagined, but by blurring the distinction in the standard of disclosure the courts are suggesting that once a procedure enters the province of doctors, it is their standard only which counts. Is there any way around this view?

The view that there is a single standard of disclosure for all interventions might be challenged from within the *Bolam* principle itself. The reasoning behind *Bolam* is that it allows for differences of opinion among the medical profession as to matters of treatment, and where there is a difference of opinion it cannot be said (at least by the courts) that one therapy is superior to another. It might be argued, however, that clinical trials are not solely about therapy, but also involve questions about the legitimate aims of research, patient autonomy and the use of patients for gaining further knowledge. These questions are not purely medical and hence not the sole province of doctors.

Support for this line of argument is to be found in a statement made by Lord Mustill in the case of *Airedale NHS Trust* v *Bland* (1993 1 All ER 821). Tony Bland suffered hypoxic brain damage after receiving a severe crushed chest injury in the Hillsborough stadium disaster in April 1989. In the three and a half years which followed he remained in a persistent vegetative state from which a consensus of medical opinion said he was unlikely to recover. The question for the court to determine was whether it was lawful to withdraw treatment, including artificial feeding, when it was known that such a course of action would inevitably lead to the patient's death. In giving judgement, the House of Lords declared that withdrawal of treatment would be lawful where responsible and competent medical opinion had formed the view that it was no longer in the best interests of an insensate patient to continue with treatment which merely prolongs life but confers no other benefit. The case demonstrated a futher application of the *Bolam* principle, yet in his own speech (on p. 895 of the House of Lords' judgement) Lord

Mustill expresses a certain reservation about *Bolam* being wholly applicable in this context:

> I accept without difficulty that this [Bolam] principle applies to the ascertainment of the medical raw material such as diagnosis, prognosis and appraisal of the patient's cognitive functions. Beyond this point, however, it may be said that the decision is ethical, not medical, and that there is no reason in logic why on such a decision the opinions of doctors should be decisive.

In other words, where a treatment decision is based solely on medical criteria there is no reason for doctors not to be the ones who make the decision, but where considerations of ethics are involved (such as withdrawing life-prolonging treatment), then there is no reason why it should be only the views of the medical profession which count. Admittedly, the context of Lord Mustill's statement is the situation presented in *Bland*, but it is still attractive as a general statement of principle for application to other types of treatment, including clinical trials, where the ethical dimension cannot be overlooked.

Assuming that clinical trials demand a standard of disclosure that is geared more to the needs of the patient than to what the doctor thinks the patient ought to know, this still leaves the question of what risks the patient should be informed about. The Department of Health (1991) guidelines on *Local Research Ethics Committees* recommend that subjects are informed of 'all known risks'. However, a discussion of these guidelines by Moodie and Marshall (1992) makes the point that, while this may be possible with established therapies, the task becomes rather more problematical with treatments that are experimental. Furthermore, should the phrase mean 'suspected risks, or risks associated with different drugs of a similar class, or what?' From the point of view of the law, the answer might be that the doctor would disclose any risk which the patient would consider to be material in deciding whether he or she wished to be entered into the trial. This in turn raises the issue of which patient is being referred to. Is it the reasonable patient, thus requiring an objective standard, or is it the actual patient in question? Picard, in *Legal Liability of Doctors and Hospitals in Canada* (2nd edition, 1984) (cited in Kennedy and Grubb 1989), suggests that the latter, subjective test is more appropriate to research. Perhaps the reasoning behind this preference is that a given risk will not bear the same importance for every patient, because each patient will assess the importance of the risk in terms of their own individual values and priorities.

Finally, to succeed in an action in negligence, the patient must also prove that the undisclosed risk occurred and that tangible harm was suffered in consequence. It is not enough for the patient merely to establish that a material risk was not disclosed, but that nothing happened as a result. Negligence, unlike battery, is only actionable on proof of damage, and the patient will need to show that a new injury has been incurred or that an existing condition has been worsened.

A large part of this discussion has focused on the extent of disclosure necessary for a doctor to avoid an action in negligence, but this is not the only way in which negligence might be alleged. It will be recalled that equipoise is an ethical requirement of a clinical trial, and it accords with the doctor's duty to offer the treatment which is in the best interests of the patient. Where there are two treatments, as in a trial, the doctor must be indifferent as to which one is the more effective. Let us imagine a situation where a doctor has a preference for one of the treatments but the patient is randomised to the other treatment, which in turn proves to be the less efficacious and gives rise to unpleasant side-effects. Alternatively, the patient is randomised to the control group and denied the chance of a cure. In each case the patient's immediate response will be that the doctor was negligent in not offering the other treatment. What is the legal position? In both cases the patient must face the obstacle presented by *Bolam* and prove that no body of respected medical opinion would have treated the patient in the same way. Bearing in mind the likely large scale of the trial, this will prove a formidable task.

The voluntariness of consent

The other aspect of informed consent which merits mention is the extent to which pressure might be brought to bear on the patient to agree to a proposed treatment. To put pressure on the patient would go against the ethical principle of allowing him or her to make an autonomous choice, and would also violate the legal requirement that consent be voluntary. So how might pressure come about? This issue was touched upon earlier in the discussion about randomising patients before seeking consent. Patients represent an attractive group of persons from which to recruit a research sample, because they are both accessible and obedient. They are accessible because they present themselves for treatment without being searched for, and the ongoing doctor–patient relationship means that they often remain in contact with the doctor after the treatment has ended, thus enabling follow-up studies to be carried out. In addition, patients are often obedient in the sense that the health-care relationship makes them dependent on the doctor and willing to do what he or she suggests. It is the question of obedience which gives cause for concern, because a patient who is ill may be eager to please the doctor, and where the condition is life-threatening, the patient may be fearful and more than usually subject to influence. Hospitalisation, too, can be an intimidating experience, and the way in which doctors are deferred to within the hospital setting may lead the patient into a mode of compliance. To summarise, the patient's dependence on the doctor, coupled with the impairing effects of illness itself, might together constitute a form of duress that negates consent.

Does this mean then that the circumstances of illness prevent a true consent from ever being given to participation in a trial? If there is a risk that patients will be exploited, should the law step in to protect patients by asserting that the circumstances of illness in themselves render consent impossible? A related line of argument was used in the case of *Freeman* v

Home Office (No 2) [1984 2 WLR 130], where it was suggested that a patient being treated in prison was incapable, as a matter of law, of giving consent because of the coercive nature of the prison environment and the inequality between the patient and the medical officer concerned. However, this argument was rejected by the court on the basis that each situation must be looked at individually in order to determine whether consent has in fact been given. This view must be correct if consent is seen to be a reflection of the right to self-determination. When the same principle is applied to the context of clinical trials, the reasoning is clear. If the law were to prevent patients from consenting to trials, then it would swallow up the very autonomy which it seeks to protect, and by implication prevent consent to routine treatment as well. Perhaps the issue of patient vulnerability can only be resolved by doctors being sensitive to the kind of pressures which patients are under when presented with treatment options.

Some concluding thoughts

There is a strong case to be made for clinical trials. As expressed at the outset, no patient wishes to receive a treatment that has not been properly tested. In the absence of a properly conducted trial, favourable results from uncontrolled studies might lead to unjustified enthusiasm for new therapies, with the result that patients are excluded from what may have been a better treatment. On the other hand, with a trial in existence it becomes easier to keep track of the side-effects of a new therapy and, should any patients be harmed, their number will be limited to those in the trial group. If the treatment brings with it unexpected results, at least these can be analysed within a scientific framework and a proper comparison made. Randomisation need not be seen simply as treatment being decided through the operation of chance, because until a treatment has been systematically proved there will always be an element of randomness as to which treatment a doctor recommends. In short, it is unethical not to carry out a trial.

The above reasons accord with the ethical principles of beneficence and non-maleficence which, when translated into the context of treatment, mean that patients ought not to be harmed, and that where there is a harmful aspect of treatment this must always be outweighed by a benefit. It is also possible to invoke the ethical principle of justice, in the sense that the risks of experimental therapy are borne by all. It would not be fair for a patient to demand an effective and safe therapy but only so long as the safety and effectiveness of the therapy had been established through prior testing on others. Furthermore, it would not be fair for a doctor to refuse to be involved in administering a trial, if the same doctor was quite happy to recommend a standard therapy which itself had already been tested and proved by a trial.

Compelling as these reasons are, they conceal a deeper conflict of ethics. The doctor as physician has an exclusive obligation to offer treatment that is tailored to the needs of the patient, but when entering a patient into a trial the doctor becomes a scientist whose aim is to produce knowledge that will benefit society in general. Schafer (1982) refers to this as the 'conflict of obligations' which a doctor confronts each time a patient is entered into a trial. The treatment which best fits the needs of the patient will take into account his or her values and preferences, but the demands of the scientific method cannot allow for these, and the patient is relegated to being a member of a statistical group. The doctor's duty of care is to keep the patient's interests paramount, but the clinical trial involves sacrificing the patient's interests to those of society. How is this conflict to be resolved?

The way in which the conflict is resolved depends very much on the particular moral framework within which the discussion is placed. For a utilitarian, where moral decision-making is aided by balancing the benefits against the harmful effects, the importance of the benefits to society of carrying out trials far outweighs the cost to individual patients of concealing information from them, although even a utilitarian would have to concede that the long-term consequence of such a practice would be a serious erosion of the trust which patients place in their doctors. On the other hand, an analysis based on patients' rights, and in particular the right to self-determination, places the emphasis on respect for autonomy and the need for information for the patient to make a fully autonomous choice. Giving priority to autonomy not only makes way for informed consent, but also goes some way towards resolving the ethical problems of equipoise, especially where decisions about what constitutes the 'best treatment' are affected by patient and doctor preferences.

Finally, there is the question of randomisation. It may be that it is not informed consent which discourages patients from being trial subjects, but the fact of randomisation and the idea that the choice of treatment is not within their control. Randomisation is considered to be an essential ingredient of a controlled study, but if it raises questions of ethical concern then it may be necessary to challenge the status ordinarily given to it. Carolyn Faulder (1985) makes the point that, even when a randomised study has been completed, there may still be dispute over the way in which the conclusions are to be interpreted. Instead of randomisation, she advocates the use of concurrent studies which match patients for certain characteristics and then allocate them to comparative treatments, taking into account any patient or doctor preferences as appropriate. Although the objection to this might be that it weakens scientific validity, this small trade-off from the scientific method might well be a price worth paying in order to maximise patients' rights.

Endnotes

8.1 Randomised controlled trials come under the heading of therapeutic research because they aim to treat the patient in addition to generating scientific data. This contrasts with non-therapeutic research which is solely concerned with collecting data from healthy volunteers or, alternatively, from patients whose medical condition is unrelated to the research in question.

8.2 For a more detailed discussion of utilitarianism, see D.D. Raphael, *Moral Philosophy* (Oxford, Oxford University Press, 1981), Chapter 4.

8.3 For a readable general introduction to the philosophy of Immanuel Kant, see D.D. Raphael, *Moral Philosophy* (Oxford, Oxford University Press, 1981), Chapter 6.

8.4 There are, of course, patients whose circumstances render them unable to agree to therapy. These include the unconscious accident victim in need of urgent attention and persons who by virtue of age or disability lack the mental capacity to give a valid consent. The law has developed separate rules to deal with these situations.

References

Baum, M. 1990: The ethics of clinical research. In Byrne, P. (ed.), *Ethics and law in health care and research*. Chichester: John Wiley & Sons, 1–24.

Burkhardt, R. and Kienle, G. 1983: Basic problems in controlled trials. *Journal of Medical Ethics* **9(2)**, 80–84.

Cancer Research Campaign Working Party in Breast Conservation 1983: Informed consent: ethical, legal and medical implications for doctors and patients who participate in randomised clinical trials. *British Medical Journal* **286**, 1117–1121.

Department of Health 1991: *Local research ethics committees*. London: Department of Health, Health Service Guidelines, **(91)5**.

Faulder, C. 1985: *Whose body is it? The troubling issue of informed consent*. London: Virago Press.

Freedman, B. 1987: Equipoise and the ethics of clinical research. *New England Journal of Medicine* **317(3)**, 141–145.

Gillon, R. 1989: Medical treatment, medical research and informed consent. *Journal of Medical Ethics* **15(1)**, 3–5.

Johnson, N., Lilford, R. and Brazier, W. 1991: At what level of collective equipoise does a clinical trial become ethical? *Journal of Medical Ethics* **17(1)**, 30–34.

Kennedy, I. 1988: *Treat me right: essays in medical law and ethics*. Oxford: Oxford University Press.

Kennedy, I. and Grubb, A. 1989: *Medical law: text and materials*. London: Butterworths.

Moodie, P.C.E. and Marshall, T. 1992: Guidelines for local research ethics committees. *British Medical Journal* **304**, 1293–1295.

Sackett, D.L. 1980: The competing objectives of randomized trials. *New England Journal of Medicine* **303**, 1059–1060.

Schafer, A. 1982: The ethics of the randomised clinical trial. *New England Journal of Medicine* **307(12)**, 719–724.

Simmons, B. 1978: Problems in deceptive medical procedures: an ethical and legal analysis of the administration of placebos. *Journal of Medical Ethics* **4(4)**, 172–181.

Vere, D.W. 1983: Problems in controlled trials – a critical response. *Journal of Medical Ethics* **9(2)**, 85–89.

Zelen, M. 1979: A new design for randomised clinical trials. *New England Journal of Medicine* **300(22)**, 1242–1245.

Social class stratification and health inequality

Moya Jolley with Abbie Perry

Introduction

The World Health Organisation in its document *Targets for Health for All 2000* made the following statement:

> Without peace and social justice, without enough food and water, without education and decent housing, and without providing each and all with a useful role in society and adequate income, there can be no health for the people, no real growth and no social development.
> (World Health Organisation 1985)

Those of a complacent disposition may think that the above message has no particular bearing on the current socio-economic situation in the UK in the 1990s. After all, this is a fairly affluent society, albeit made uncomfortable for some by prolonged economic recession and rising unemployment. We have equal-opportunity legislation, state education for all, a National Health Service providing for the care and rehabilitation of the sick in body and mind, and a social security system designed to minimise the worst effects of poverty (whatever its origin).

This is perhaps the 'comfortable' view of things. There is increasing research evidence which contradicts such complacency. Most social investigators accept, even if they deplore, the fact that the UK remains in many ways a class-divided society, despite the social upheavals that have taken place throughout the 20th century.

The Victorian attitude of intolerance towards those less well off was often accompanied by a belief that poverty was largely a self-inflicted problem. This attitude is not dead; it is embodied in official 'back to basics' rhetoric. The often tardy responses by government to various health and welfare reports in the past two decades, and the failure to implement many of their recommendations at either local or central levels, may be a distant reflection of such entrenched social attitudes and values.

We are not dealing with illusions. We hope to examine a powerful social phenomenon which has the potential to enhance or diminish the individual across a wide spectrum of life experiences. For instance, differential mortality rates show that, in terms of health: 'British society is stratified to a fine grain from top to bottom' (Davey Smith *et al.* 1990). When some people have more resources than others, they gain an advantage derived from their social position. Of the factors contributing to structured variations (patterns) in life and death, *social class* is the most significant.

Social class, for good or ill, influences the norms of family life and the transmission of attitudes, values and beliefs. It has a central role in determining success or failure in education and, subsequently, job market chances and career progression. All areas of social life are affected. It would be unwise to speculate that health and health care might somehow have remained unchallenged. On the contrary, research indicates that they have not.

Medicine defines health needs primarily in relation to biology, or more explicitly, pathology. Social researchers use an alternative or contrasting approach (Mechanic 1992). They measure well-being, illness and health provision on the basis of a person's social class (occupational) position. This is an important approach for health care professionals who are concerned with providing an appropriate and acceptable service. If a person's health status is seen to be largely a product of social circumstances rather than inherited temperament or genetic predisposition, then improvements must lie in the direction of social reform and not just individual behavioural change. Not everyone agrees on what these reforms, levels of individual responsibility or funding for health should be. It is hardly surprising to learn that this is a highly contentious area among sociological thinkers as well as politicians and economists (see Chapter 2).

This chapter will present sociological explanations of the relationship between social class and health status, a major dimension of continuing *structured inequality*. Relevant reports will be cited in the discussion.

Stratification: forms and features

Stratification on the basis of social class is an area of sociology that is alive with controversy. Social class has been viewed over the years by sociologists of various persuasions in both negative and positive terms. Different perspectives provide contrasting explanations of the purposes and underlying functions of social class divisions in a capitalist society such as modern Britain. Many of these views are irreconcilable in their differences of outlook.

The study of *social stratification* '(. . .) is probably the most difficult and confused area within sociology, not least because there is no general agreement about what constitutes class' (Haralambos and Holborn 1990, p.109). Similarly, Dahrendorf (1976), in his incisive study of class and conflict, observes that the concept of class is

> (. . .) one of the most extreme examples of the inability of sociologists to achieve (. . .) a minimum of consensus even in the modest business of terminological decisions.
>
> (Dahrendorf 1976, p.74)

Sociologists, by virtue of being an integral part of the subject they study, inevitably experience problems relating to neutrality and objectivity. All observation must, to some extent, be influenced by personal attitudes and values as well as individual life experiences. Only too often one may 'see what one wants to see' and fail, in the process, to achieve an element of impartiality. Indeed, it has been argued that the major theoretical perspectives, to be addressed later in terms of social class, far from being value-free are themselves ideologically slanted (Haralambos and Heald 1980, p.95). Social stratification may be a crucial and fascinating area in contemporary sociology, but it is one where science and politics have become inextricably entangled (Saunders 1990, p.vi). When applied to health care in the prioritising of certain needs over others, the problem of how to distinguish between science and political ideology becomes apparent. Consequently, sociologists may openly acknowledge this problematic, stating a direct connection between theories of stratification and political ideologies, and making no secret of their own commitment to particular values (Haralambos and Heald 1980, p.96). For this among other reasons, their views are not necessarily welcomed by health policy makers (see Chapters 2 and 10).

The term 'stratification', borrowed from geology to describe layered rock formations, refers to the inequalities between different groups as social and not natural products. However, the analogy can be misleading, as geographical strata (layers) possess a degree of permanence, whereas in the social context these change over time, albeit sometimes only slowly.

History and cross-cultural anthropology reveal that inequalities have existed in all forms of human society. What varies across time and place is the criteria used to discrimate between individuals and groups. Thus, social stratification theorists have concentrated on differences based upon class, gender, race, ethnicity, age, caste or religious affiliation. Race, for instance, as a stratifying factor has a long history extending far back to ancient slavery. Gender operates in discriminatory ways in modern societies, the UK included, as the women's movement bears eloquent witness (Abbott and Wallace 1990).

Jones and Jones (1975) identified caste and class as two major and contrasting *systems of stratification*. While caste is seen to be a 'closed' system in which no movement is possible except in rare instances, class is 'open', allowing for both upward and downward social mobility. The authors define social stratification as 'the way individuals are ranked on a scale of superiority/inferiority which results in differences between them of privileges, rewards, obligations and restrictions' (Jones and Jones 1975, p.63). Along the same lines, Turner (1986, p.29) sees stratification as 'social differentiation plus evaluation in terms of reputation, status or wealth'.

Modern history provides numerous examples of these ranking systems in practice, by means of race in South Africa, caste in India, ethnic differentiation in Nazi Germany and currently in what was Yugoslavia. Racial and ethnic identity are often fundamental in structuring access to social resources such as housing and employment, while religious affiliation is significant in the social context of Northern Ireland and the Middle East (Saunders 1990). These social divisions engender potential conflict, hostility, alienation and untold human suffering, as differing groups confront the effects of inequalities in political power, social status/prestige, and economic rewards. These are the core elements in any system of stratification, dramatically affecting the well-being, development and self-actualisation of the individual throughout the life cycle.

It can be seen, therefore, that strata constitute groups. These groups share a common identity and lifestyle, and have common interests, beliefs and values which distinguish them from others. In advanced market-orientated societies, grouping according to socio-economic position or social class is the system of stratification, in the case of Britain having its roots in the period of the industrial revolution. For better or worse, an individual's social class position will influence his or her 'life chances', educational and occupational opportunities, as well as the capacity to enjoy and maintain positive health over his or her life span. Social class has a significant relationship to health and access to care; it needs to be considered in some depth.

Dahrendorf (1976) draws attention to the shifts of meaning that have accompanied the concept of class throughout its history. A brief consideration of *functionalist* and *Marxist* viewpoints bears this out.

As far as sociological thinking on social class is concerned, the ideas of Karl Marx have been highly influential. Indeed, many sociologists see Marx's contribution as the most explanatory theory of the phenomenon of class in *capitalist* societies. For at the 'centre of Marx's theory of society and history is the notion of a gradually unfolding conflict in which the primary units are not individuals, nor localised associations, but classes' (McAll 1990, p.19). Classes are taken to be hostile, opposing interest groups and exploitation an objective fact, integral to the capitalist system. According to Marx, whoever controlled the means of economic production also controlled the dominant prevailing value system within society, referred to as 'ruling class ideology'. These ideas have been further developed by contemporary Marxist thinkers (Braverman 1974; Hayes 1994).

For Marxists, classes are groups sharing the same relationship to the means of production – the bourgeoisie or owners of production, and the proletariat with only their labour to sell. The economic base or infrastructure shaped the social superstructure where relationships to production, as owners or non-owners, would again be reflected and reproduced. In the Marxian view, political power derived from economic power, and reflected ruling class interests, projecting a distorted view of reality. *Class struggle* is identified as the driving force of social change.

A Marxist concept of social class is one of conflict, exploitation and oppression of one group by another, resulting in relationships which are potentially disruptive and injurious to society as a whole, and carrying within them the seeds of their own destruction (Haralambos and Heald 1980, p.38; Giddens 1989, p.209).

This approach is not adhered to by all sociologists. Indeed, structural functionalists take an opposing stance, arguing that stratification by social class is highly functional for society in general. From this perspective, society is seen to consist of interdependent groups working together in co-operation, within an overall relationship of reciprocity. Functionalists recognise that the division of labour inevitably leads to inequality, in terms of both power and prestige but, as leading theorist Talcott Parsons (1951) suggested, such inequality ultimately benefits all members of society as it serves to further collective goals based on shared values (Haralambos and Holborn 1990).

Stratification is seen to be a key mechanism for ensuring *effective role allocation*, so that the most important positions are conscientiously filled by the most qualified persons (Davis and Moore 1966). For functionalist theorists, stratification solves the problem of placing and motivating individuals in society. It is seen as an inevitable feature of advanced industrial societies, beneficial and functional for society as a whole. Not surprisingly, this viewpoint has been heavily criticised by both Marxist sociologists and those of a non-Marxist, liberal persuasion.

Whatever way stratification systems are analysed, in terms of conflict as in the Marxist framework, market position as in the work of Weber, or based on a theory of social action as in the work of Parsons, what is not in question is that they involve socially structured inequalities.

Turner (1986, p.30) suggests that 'the existence of social inequality is the product of sanctions, norms and power relations'. These inequalities in modern capitalist society emerge from a complex relationship between politics and economics. Although government attempts to 'play down' increasing demands for welfare, health and education services, the economic requirement and coercive influences of a capitalist economy have to be addressed. This contradiction between politics and economics can constitute a de-stabilising factor in society. This may be as true in socialist societies as it is in capitalist ones (Haralambos and Heald 1980, p.91; Giddens 1989, p.331).

In modern British society, these inequalities may be considerable, involving power differentials, inequality of opportunity, inequality of access to, and failure in, social justice. These dimensions of social inequity will now be addressed in relation to health and health care provision.

Social class and occupational structure

A social class, according to Jones and Jones (1975), is a section of the general population which sees itself, and is seen by others, as distinct from others in the population, in terms of value orientations, possessions and prestige, as well as education, lifestyle and occupation. Class membership influences social and sexual attitudes and behaviours, language acquisition, leisure activities, and many other facets of life. According to McAll (1990):

> British society is divisible into classes, both in the strict sense of relations of production, and (. . .) in the loose descriptive sense (. . .) of class endogamy, class dialect, class housing, class culture, class education and most strikingly, class patterns of consumption.
>
> (McAll 1990, p.139)

The author concludes that:

> (. . .) to grow up in a British town is to grow up in an already rigidly divided class landscape and one in which contemporary class divisions have only slowly evolved out of class divisions in the past.
>
> (McAll 1990, p.144)

Initially, *class consciousness* may be dependent upon the physical environment in terms of place of residence, type of housing, and marginalised contact with other classes. Each class group has its own norms, relationships and life experiences. Very early in life children are socialised into their own particular class-related culture. The education system tends to reinforce these experiences for many children, and in so doing, reproduces class relations. The history of mass education in this country, since its inception over 100 years ago, amply demonstrates this process.

> (. . .) class in Britain is reducible (. . .) to closed universes of action and meaning. To emerge from childhood and adolescence is to be thoroughly familiar with one's own class domain and to be aware of where the boundaries lie between that domain and those above and below it, but to have little knowledge of what lies beyond those boundaries.
>
> (McAll 1990, p.145)

It appears that problems develop when different classes interact in the wider societal context. Some years ago, Bernstein (1962) showed how differences in language acquisition could result in learning problems at school, where middle-class teachers endeavoured to communicate with working-class children in inner-city schools. Educational research continues to demonstrate that when teachers and pupils from differing social backgrounds encounter each other, the result may be breakdown in communication, failure of expectation on both sides, or the labelling of pupils by teachers, with all the potential that contains for the realisation of self-fulfilling prophecies (Sharp and Green 1975).

McAll (1990, p.149) reminds us that 'Prejudice and identity, class culture mechanisms of exclusion, coercive force, are all part of what class means'. It would be naïve, therefore, to think that these problems are not replicated in the health care context.

Stratification systems are not static, and change in the distribution of wealth and income occurs constantly. What is of interest is the direction that these changes take, and their impact in society across the class spectrum. The Report of the Royal Commission on the Distribution of Income and Wealth 1979 showed that redistribution benefited middle- rather than low-income groups. Furthermore, tax changes in the 1980s resulted in overall gains to those who were already well off. In fact, that particular decade saw an increase in income inequality and a strengthening of class divisions.

Occupational class structure

For the purpose of data collection required for government censuses and surveys, the schema devised by the Registrar General is that most commonly used (*see* Table 9.1). First developed in 1911, this scale has been used for much empirical social research ever since. The ranked social groupings have been subject to change over the years, and in 1981, for census purposes, individuals were allocated to one of six classes on the basis of occupational and employment status.

The system of rank ordering, according to levels of occupational skill and perceived status in the community, has inherent weaknesses. For example, the classification of married women under their husband's or partner's occupation rather than their own tends to be misleading. Similar problems exist in relation to the 'occupational status' of retired people. The scale is also

Table 9.1 The Registrar General's social class classification

Social Class	Description	Type of occupation
1	Professions	Lawyer, lecturer
	Business	Large employer
2	Lesser professions	Teachers, nurses
	Managerial/trade	Shopkeepers, office managers
3 NM	Skilled non-manual	Clerical workers, supervisors
3 M	Skilled manual	Miner, electrician
4	Semi-skilled manual	Farm workers, machine operators
5	Unskilled manual	Building labourers, kitchen staff

Adapted from Blane (1982, p.117)

vulnerable to inaccuracy when social changes such as increasing home ownership, single parenthood, second incomes and mounting unemployment are taken into account. These categories cut across the traditional relationship between a man's occupation and his family's resources. Stacey (1976, p.82) referred to the Registrar General's scale as 'more of a blunderbuss than a carefully calibrated instrument'.

For these reasons, researchers such as Goldthorpe, Hall-Jones and Halsey (compare Jones and Jones 1975) devised more precise scales for use in their own investigations. However, much large-scale research continues to be based on data collection employing the Registrar General's classification scheme.

The reader, in examining the statistics relating to health and illness should, perhaps, proceed with caution. In addition to the points noted above, the comments of Slattery (1986) could usefully be borne in mind:

> All forms of social knowledge represent power: power to inform or mislead, the power to illuminate or manipulate. Whoever controls the definition of official statistics controls public debate (and criticism); whoever has the power to withhold official data (or not collect it in the first place) has the power to prevent public discussion from arising.
>
> (Slattery 1986, p. 11)

Official reactions and responses to reports on health inequality (to be discussed later) tend to confirm Slattery's contentions.

At this point, it is necessary to consider briefly another major element in the prescribed subject area of this chapter, that of health. Although health professionals, including students of nursing, may reasonably feel that they already possess considerable knowledge of this concept, the sociological contribution will serve to extend their existing insights.

Concepts of health

McBean (1991, p.58) suggests that 'to define health would be to deny its breadth as an issue'. Few would argue as to the breadth of health as a subject for debate; despite this, many writers have searched for, and endeavoured to elaborate, its true meaning and definition. If, as Noack (1987) believes, health professionals cannot evaluate their work if health itself cannot be defined, then possible definitions need to be sought.

Health does not exist in isolation but within a specific socio-political, cultural and interactive framework (Jones 1991). Concepts of health are never static entities, but change in relation to time, place and individual age. The range of definitions, therefore, will vary accordingly. At certain times and in particular instances, the absence of physical disease may be uppermost; at others, the emphasis may be on well-being and self-actualisation.

The World Health Organisation's (1946) all-encompassing view stems from its conviction that appropriate health care provision should be available to every individual across the globe (Saunders and Carver 1985, p.vii). For this reason it is often taken to be almost too general, idealistic and static:

> Health is a state of complete physical, mental and social well-being, and not merely the absence of disease and infirmity.
>
> (World Health Organisation, 1946)

Instead, health may be seen predominantly in terms of its functional importance for society in the maintenance of individual role performance (Parsons 1972), or it may be defined as a commodity, something that can be bought and sold (Tawney 1931). Dubos (1979), however, viewed health in terms of personal strength and the ability to adapt to life's circumstances. He suggested that perfect health was neither possible nor particularly desirable. First, no formula devised would be broad enough to fit the requirements of a writer, a boxer, a New York bus driver or a contemplative monk. Secondly, 'Unless men become robots, no formula can ever give them permanently the health and happiness symbolised by the contented cow' (Dubos 1979).

An holistic view of health puts a high value on human experience or the quality of a person's life; this is much more than just the absence of disease pathology. In this view, health is a continuum where even the deprived or handicapped may achieve satisfactory levels. This conception is perhaps encapsulated in the romantic definition of the novelist Kathryn Mansfield:

> By health I mean the power to live a full, (. . .) life in close contact with what I love (. . .) I want to be all that I am capable of becoming (. . .) to learn, to desire, to know, to feel, to think, to act. This is what I want. And nothing less.
>
> (Mansfield 1977, p.278)

Health can mean many different things, and as Seedhouse (1986a) reminds us, definitions can never be the 'last word' because these are informed by theories which change over time. He suggests that 'health does not have a core meaning waiting to be discovered. There is no undisputed example of health' (Seedhouse 1986a, p.53).

Lay beliefs about health are varied and can often be seen to be class-related. Research carried out by Blaxter and Paterson (1982) revealed the prevalence of a functional view or 'the ability to cope' among their respondents (a sample of two generations of working-class mothers). They found that health, in the working class generally, was regarded very much as a matter of being able to 'get through the day'. Many saw themselves and their children as 'healthy', despite the presence of illness in some instances. By way of contrast, middle-class people tend to view health in terms of broader issues, as a positive sense of well-being, energy and vitality, similar perhaps to Mansfield's definition (see above).

If, as Seedhouse (1986a) suggests, the writings on health constitute 'an indigestible spaghetti of confusion', it nevertheless emerges as a multi-faceted phenomenon, and a subject much talked and written about. Indeed, Newman (1986) comments that the concern is now little short of idolatrous. This is, no doubt, in part because health does not constitute an

absolute fact but a relative or cultural value as well as a biological con
It is not, therefore, the sole property of the medical profession or prof
allied to medicine but 'a universal concern which cannot be separate
issues of life' (Seedhouse 1986b).

For sociologists, health is very much a political as well as a social iss
politicians, it is viewed more in economic terms based upon a defini
being 'disease-free'. Current debates on health in the political arena t
revolve around the gap between expected levels of personal respons
and the costs of maintaining acceptable standards of service provisio
as Robbins (1987) comments, the determinants of health tend to lie o
the health service:

> Health is gained, maintained or lost in the worlds of work, leisure,
> home and city life.
>
> (Robbins, quoted in McBean 1991, p.69)

The medical profession itself has been heavily criticised by social investigators in terms of its role in health care and illness prevention; there are links
here with Robbins' statement above. Illich, writing in 1975, suggested that
the medical establishment had become a major threat to health due to the
dominance of a technological, deterministic model and its disregard of the
qualitative aspects of individual health, such as emotional and cultural life.
He believed that medical activity could seriously undermine the autonomy
of individuals, communities and whole societies; people would lose their
ability to self-care as a result of the processes of clinical, social or cultural
'iatrogenesis' (the 'ills' of society are exacerbated rather than 'cured' by
technological medicine). Other writers, concerned to evaluate the nature
and extent of medicine's social power, have explored the concept of a
'medicalisation' of everyday life (compare Navarro 1975; Strong 1979; Hillier
1982; Cornwell 1984; Elston 1991; Riessman 1992).

It can be seen, therefore, that this is a highly contentious subject area, and it
may well be true that 'the idea of health as a specific, definable, fully describ-
able state to which everyone can aspire equally is nonsense' (Seedhouse
1986a, p.56). If health, as measured by mortality and morbidity rates, indicates anything it is an ever increasing and unacceptably high correlation
between poverty, illness and premature death rates (Blackburn 1991).

In order to address these disturbing trends, we need to consider *health
inequalities* within the context of capitalist society. According to researchers
in this area:

> The sociological contribution is (. . .) to increase understanding of the
> social and socio-economic factors which play a part in the promotion of
> health, and the causation of disease, and in part to take the natural next
> step and relate these factors (. . .) to the broader social structure.
>
> (Townsend *et al.* 1990, p.36)

In other words, in order to find out what makes us sick, we must turn to
an analysis of the economy and politics.

Political influences in illness and health

A large component of adult physical pathology and death is a measure of the misery caused by social and economic organisation. This approach is confirmed by Doyal and Pennell (1979) in their analysis, *The Political Economy of Health*. They argue that little sense can be made of patterns of health and illness outside the context of the mode of production in which these occur. The distribution of illness in society is seen to follow closely the distribution of income and wealth; level of income determines to a great extent standards of housing, type of local environment and other factors such as diet, clothing and overall quality of life. Many writers would concur with this viewpoint, seeing the capitalist economic system as a powerful, underlying cause in matters of mortality and morbidity. The ensuing problems which emerge are not related just to what is produced, but also to how production is organised. For instance, high wages may not always compensate for soul-destroying or 'mindless' work, nor redundancy payments for a sense of rejection and being on the 'scrapheap' of society.

Such factors may be highly injurious to both physical and mental wellbeing. It also needs to be borne in mind that the social relations of capital exist not only in the industrial context, but in other areas of the social superstructure, including schools, hospitals and government departments. McKinlay (1984) draws attention to the fact that decision-making under capitalism is seldom influenced by an awareness of collective needs, or the social costs likely to be involved. Instead, the 'inexorable requirement of profitability' always dictates the criteria or priorities; this is the 'fundamental and defining characteristic of capitalism' (McKinlay 1984, p.3). Health care professionals, trying to cope with numerous changes in structure, policy and modes of accountability, may be only too painfully familiar with the problem McKinlay enunciates.

The Marxist theorist Navarro (1986) clearly shares the views described above:

> (. . .) the crisis of medicine under capitalism is the crisis of medicine in capitalism.
>
> (Navarro 1986, p.2)

In this framework, the institutions of science and medicine are not neutral because their knowledge and practices reproduce class, race, sex and other forms of oppressive relations. Along with Doyal and Pennell (1979), Navarro sees capitalism as both directly and indirectly implicated in the causation of disease via working conditions and practices, environmental and atmospheric pollution, and patterns of consumption, to name but a few powerful influences. Marxists also take into account threats to mental health in terms of economic instability and ever-present risks of unemployment, lack of personal fulfilment in work, the lack of control over work itself, and an increasing sense of alienation. The working class are particularly vulnerable in these respects, including mothers isolated in the home with young children (Brown and Harris 1978). Mangen (1982), for example, draws attention to the sharp class gradient in suicide and parasuicide, where admissions to hospital were shown to be eight times greater in social classes 4 and 5 than in classes 1 and 2.

Medicine, it has been noted by many theorists, is not only a scientific endeavour, but also an enterprise or business. Considering its role in capitalism, McKinlay (1977) viewed the profession's connections to the highly profitable pharmaceutical industry, scientific and technological equipment suppliers and the development of the private health sector. The organisation of medical care, therefore, can provide a profitable area for capital accumulation. It can also conflict with the need to reduce health service costs, thus necessitating cut-backs in expenditure. A matter for fierce debate in the 1990s, health policies are not necessarily the rational responses of a benevolent state (Doyal and Pennell 1979). The pursuit of health and the pursuit of profit may constitute a contradiction within a capitalist economy (see Chapter 6).

Social class membership and health status

The growth of statistical evidence, built up over the last 50 years, demonstrates an inverse relationship between an individual's class position and his or her state of health. In other words, the more one descends the social scale, the higher the prevalence of ill health; conversely, the more affluent people are, the more likely they are to be healthy. Mortality and morbidity rates (*see* Fig. 9.1) reveal a class pattern, which applies to men and women, and bears on us from before we are born until long into retirement (Lynch and Oelman 1981; Mitchell 1984;. Townsend *et al.* 1990).

The relationship between *social class, life and death*, has, of course, been known since the early work of William Farr in the mid-19th century, and indeed can be traced back even further. Many researchers utter words of caution at this point, because mortality and morbidity rates as health status indicators need to be interpreted critically (Doyal 1979). Crude mortality rates, for example, do not provide information concerning age, ethnic origin or geographical distribution. Cause of death, as most coroners would agree, is notoriously difficult to ascertain and to attribute to a single disease process. Furthermore, morbidity rates for particular conditions may be biased by subjective factors because they are compiled from a wide range of source material, such as general practice and hospital attendance records, self-report studies on illness behaviour, and statistics of absences from work due to sickness or disability.

Despite these constraints on accuracy, the causes of perceived differences up and down the class hierarchy continue to be a matter of intense, if not bitter, debate. As previously mentioned, class is analysed as the product of a complex interplay of power, status, wealth and economic position. It is a 'useful summarising concept which permits sociologists to make reasonable predictions about an individual's way of life, opportunities, and life

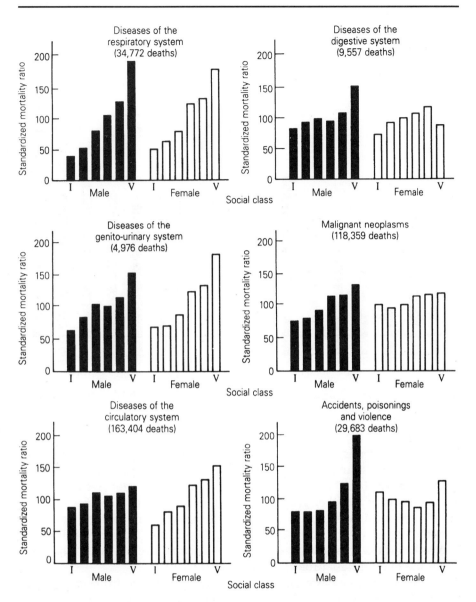

Figure 9.1 Occupational class and mortality in adult life (men and married women 15–64 years of age) by husband's occupation. (*Source*: Office Population Censuses and Surveys 1978.)

experiences (. . .) it is a sub-culture existing beneath the general national culture' (Mangen 1982, p.63). The pervasive influences of social class in matters of health have long interested sociologists: 'Class differences in health represent a double injustice: life is short where its quality is poor' (Wilkinson 1986, p.2). Problems of ill health become cumulative as the social

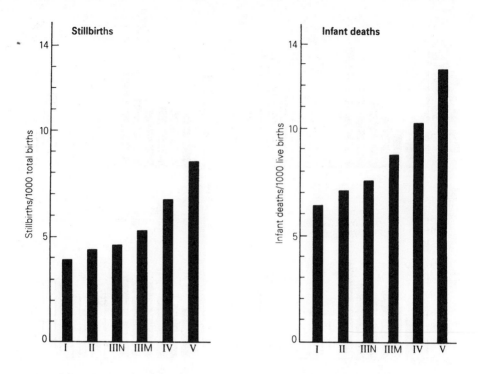

Figure 9.2 Outcome of pregnancy by social class of father, England and Wales, 1984. *Source*: Whitehead (1987, p. 10)

class scale descends, with those in Social Class 5 showing some of the highest levels of sickness and death. In terms of life span, research indicates that in Social Classes 1 and 2 individuals may experience longer lives than their counterparts in all other groups. Babies born to parents in Social Classes 4 and 5 are four times more likely to die in the first year of life than those with parents higher up the scale (*see* Fig. 9.2). In addition, lower working class males have less chance of living to a pensionable age (65 years) than men from the middle-class professions (Power *et al.* 1991).

It is clear from the examples above, which are drawn from an extensive body of research, that marked inequalities occur at every stage of the life cycle (Cornwell 1984; Mitchell 1984; Arber 1987). There appears to be no firm evidence at the present time that *class differentials* in health are narrowing. Up to the decade commencing in 1980, however, it was thought that society was generally becoming more egalitarian, with less emphasis being placed on social differences. This view was soon to be challenged.

The Black Report on *Inequalities in Health* was published by the Department of Health and Social Security in 1980. It received a less than enthusiastic reception from the prevailing Tory government. This was hardly surprising, given the hard-hitting nature of the report's findings and the perceived economic costs of implementing its many recommendations. The Secretary of State for Health and Social Security at the time made it clear that 'additional expenditure on the scale which could result from the report's recommendations – upward of £2 billion a year – is quite unrealistic' (quoted in Townsend *et al*, 1990).

The report drew attention to social class differences for most causes of death, demonstrating an inverse relationship between mortality rates and occupational rankings, using the *Registrar General's scale* (*see* Table 9.1). A similar picture emerged in relation to a wide range of physical and mental diseases. Why such class-related inequalities continued to exist, nearly half a century after the establishment of the National Health Service and against an overall improvement in the health of the population, became a matter of political debate.

The Black Report (Department of Health and Social Security 1980) provided four possible explanations for the causes of continuing inequalities: artefactual, natural, materialist or cultural. Artefactual causes relate to the statistical problems encountered when comparing groups with each other over a period of time. We have to consider not only that the Registrar General's schema has been subject to variation, but also that occupations have undergone change as well. Whitehead (1987) notes that subsequent studies attempting to control these factors have tended to show that the Registrar General's scale may have considerably underestimated class gradients in both mortality and morbidity, thus constituting an insensitive measure of hierarchical differences.

Interestingly, natural or social selection explanations suggest that health inequalities influence social mobility, the healthy tending to be upwardly mobile, while the unhealthy drift downwards. The materialist or structuralist explanation emphasises the importance of differences in material constraints, such as living and working conditions throughout class groupings, seeing them as major determinants of health. Finally, the cultural or behavioural explanation draws attention to the importance of individual responsibility and free will. Ill health is taken to be a direct result of a person's own actions and health beliefs. Smoking and drinking habits and the 'uptake' of preventive services come into this category.

Researchers working on the investigation expressed a preference for the materialist explanation. Blane (1985) suggests that this is the only way to account for the overall improvement in the health of the population, at the same time as social class differences are maintained. According to this approach, income distribution, poverty, access to education, housing or working conditions are seen as contributory, causal factors.

The report did not overlook inequalities in health care provision, particularly in the use of *preventive facilities*. It emerged that middle-class people were generally better served than their working-class counterparts. Indeed, health service institutions were seen to be related to the values and preferences of the middle-class 'consumer', to the detriment of those less articulate in expressing their needs and less able to command resources of time or money. The research clearly indicated that health was strongly related to socio-economic circumstances. Henceforth, the study of health education and promotion shifted slightly (but significantly) from an exclusive focus on individual responsibility to consideration of social structures (known as the 'new' public health; see Chapter 10). The fact that had been frequently ignored was that many people were simply not in a position to choose a healthy lifestyle (Cornwell 1984). Those from Social Classes 4 and 5 were likely to be exposed to potential health hazards in both home and work environments, and to social pressures that encourage habits injurious to health, such as smoking and drinking, in order to relieve stress (Mitchell 1984).

Despite the above findings, little was done by the government to implement the Black Report's recommended policies. The justification given made it clear that a lack of knowledge and hence misuse of services by the poorer groups in society was the real problem. It was their personal inability to cope with life, rather than any failing on the part of the health services available, which was to blame (Crombie 1984).

Writing 10 years later, Davey Smith *et al.* (1990) found the situation to have worsened. Social class differences in life expectancy and mortality between those at the top and those at the bottom of the scale were widening. This trend had been investigated by the Health Education Council (Whitehead 1987). While the author accepted that natural differences in health do occur within the population, she was concerned with unfair or unjust levels of inequality and the means by which equality of access, treatment and quality of care could be promoted. Such considerations took into account not only social class membership but also ethnicity, gender and location factors.

It has been calculated that every 1 per cent rise in unemployment contributes to 5000 deaths (Navarro 1993, p. 27). These figures apply to the USA. For a consideration of the UK equivalent, the reader is referred to *The forsaken families* (Fagin and Little 1984). Victorian values, it seems, die hard and the poor still experience *stigmatisation* and are seen in some quarters to be feckless, thriftless, and lacking in initiative. Social attitudes remain to some extent 'anti-poor', and influence those who make the policy and take the major health care decisions.

Perceptions and relationships: carers and clients

Health professionals generally, and the medical profession in particular, tend to be highly concerned with the objective, physical aspects of treatment and care, and rather less with the psycho-social elements or the 'affective domain'. This approach is consistent with the continued influence of the medical treatment model. There are variations in how sociologists view the function of the medical profession and the way in which it has changed over time. To Parsons (1951), a leading functionalist theoretician, medicine is a benign and integrative force in society, a servant of the common good. On the other hand, Zola (1977) argues that it exercises a powerful monopoly in matters of health, as well as a degree of social control. For instance:

The medical profession has first claim to jurisdiction over the label of illness and anything to which it may be attached, irrespective of its capacity to deal with it effectively.

(Zola 1977, p. 52, quoting Freidson 1970)

Kennedy (1981) asserts that illness now constitutes an indeterminate concept, being the product of fluctuating social, political and moral values (see Chapter 5).

If illness is a judgement, the practice of medicine can be understood in terms of power. He who makes the judgement wields the power.

(Kennedy 1981, p. 7)

In this view, illness is a status rather than a state, granted or withheld by those having the power to do so. Kennedy cites the French theorist, Foucault, who argued that 'in the modern world there is no clear line between concern for the welfare of others and coercive control over their lives' (compare Kennedy 1981, p. 6) The expert can become society's agent, the enforcer or 'thought policeman'.

It appears that doctors have both socialising and coercive powers at their disposal, and that these are utilised in such a way as to ensure that the prevailing social and political values of society are upheld and reinforced (Foucault 1973a, 1973b; Zola 1977). As doctors and other health care professionals come from, or are socialised into, the middle classes, this is hardly surprising. If structures of reality, life experiences, communication and language vary across different class groups, then the scene is set for conflict and misunderstanding between the providers of care and those who have the greatest need – the socially disadvantaged.

According to Dr Julian Tudor Hart (1975), 'The availability of good medical care tends to vary inversely with the need for it in the population served. This *inverse care law* operates more completely where medical care is most exposed to market forces, and less so where such exposure is reduced' (my italics). This is an interesting comment in the light of current government policy within the National Health Service. Thus, in:

areas with the most sickness and death, general practitioners have more work, longer lists, less hospital support (. . .) and hospital doctors shoulder heavier case loads with less staff and equipment, more obsolete buildings, and suffer recurrent crises in the availability of beds and replacement staff.

(Tudor Hart 1975, p. 205)

Earlier, Titmus in his 1968 study, made the point that:

higher income groups know how to make better use of the NHS; they tend to receive more specialist attention; occupy more of the beds in better equipped and staffed hospitals; receive more effective surgery; have better maternity care; are more likely to get psychiatric help and psychotherapy than low income groups – particularly the unskilled.

(Titmus, quoted in Stacey 1976, p. 77)

Further research has produced little evidence to show that this situation of socially maintained injustice has in any way radically changed. The fact that the middle classes obtain greater benefit from the available health services is related to their enjoyment of advantages in income and wealth, education and environment, and the power to command resources. These factors influence not only the uptake of resources but also relationships in the health care context.

The relationship between doctor and patient is redolent of uncertainty on both sides, consisting as it does of differing role expectations, rights and obligations. The middle-class patient's perceptions and expectations may well be critical, demanding and knowledgeable, viewing the doctor as a peer, and sharing a similar mode of language and social class culture. This may place him or her in an advantageous position compared with working-class patients (Stacey 1976).

Doctors inevitably bring to their practices the values, attitudes and assumptions relative to their class location, and the same applies to nurses (see Chapter 1). Social class stereotypes may well influence patient perception, treatment, and levels of attention given (Cartwright and Anderson 1981).

Cornwell's study (1984) in the east end of London, a traditional working-class area, found that a constant theme emerged of the perceived power of the doctor and the *social distance* created by it. The patients interviewed felt that they were in an unequal context or contest, and emotions were aroused relating to their undignified and *subordinate position* (see Chapter 3). Although in general there was respect for hospital doctors and other health professionals, relationships with general practitioners were less happy, while views of maternity and community services were sharply critical. The quality of doctor–patient interactions affects anxiety levels and the instilling of confidence, as well as the transmission of information. The perception a patient has of his or her doctor may itself enhance or inhibit communication.

Freidson's (1970) perception of the doctor–patient relationship was one of potential conflict. 'It is my thesis that the separate worlds of experience and reference of the layman and the professional worker are always in potential conflict with one another'. Such conflict could arise, according to Freidson (1970), from a desire to maintain *professional control* on the part of the doctor, or from differences of viewpoint between the doctor and patient regarding the nature of the patient's problems. It may rarely become overt; instead, strategies designed to influence, such as non-verbal behaviours, persuasion and bargaining, may be employed. In these situations, the doctor is at a considerable advantage in terms of knowledge and power (Tuckett 1976). Illness is not, therefore, a purely biological problem, it is:

(. . .) problematic and socially defined for the ways in which patients and physicians define and act towards illness are only partly determined and shaped by the 'primary' underlying disease process by which the illness is produced.

(Field 1976, p. 360)

Doctors play a crucial role in the legitimation of the validity of an individual's illness. They may help or hinder in terms of the power to grant or refuse certificates of sickness, to seek aid for patients needing rehousing, or be able to assist in the provision of other needed resources. The medical control of illness is pervasive, but increasingly the Department of Health or the Department of Social Security and Local Authority Housing departments, devise their own bureaucratic definitions of hardship, disability and impaired mobility (see Chapter 5).

Stacey's (1976) research indicated that general practitioners tended to know their middle-class patients better than those of the working class, and to allow them more consultation time. Mitchell (1984) found much discontent expressed by working-class patients at the attitudinal responses of doctors and other health care professionals. These included failure to respond to requests for information, failure to explain treatment being given, personal derogatory remarks in the patient's presence such as 'she is not very intelligent you know', and the ignoring of relatives. Indeed, many expressed a range of feelings when speaking of their doctors, extending from discomfort to outright distress (Mitchell 1984, p. 161).

In general practice and in hospitals, staff responses appear to be influenced frequently by perceived 'social worth'. Mitchell (1984, p. 162) quotes one doctor as saying: 'All my Social Class 1 and 2 patients have cut down on smoking, but it is impossible to get through to classes 4 and 5'. Such responses, of course, do not relate to the class factor alone but to other attributes of persons as well, for example, gender, age and ethnic origin. The young may be seen to have greater value than the old. Some ethnic groups may be thought to have low pain thresholds, or to complain too readily, while the fact of their social conditions, and their experiences of racial discrimination are rarely taken into account. Those who present with self-inflicted problems such as drunkenness or attempted suicide may receive the least sympathy of all. Stereotypes, therefore, play their part in influencing both attitudes and treatments.

These problems are exacerbated in the current health context. The organising principles of modern hospitals stem from the values of the world of business management, which pervade all working levels and practices, as well as policy decisions (Mitchell 1984). Quantity, not quality, and management pressure to increase patient throughput, and therefore workload, result in stress and soaring sickness rates among staff, in addition to the ever-present danger of error induced by work overload. This is a familiar situation to many readers, no doubt. Rigid, bureaucratic and hierarchical organisation within the working structure discourages questioning or challenges to the status quo. Long ago Florence Nightingale described hospitals as, 'Not only a dismaying reality, but also a didactic microcosm illustrating the interdependence of health and order in the larger society' (compare Fox 1979). We may reflect, at this point, on how much has really changed since that comment was made.

Many researchers (Katz 1969; McClure 1978; Clay 1987; Mitchell 1984) suggest that nurses tend to express their views not overtly but indirectly by means of the *doctor–nurse game* (Stein 1967). Nurses still experience problems of relative powerlessness and own to a sense of being undervalued, even though they are centrally involved in continuous patient care. As a group, particularly if they are in any danger of believing in their 'angel' image, nurses do not see themselves in terms of bigotry, prejudice or discrimination. Nurses care for the sick, irrespective of class, creed, colour or nationality, and the quality of that care is presumed to be uniform throughout. A glance at some of the findings of nursing research, from *The Unpopular Patient* (Stockwell 1972) onwards, should at least give nurses pause for thought. As Alonso (1985) reminds us, hackles rise when a patient questions treatment, grumbles are heard concerning 'another overdose', and complaints are made about a ward 'full of Grans'. Prejudiced opinions about male nurses or those from ethnic minority backgrounds, not to mention enslavement to a rigid professional hierarchy, should serve to convince most nurses that doctors are certainly not the only group to be influenced by preconceived values, beliefs, assumptions and attitudes.

Price, writing in 1985, showed that nurses' behaviour could be influenced by their perception of the patient's class status. Nurses, in this particular piece of research, were inhibited from taking an assertive or moderately assertive stance with higher ranking patients, and felt much more able to be forthright with those patients who they perceived to be of a lower status. Sayer (1992) warns of the danger that: 'Individuals may be seen as representative of a race, age group, gender, occupation, or disability. They will then be given the characteristics we believe people in that group have'.

Examining nurses' unfavourable attitudes towards patients from ethnic minority backgrounds, Kem Louie (1990) found that these could lead to less than optimum care for the patients concerned. Similar studies on geriatric provision showed that nurses with negative attitudes towards the elderly adopted a custodial rather than a therapeutic approach in the care they delivered. Thus, a lack of knowledge and understanding about a patient's culture may lead to a completely inappropriate model of treatment (Perry 1988). These examples, taken from a considerable body of research, illustrate that nurses 'are not beamed down as well-rounded human beings, uncontaminated by the bigotry in the wider world' (Wright 1988). However, in the current context of health organisation, training in cognitive competencies is more likely to take precedence over a political education concerned with equal opportunities.

Conclusions

The foregoing account has served to indicate the powerful effects of stratification factors in the identification of needs and care provision. These influences permeate every level and context in the health system, either enhancing or diminishing the well-being of clients and the effectiveness of carers. In *Disabling Professions*, Illich *et al.* (1977) show that professional relationships, including contestations over status at work, are not 'outside' these processes. At the micro-level, practitioners confront these influences in the daily activities of care-giving. At the macro-level, while pharmaceutical and insurance industries continue to profit,

> society is left with the uncomfortable phenomenon of a portion of its population living, and living well, off the sufferings of others and to some extent even unwittingly having a vested interest in the continuing existence of such problems.
>
> (Illich et al. 1977, p. 66)

The authors here are referring to the American health context, but the message has relevance to us in the UK. The NHS that we took for granted no longer seems to exist, and the ideology behind its creation has been almost discredited.

> The essence of a satisfactory health service is that the rich and poor are treated alike, that poverty is not a disability and wealth not advantaged.
>
> (Bevan 1952)

Readers may consider whether health care in the 1990s is moving towards, or away from, its original ideology.

References

Abbott, P. and Wallace, C. 1990: *An introduction to sociology: feminist perspectives.* London: Routledge.

Alonso, R. 1985: Discriminate? Not us! *Nursing Times* **81(9)**, 41.

Arber, S. 1987: Social class, non-employment and chronic illness: continuing the inequalities in health debate. *British Medical Journal* **594**, 1069–1073.

Bernstein, B. 1962: Social class, linguistic codes and grammatical elements. *Language and Speech* **5**, 221–240.

Bevan, A. 1952: *In place of fear.* London: Quartet Books.

Blackburn, C. 1991: *Poverty and health.* Milton Keynes: Open University Press.

Blane, D. 1982: Inequality and social class. In Patrick, D. and Scambler, G. (eds), *Sociology as applied to medicine.* London: Bailliere Tindall, 113–124.

Blane, D. 1985: An assessment of the Black Report's explanations of health inequalities. *Sociology of Health and Illness* **7(3)**, 423–445.

Blaxter, M. and Paterson, E. 1982: *Mothers and daughters: a three generation study of health attitudes and health behaviour.* London: Heinemann.

Braverman, H. 1974: *Labor and monopoly capital: the degradation of work in the twentieth century.* New York: Monthly Review Press.

Brown, G. and Harris, T. 1978: *The social origins of depression.* London: Tavistock.

Cartwright, A. and Anderson, R. 1981: *General practice revisited: a second study of patients and their doctors.* London: Tavistock.

Clay, T. 1987: *Nurses, power and politics.* London: Heinemann.

Cornwell, J. 1984: *Hard-earned lives: accounts of health and illness.* London: Tavistock.

Cox, C. and Mead, A. (eds) 1975: *A sociology of medical practice*. London: Collier-Macmillan.

Crombie, D. 1984: *Social class and health status*. McGonaghey Memorial Lecture. London: Royal College of General Practitioners.

Dahrendorf, R. 1976: *Class and class conflict in industrial society*. London: Routledge and Kegan Paul.

Davey Smith, G., Bartley, M. and Blane, D. 1990: The Black Report on socio-economic inequalities in health 10 years on. *British Medical Journal* **301**, 18–25.

Davis, K. and Moore, W.E. 1966: Some principles of stratification. In Bendix, R. and Lipset, S.M. (eds), *Class, status and power*, 2nd edition. London: Routledge and Kegan Paul, 47–53.

Department of Health and Social Security (DHSS) 1980: *Inequalities in health. Report of the research working group (Sir Douglas Black, Chairman)*. London: Department of Health and Social Security.

Doyal, L. 1979: A matter of life and death: medicine, health and statistics. In Irvine, J., Miles, I. and Evans, J. (eds), *Demystifying social statistics*. London: Pluto Press, 237–254.

Doyal, L. and Pennell, I. 1979: *The political economy of health*. London: Pluto Press.

Dubos, R. 1979: *The mirage of health*. New York: Harper Row.

Elston, M. A. 1991: The politics of professional power: medicine in a changing health service. In Gabe, J., Calnan, M. and Bury, M. (eds), *The sociology of the health service*. London: Routledge, 58–88.

Fagin, L. and Little, M. 1984: *The forsaken families: a timely and disturbing report on the effects of unemployment on family life in Britain*. Harmondsworth: Penguin.

Field, D. 1976: The social definition of illness. In Tuckett, D. (ed.), *An introduction to medical sociology*. London: Tavistock, 334–366.

Foucault, M. 1973a: *The birth of the clinic*. London: Tavistock.

Foucault, M. 1973b: *Madness and civilization: a history of insanity in the Age of Reason*. New York: Vintage Books.

Fox, R. 1979: *The sociology of medicine*. New Jersey: Prentice-Hall.

Freidson, E. 1970: *Profession of medicine: a study in the sociology of applied knowledge*. New York: Dodd-Mead.

Giddens, A. 1989: *Sociology*. Cambridge: Polity Press.

Haralambos, M. and Heald, R.M. 1980: *Sociology: themes and perspectives*, 1st edition. Slough: University Tutorial Press.

Haralambos, M. and Holborn, M. 1990: *Sociology: themes and perspectives*, 3rd edition. London: Unwin Hyman.

Hayes, M. 1994: *The new right in Britain: an introduction to theory and practice*. London: Pluto Press.

Hillier, S. 1982: Medicine and social control. In Patrick, D. and Scambler, G. (eds), *Sociology as applied to medicine*. London: Bailliere Tindall, 175–184.

Illich, I. 1975: *Medical nemesis: the expropriation of health*. London: Marion Boyars.

Illich, I., Zola, I., McKnight, J., Caplan, J. and Shaiken, H. 1977: *Disabling professions*. London: Marion Boyars.

Jones, R.K. 1991: *Sociology of health and illness*. Kenwyn: Juta & Co.

Jones, R.K. and Jones P.A. 1975: *Sociology in medicine*. London: English University Press.

Katz, F. 1969: Nurses. In Etzioni, A. (ed.), *The semi-professions and their organisation*. New York: Free Press, 54–81.

Kennedy, I. 1981: *The unmasking of medicine*. London: Allen and Unwin.

Louie, K. 1990: Empathy, anxiety and transcultural nursing. *Nursing Standard* **5(5)**, 36–40.

Lynch, P. and Oelman, B. 1981: Mortality from coronary heart disease in the British Army compared with the civil population. *British Medical Journal* **283**, 405–407.

McAll, C. 1990: *Class, ethnicity and social inequality.* Montreal: McGill-Queens University Press.

McBean, S. 1991: Health and health promotion in nursing. In Perry, A. and Jolley, M. (eds), *Nursing: a knowledge base for practice.* London: Edward Arnold, 52–92.

McClure, M. 1978: The long road to accountability. *Nursing Outlook* **26(1)**, 47–50.

McKinlay, J. 1977: The business of good doctoring or doctoring as good business: reflections of Freidson's view of the medical game. *International Journal of Health Services* **7(3)**, 459–483.

McKinlay, J. (ed.) 1984: *Issues in the political economy of health care.* New York: Tavistock.

Mangen, S. 1982: *Sociology and mental health.* Edinburgh: Churchill Livingstone.

Mansfield, K. 1977: *Letters and journals.* Harmondsworth: Pelican.

Mechanic, D. 1992: Health and illness behaviour and patient–practitioner relationships. *Social Science and Medicine* **34(12)**, 1345–1350.

Mitchell, J. 1984: *What is to be done about illness and health?* Harmondsworth: Penguin.

Navarro, V. 1975: The industrialization of fetishism or the fetishism of industrialization: a critique of Ivan Illich. *International Journal of Health Services* **5(3)**, 351–371.

Navarro, V. 1986: *Crisis, health and medicine.* London: Tavistock.

Navarro, V. 1993: *Dangerous to your health: Capitalism in health care.* New York: Monthly Review Press.

Newman, M. 1986: *Health as expanding consciousness.* St Louis: Mosby.

Noack, H. 1987: Concepts of health promotion. In Abelin, T., Brzezinski, Z. and Carstairs, V. (eds), *Measurement in health promotion and protection: World Health Organisation, European Series No. 22.* Copenhagen: World Health Organization Regional Publications.

Office of Population Censuses and Surveys (OPCS) 1978: *Occupational mortality 1970–72. Decennial Supplement.* London: HMSO.

Parsons, T. 1951: *The social system.* New York: Free Press.

Parsons, T. 1972: Definitions of health and illness in the light of American values and social structure. In Jaco, E.G. (ed.), *Patients, physicians and illness*, 2nd edition. London: Collier-Macmillan, 107–127.

Perry, F. 1988: Far from black and white. *Nursing Times* **84(10)**, 40–41.

Power, C., Manor, O. and Fox, J. 1991: *Health and class: the early years.* London: Chapman Hall.

Price, R. 1985: The confidence to educate? *Nursing Mirror* **161(17)**, 39–42.

Riessman, C.K. 1992: Women and medicalization: a new perspective. In Kirkup, G. and Smith, L.S. (eds), *Inventing women: science, technology and gender.* Milton Keynes: Open University Press, 123–144.

Robbins, C. (ed.) 1987: *Health promotion in North America: implications for the UK.* London: Health Education Council and King Edward's Hospital Fund.

Saunders, D. and Carver, R. 1985: *The struggle for health: medicine and the politics of underdevelopment.* London: Macmillan.

Saunders, P. 1990: *Social class and stratification.* London: Routledge and Kegan Paul.

Sayer, L. 1992: Prejudice pre-empted. *Nursing Times* **88(37)**, 46–48.

Seedhouse, D. 1986a: *Health – the foundations for achievement*. Chichester: John Wiley.

Seedhouse, D. 1986b: A universal concern. *Nursing Times* **82(4)**, 36–38.

Sharp, R. and Green, A. 1975: *Education and social control: a study in progressive primary education*. London: Routledge and Kegan Paul.

Slattery, M. 1986: *Official statistics*. London: Tavistock.

Stacey, M. 1976: Sociology of the National Health Service. *Sociological Review Monograph No. 22*. Keele: University of Keele.

Stein, L. 1967: The doctor–nurse game. *Archives of General Psychiatry* **16**, 699–703.

Stockwell, F. 1972: *The unpopular patient*. London: The Royal College of Nursing.

Strong, P.M. 1979: Sociological imperialism and the profession of medicine: a critical examination of the thesis of medical imperialism. *Social Science and Medicine* **13A(2)**, 199–215.

Tawney, R. 1931: *Equality*. London: Allen & Unwin.

Titmus, R.M. 1968: *Commitment to welfare*. London: Allen and Unwin.

Townsend, P. and Davidson, N. 1982: *Inequalities in health: the Black Report*. Harmondsworth: Penguin.

Townsend, P., Davidson, N. and Whitehead, M. 1990: *The Black Report 1980 and the health divide*. Harmondsworth: Penguin.

Tuckett, D. (ed.) 1976: *An introduction to medical sociology*. London: Tavistock.

Tudor Hart, J. (1975): The inverse care law. In Cox, C. and Mead, A. (eds), *A sociology of medical practice*. London: Collier-Macmillan, 189–206.

Turner, B. 1986: *Inequality*. London: Tavistock.

Whitehead, M. 1987: *The health divide: inequalities in health in the 1980's*. London: Health Education Authority.

Wilkinson, R. 1986: *Class and health*. London: Tavistock.

World Health Organisation (WHO) 1946: *Constitution of the World Health Organisation*. Geneva: World Health Organisation.

World Health Organisation (WHO) 1985: *Targets for Health for All 2000*. Copenhagen: World Health Organisation.

Wright, S. 1988: Prejudice? Not me! *Nursing Standard* **2(49)**, 42.

Zola, I.K. 1977: Healthism and disabling medicalization. In Illich, I., Zola, I., McKnight, J., Caplan, J. and Shaiken, H. (eds), *Disabling professions*. London: Marion Boyars, 41–67.

What is the sociology of knowledge? The example of health education and promotion

Nicki Thorogood

Introduction

Sociology is a *critical* discipline, in the sense that it suggests that nothing is simply 'just there', but is always the consequence of social processes which can be unravelled from this perspective. Sociology, then, is interested in the social processes which constitute the 'commonsense' and the 'taken for granted'.

This chapter takes a brief but critical look at the idea of knowledge. Far from being taken for granted, the concept of knowledge is highly problematic.

Where does knowledge come from? How do we distinguish what is true from what is not? For health care workers in professions which claim knowledge of what is good for us, and who make recommendations about quite intimate aspects of daily life and routine as a consequence, this is surely a crucial area. A critical analysis of *knowledge* is then a central concern for sociology, but it is also of vital importance for those training and working in professions whose bodies of knowledge might otherwise remain unquestioned, as taken for granted truths. Nursing, for example, is increasingly becoming concerned with the prevention of illness and disease and the promotion of good practice and healthy lifestyles. General practice nurses, in particular, are developing health education and promotion as key aspects of the primary care services that they provide (Ross *et al.* 1994). It seems, therefore, that it is important to address the area of health promotion from a critical (sociological) perspective; this necessarily implies asking questions about the knowledge which creates this.

First, I will outline the main parameters of the debate regarding knowledge. Then I will explicate in more detail one particular approach to knowledge which, I suggest, offers a useful insight into the practices of health education and promotion. Finally, I shall examine health education and promotion in more detail, taking the issues raised by HIV/AIDS as an example.

The concept of knowledge

What is knowledge? This is a thorny question which has vexed many an academic discipline, indeed it is the centre of many philosophical debates. The aspect of philosophy concerned with the theory of knowledge is called *epistemology*. This explores what can be known, centrally posing the question of language. Is it possible to know something without first having the language? Is there any reality outside of language? Empiricist philosophers (e.g. Popper 1968) suggest that the evidence of the senses is real and that knowledge (in the form of scientific progress) can only be gained through empirical investigation and experiment. By contrast, philosophers like Nietzsche (1969) argue that we can only 'see' what we are trained to see, that is, what we have language for. An example of this might be X-rays, which appear as incomprehensible 'photographs' to the untrained eye, but which reveal vital information and knowledge to those who have been trained.

The concept of knowledge from a sociological perspective is concerned with the use and distribution of knowledge within a society – for example, how people in privileged positions will have access to knowledge which further maintains their privileged positions or how the education system is structured by class, race and gender. Another aspect of the sociological perspective is concerned with the creation or *construction* of that which is called knowledge and the different statuses attached to it; for example, 'first aid' vs. 'old wives' tales' for treating minor ailments, or a newspaper report and an academic research report of a new scientific finding. For sociology, then, *knowledges* are belief systems, and we must look to the social context in which they are produced in order to understand them. Since understanding a belief system requires that we apply our socially constructed thinking, we quickly get caught in a relativist trap. How do we know what we know? And why is it any more valid than what anyone else knows? This should not, however, daunt us. These are still questions worth asking, and whilst we may have to renounce the idea of any one externally given standard of true knowledge, we can instead ask questions about the formation of belief systems. These questions would entail an examination of the social institutions which produce and are produced by these systems, e.g. religion, medicine, politics, education, science, and mass media.

These aspects of social life all adhere to belief or knowledge systems which purport to explain the world, to answer questions about what is right and true. 'Experts' in these areas are those with claims to special abilities or talents for discovering these answers. This clearly implies a certain amount of prestige and status, which in turn suggests the exercise of power. For example, experts can seek out ideas or knowledge which support or maintain their position. They may also undermine competing or unorthodox ideas (Bilton *et al.* 1987, p. 401). Crucially, experts determine what *is* knowledge and what is not. Knowledge, then, is highly stratified and is a key element in *power relations*.

This fundamental relationship between knowledge and power is a central concept in the work of the French philosopher Foucault, best known for his radical reconceptualisations of *power* and *knowledge*. Traditionally, power has been thought of as an entity, as something to be possessed, wielded and used as a means of domination (Bilton *et al.* 1987). Foucault's notion is of a medium which may be both productive and repressive, a lighter, more flexible concept. For Foucault, what we call knowledge and power are inextricably linked; the one implies the other. It is worth considering this in a little more detail. Foucault's analysis of power is subtly different from other conceptions found in social science. For him, power is not an entity to be held or fought for, but a *relation*, a medium, a vehicle. Power

> (. . .) is not conceived as a property or possession of a dominant class, state, or sovereign but as a strategy; the effects of domination associated with power arise not from an appropriation and deployment by a subject but from 'manoeuvres, tactics, techniques, functionings'.
>
> (Smart 1985, p. 77)

Thus power can only be exercised, not possessed. The exercise of power produces certain forms of knowledge:

> Mechanisms of power have been accompanied by the products of effective instruments for the formation and accumulation of knowledge – methods of observation, techniques of registration, procedures for investigation and research, apparatuses of control. Thus the exercise

of power necessarily puts into circulation apparatuses of knowledge, that is, creates sites where knowledge is formed.

(Smart 1985, p. 80)

The reason for concentrating in some detail on Foucault's analysis is that it provides a sophisticated analytical tool for looking at the arenas of health and medicine, particularly health education and promotion. Taking a Foucauldian perspective, this chapter will focus on the construction of knowledge in the discourses of health and medicine, using public health as a specific example. In order to understand this, we need to address the production of these discourses within a paradigm of science and rationality.

The scientific paradigm

To begin with, the concepts of *paradigm* and *discourse* must be clarified. It is commonly held that we are living in a scientific age. This implies that the dominant explanatory mode is that of science and rationality. Other viewpoints, or explanations of the way things are, are not held in such esteem (e.g. religion, fate, the paranormal). The pre-eminence given to rationality and science has been the focus of many major philosophical debates in the works of Weber, Nietzsche, Foucault, Marx and Kuhn.

According to Kuhn (1970), 'Paradigms embody a particular conceptual framework through which the world is viewed', and the dominant contemporary conceptual framework is science, whereas in the past the dominant paradigm might have been religion and in the future it may be something else. This position privileges science and its methods, and defines the boundaries within which research can take place. For example, in Mulkay's (1979) consideration of the status of parapsychology he points out that:

For the critics of parapsychology, the central assumption that paranormal phenomena do not exist was never in question. Rather it persuaded and gave meaning to the whole armoury of formal arguments which they employed. It ensured that, for these critics, every item of evidence and every claim of reasoning provides further grounds for rejection of the deviant views.

(Mulkay 1979, p. 91, quoted in Bilton *et al.* 1987, p. 413)

Thus knowledge and therefore power are currently exercised within a scientific paradigm:

Scientific expertise brings with it the power to define reality. One way is to distinguish lay from scientific (expert) knowledge. Scientists are credited with access to knowledge denied ordinary mortals.

(Kitzinger 1987, p. 10)

Scientific knowledge is no more neutral, objective or value-free than the knowledge of any other belief system. It is not a thing which pre-exists society; it is a product of the people who do it and the practices they employ.

Science does, however, lay claim to objectivity and the notion of progress, both of which may be understood as techniques for maintaining its dominant position among stories to explain the world. This *world view* may be called a paradigm, and the techniques and practices by which it is produced a discourse.

There are a number of scientific fields of enquiry, but central to the scientific project is medicine – and medicine (but not necessarily health) exists entirely within the scientific paradigm. Medicine can be said to be a scientific discourse. The term discourse refers to more than just words. The terms 'discourse' and 'discursive practices' encompass a whole assemblage of activities, events, instruments and settings. If the scientific world view is a paradigm, the techniques and practices by which it is produced are a discourse.

Nursing is currently located within this paradigm, although it also draws upon the techniques and practices of emotional or care work (James 1989; Smith 1992). Whilst it would be interesting to consider the construction of nursing knowledge more widely, it is perhaps timely to direct our attention to *health education and promotion* as a project. Contemporary nursing is distancing itself from the 'handmaiden to the doctor' stereotype, and claiming for nurses a distinct contribution to health care. This stems from the unique relationship between nurse and patient, and the forms of health care practice that this allows. Perhaps the most recently recognised aspect of the nursing process is a responsibility for health education and promotion, particularly in the light of the recent 'Health of the Nation' targets. Health education and promotion now form an integral part of all NHS contracts, and are widely accepted as being beneficial. This is increasingly relevant to nursing, particularly in its role in general practice (Stilwell 1991; Peter 1993; Ross *et al.* 1994). This chapter advises caution and a more considered approach to the wholesale adoption of health promotion goals.

For our purposes, I am focusing on one aspect of the scientific paradigm, the discourse of public health and the discursive practices of health education and promotion, particularly in relation to HIV/AIDS. One reason for this focus is that, despite the dominance of public health medicine, attempts to reduce the spread of HIV infection have had limited success. This leads us to question *why* these policies have not been more successful, and to assess this discourse critically. One explanation might be that, although public health has become increasingly sophisticated and has adopted a new and 'progressive' rhetoric, it nevertheless remains within the medico-scientific paradigm. A critical perspective, such as that developed by Foucault, suggests that this reliance on rational discourse has created a one-dimensional health education which cannot accept or engage with alternative discourses.

The development of public health medicine

In practice, what does this one-dimensional health education mean? To begin with, we should consider briefly the historical development of public health.

According to Foucault (1979a), the emergence of the concept of *the population* coincided with the development of the concept of public health. These notions indicate a shift away from a 19th century understanding of power which was exercised by the sovereign (king) through the (male) head of the family, towards a more subtle form of the play of power. This is exercised through the population and those segments of it – individuals, families and communities – which constitute it but no longer represent it. This knowledge pertaining to the population, its patterns and statistics, is central both to the project of public health and to the new techniques of power identified by Foucault (1979b) as discipline and surveillance. A Foucauldian analysis suggests that a discourse such as public health is just such a disciplinary technique and could, therefore, only emerge within a disciplinary society (Nettleton 1992; Armstrong 1993). This perspective places public health at the centre of the construction of social life. We can then explore how certain aspects of society are maintained and reproduced through health education and promotion practices.

The discourse of public health has a range of discursive practices. It has become the *epidemiological* branch of medicine, concerned with classifying disease, establishing aetiology and recommending medical intervention to prevent the occurrence of disease. Public health has also incorporated notions of the ecological and social contexts of health. However, the pre-eminence of the epidemiological model has, on the whole, reduced the broader perspective to a more sophisticated socially aware epidemiology. Government, therefore, through public health investigates the lives and health of the population. For Foucault, it goes further, and the health of the population as a whole becomes a legitimate object of government, to be achieved

> Either directly through large scale campaigns or indirectly through techniques that will make possible, *without the full awareness of the people*, the stimulation of birth-rates, the directing of the flow of population into certain regions or activities, etc.
>
> (Foucault 1979a; my italics)

Sex and public health

Historically, sexual practices have not been an area of major interest for public health. There are, of course, exceptions to this, particularly the 19th century Contagious Diseases Acts which attempted to control sexually transmitted disease (Mort 1987), and, in this century, HIV/AIDS. These exceptions serve to confirm that, for public health, 'sex' takes limited forms. For public health, focusing on sex is potentially problematic because of the tension between its socially constructed private nature (Foucault 1979c; Weeks 1989) and the medical need to control sexually transmitted disease – the more so in the face of an HIV/AIDS epidemic. Until recently the consequences of 'wrong' sexual behaviours have rarely been fatal; it has been lower priority to a public health focused almost exclusively on preventable mortality. Prior to the recognition of HIV, sex was dealt with in terms of outcomes of sexual behaviour, through an approach in which different behaviours were identified and labelled as pathological, e.g. homosexuality and promiscuity. Specific consequences such as cervical cancer, herpes or unwanted pregnancy were addressed in isolation. Sex as the unifying factor has never been the focus.

HIV/AIDS alters priorities

HIV/AIDS has radically altered priorities for public health, which is obliged to address sexual behaviour more closely. It began in the usual medical way by describing the disease and classifying groups in the population deemed to be at risk, and to which preventive interventions should be addressed. Strictly medical approaches (screening, immunisation) were, however, inappropriate. Increasingly, health education, the social arm of public health, became seen as a principal weapon against the advancing disease. In this model, sex is therefore an instrumental act, a particular behaviour amenable to change, like smoking or drinking.

As noted elsewhere (Thorogood and Jessopp 1990), government policy towards sex education is limited; sex education has not been a major focus for health education. The advent of AIDS in the early 1980s as a public health issue has, however, raised contradictions for public policy. This arena is currently dominated by rhetoric upholding 'traditional family life and values'; this can be given additional support by associating AIDS with marginalised 'deviant' groups. On the other hand, concern about the epidemiology of HIV/AIDS has demanded education around sexual behaviour as a primary prevention strategy. This tension is reflected in early information and prevention strategies. For example, Central Office of Information leaflets about AIDS were sent indiscriminately to every household in the country. These gave little practical information and did not go beyond generalised hints. The tone was apocalyptic, suggesting that everyone had a responsibility to be aware of the 'facts' of transmission so as not to 'die of ignorance'. By any standards, it was a crude attempt at control without opening the private domain of sexual behaviour to public scrutiny.

Sex, I suggest, is a special case in that it is constructed in a matrix of different discourses, all of which must be recognised for public health education/promotion messages to be relevant. The issue of sex crystallises all the dilemmas of public health, since sex carries the symbolic representation of all that should remain hidden from the public gaze. It represents the core of intimate relations, those that should be most jealously guarded from the intrusions of state regulation. These intimate relations are the key to achieving public health's goals – control and surveillance of infectious disease.

Sex, then, highlights the central problematic of public health, which is the relationship between individual liberty and the public good, because to make sex education effective, for it to achieve public health's targets of reducing unwanted pregnancies, HIV, etc., the empowering techniques of the *new public health* would have to be employed. This creates a tension for public health between the use of more effective techniques for promoting the healthy choice, and the possibility that such techniques may facilitate the making of the 'wrong' choice.

In terms of the sociology of knowledge, we might be asking what informs the concept of 'healthy', or indeed 'choice'. Furthermore, we might take a critical view of the construction of HIV/AIDS as a sexual disease, and therefore a public health problem. Within a different paradigm it might be understood as a moral problem. Indeed, to a lesser extent this alternative conception prevails; HIV/AIDS nevertheless retains the identity of a disease, albeit a disease with moral connotations.

The next section examines in more detail the development of the new public health, and some issues it raises for health care practitioners.

The 'new public health' and health education

During the 1980s, public health has been developing a new model now known as 'the new public health' (Ashton and Seymour 1988), which attempts to integrate medical/social aspects and the 'progressive' critique of traditional health education methods. Such methods originated within the discipline of health education, and from community development. The new public health rhetoric draws on the World Health Organisation's broad definition of health, and the 'Health for All' programme of intersectoral responsibility and public participation.

This new public health sees as its legitimate object areas of public life that were previously marginalised or excluded. It addresses, among other things, economic, political and environmental targets, not limiting itself to social/ medical ones.

Part of this broadly based, holistic approach involves eschewing didactic models of health education, to promote instead models drawn from education theory and community development. These promote participative techniques in which people are invited to work at their own pace, and to prioritise and contextualise the information given (see Chapter 6). The most progressive techniques also emphasise the importance and relevance of the knowledge already held by the community we are addressing.

For clarity, we shall refer to the techniques of this general approach as *empowerment*; we shall examine further how this concept has been taken up in health education. Health education/promotion might be described as having three basic models of practice (Tones 1986, p. 7) which should not be mutually exclusive, but may elicit varying degrees of conflict between their proponents. The first is the traditional information-giving preventive model which seeks 'to persuade the individual to adopt a particular lifestyle' (p. 7). The second model is the education-based approach which prioritises rationality and free choice (Tones 1986). The third model, the radical one, acknowledges the socio-political constraints on free choice and concentrates on 'critical consciousness-raising' (p. 8) as a means of empowering communities to take collective social and political action. The persuasion approach loosely adheres to the medical model. This suggests that professionals have privileged knowledge and must persuade lay people (through shock tactics, bullying or encouragement) to adopt the recommended ways. The main criticism of this approach is that it may lead to victim blaming; if people do not act on the experts' advice, they have only themselves to blame. The education model, however, suggests that people should be educated to understand that professional knowledge will enable them to make the healthy choice. This chain of reasoning is referred to as 'K-A-B' (knowledge-attitude-behaviour change), which is well documented as a rather less-than-accurate representation of what actually happens. The major criticism of this approach is that knowledge alone does not lead to behaviour change, as there are other barriers to be taken into account, such as the relevance, practicality or accessibility of the recommended changes. This model makes assumptions about the nature of choice. It probably remains the most widespread approach to health education. The third, radical/political approach might be seen as a response to the problems encountered with the other models. It is broadly termed health promotion, and encompasses a wider view of health issues, for example, lobbying for taxes on alcohol and smoking, or campaigning for local housing improvements. In practice, health promotion/education is likely to consist of a pragmatic mix of (often unarticulated) approaches.

Several theoretical tangles remain which should be addressed here. For instance, there is a potential conflict between the individual free choice of the education model and the radical/political proscriptive model. What if your free choice would not have been the same as the goals of the health promotion campaign, for instance wearing seat belts or reducing cholesterol in your diet? It has been suggested (Tones 1986) that the solution to these possible contradictions is through self-empowerment:

> Self empowerment strategies, then, seek to facilitate decision-making by modifying the individual's self-concept and enhancing his or her self-esteem. Attempts are made to achieve this by equipping people with a variety of 'life skills' which not only modify self images but also prove useful in their own right for the attainment of *specific* goals.
>
> (Tones 1986, p. 9; my italics)

These techniques meet not only political and ideological requirements, but also educational goals. They are demonstrated to be effective ways of learning on the grounds that more information is retained, and that the information retained is more likely to be acted upon. It would seem appropriate for those in the field of public health and health education/promotion to adopt these techniques on a large scale. Why then are the techniques not in more widespread use?

This question is expecially relevant to HIV/AIDS initiatives, as these educational methods are particularly suited to a subject which necessitates discussion of intimate behaviours – areas of life generally deemed to be private and personal. Although many locally based initiatives have taken this approach, they are not endorsed on a national basis (Ashton and Seymour 1988). Empowering techniques encourage the examination of attitudes and values whilst leaving the disclosure of personal information under the participant's control, in theory at least. Why are these methods not central to national public health strategies?

Rhodes and Shaughnessy (1988) have pointed out the Health Education Authority's failure to produce effective safer sex education; they contrast this with the Terrence Higgins Trust's more client-centred approach. Others note the failure of the HEA's AIDS campaign to take gender relations into account, thus rendering much of their safer sex advice irrelevant to young women (Holland *et al.* 1990a, 1990b; Wilton *et al.* 1990). The World Health Organisation in 1946 recognised the importance of situating health information and advice in the context of people's lives. Why then does national public health education fail to encompass these dynamic, pluralistic processes, which would be more effective techniques for achieving behaviour changes, particularly in matters involving sex? There are three key ideas which may explain this: first, the notion of choice; second, the obscuring of values by science; and third, the assumption of rational behaviour.

Choice

One reason I suggest may be the issue of free choice. The political contradictions inherent in sex education referred to earlier may partially explain the failure to adopt empowerment techniques on a wide scale. More pertinent may be the potential of empowerment techniques for *really* allowing the subjects' choice.

There are two points which need to be followed up here: first, the notion of empowerment itself; and secondly, the potential of empowerment techniques. We have already discussed how health education has incorporated empowerment in the radical approach. This concept requires further unravelling. Semantically, empowerment implies the transfer of power from one party to another, from health educator/promoter to 'communities' – from 'us' to 'them'. It would no doubt be argued by educators/promoters that they do not intend this to be the case. However, the meaning is embedded in the language. Leaving semantics aside, there remain unresolved problems with empowerment as a model. The central question, surely, is empowerment for what? Health promotion 'works through effective community action. At the heart of this process are communities having their own power and having control of their own initiatives and activities'. Furthermore, it is intended to support 'personal and social development through providing information, education for health and helping people develop the skills which they need to make healthy choices' (Ashton and Seymour 1988, p.

26). These are laudable intentions, indeed ones which we pursue in the course of our daily work, but we should examine the rhetoric more closely. This same phrase 'making healthy choices' recurs again and again. What are these healthy choices and who defines them?

Whilst socio-economic constraints on choice may be recognised, the value loading of choices is largely unacknowledged. Unresolved, and mostly unaddressed, is the problem of the freedom to make the 'wrong' choice. The inherent difficulties and contradictions of advocating this approach are apparent in Tones' (1986) paper. Self-empowerment must also embody the spirit of voluntarism:

> For those seeking to promote self empowerment, the capacity to freely choose is success enough even if an individual should choose not to reduce his risk of coronary heart disease or steadfastly refuses to participate in political activism to close down a factory having a poor safety record.
>
> (Tones 1986, p. 11)

Here is the core problem. Are we really to believe that health education/promotion, and its disciplinary framework, public health medicine, will be content to measure its success as the capacity to choose freely? As we have said, educational models of health do acknowledge social constraints on choice, but these constraints are related to social class. Tones argues, for example, that 'free choice' may be curtailed by socialisation (e.g. the 'culture of poverty') or by social inequality (see Chapter 9).

Interestingly, no link is made between socialisation and social inequality. It seems to be suggested that cultural/behavioural patterns are separate from the social context in which they are related. It is also implied that those socialised in the culture of poverty are inferior to those

> Whose socialisation has provided them with self empowering skills and experiences [and who] have a much greater degree of genuine choice.
>
> (Tones 1986, p. 8)

Self-empowerment then is really about making 'middle-class' skills and experiences available to the culture- and health-impoverished working class. There is, after all, such a concept as genuine choice. Implicit within this is the assumption that empowered people will, for the most part, make previously defined healthy choices. Thus critics of the education model maintain that, 'Any attempt, therefore, to educate people to make informed health choices in such [constrained] circumstances is not only ineffective but unethical . . .' (Tones 1986, p. 8). We are offering people something they have no hope of achieving.

This more sophisticated health education, which takes social circumstances into account, further obscures the value-laden agenda.

Empowerment facilitates decision-making and opens up the issue of choice – how it is constructed and constrained. In the process of allowing health education/promotion messages to be deconstructed and made relevant to their target audience, underlying moralities and values are also made visible. Sex education is a clear example. In general, this is a euphemism for education to prevent unwanted pregnancies and sexually transmitted diseases. The moral agenda is that these are undesirable occurrences. With an 'empowering' perspective it has to be acknowledged that this is only one view, and that it has no greater validity than any other. Public health educators must then be committed to supporting other choices, or forced to acknowledge that they prioritise their own moral perspective as the healthy choice.

The presence of this tension in public health education and promotion is, I suggest, a major reason for the lack of any widespread use of empowerment techniques. Although these are effective learning techniques, they might also have the potential to render visible the moral aspects of public health or to facilitate the making of unhealthy choices.

Rational choice

There is a further difficulty. Progressive rhetoric holds that there is no 'wrong' choice (see above). Yet underlying this is the assumption that, once in possession of the information, the decision-making skills and with socio-cultural barriers removed, any rational person would make 'the healthy choice'. This suggests that a critical appraisal of the discourse of rationality might be in order. It is the location of public health education and promotion within the discourse which is considered next.

One effect of the reliance on rationality is the implicit consensus that health education has access to knowledge or information which it must seek to promote amongst the public, either as individuals or as 'communities', for the benefit of the recipients.

Health education/promotion is then charged with using the most effective methods to achieve this transmission. Indeed, the semantic shift from education to promotion is seen as evidence of a progression to more effective techniques (Rodmell and Watt 1986; Tones 1986). While the pursuit of public health goals has taken a number of forms, it remains locked within a rational discourse which assumes that, in an ideal world, increased knowledge leads to changes in attitude and hence to behaviour change.

My contention here is that public health is bound to be ineffective in its objectives because it is locked within a form of knowledge, the scientific paradigm, which privileges rationality. The object of public health, the population (and within that individuals, families and communities) is deemed to act rationally. It is of course recognised that there are many obstructions to the smooth flow of rational choice and decision-making, but in an ideal world rationality would be the natural state. It is from within this paradigm that the concept of a healthy choice arises. The healthy choice is the rational choice, the medico-scientific choice, the choice that avoids disease and discomfort as defined within medical science. This focus has failed to acknowledge the shifting nature of rationality and has obscured other discourses.

We are all aware that rationality is contextual and relative. Teenage pregnancy, for example, is problematised in most industrialised societies and normalised in many contexts. There is not a *single* rationality, even within the discourse of health. Graham (1993) makes this case forcefully in her work on smoking amongst mothers of young children.

Whilst public health education/promotion is premised on rationality, it takes no account of other discourses which construct social interaction. Central to these would be, for example, risk, pleasure and danger. Currently, public health presents the healthy choice, based on rational discourse. This is constructed as natural, neutral and objective. Discourses such as pleasure and danger are constructed not as valid alternatives, or indeed as coexisting facets of experience, but as moralities, or rather immoralities. The 'healthy choice' of public health thereby conceals its own morality by harnessing 'healthy' to rational, and this becomes synonymous with the sensible and correct choice.

As noted earlier, this is clear in relation to sex which is addressed only in the domain of disease. Whilst other possible formulations of experience are unacknowledged, the message remains ineffective; again the work of Wilton *et al.* (1990) and Holland *et al.* (1990a, 1990b) in relation to HIV demonstrates how discourses of gender and sexual penetration should be taken into account. It is only by theorising these areas that we begin to see any possibility for relevant health education.

Conclusion: the choices for public health

How then should public health education/promotion respond to the possibility of making the 'wrong' choices? How should it weigh up individual freedom of choice against the public good?

One solution might be in the use of empowerment techniques. As we have suggested here, 'empowerment' too has elements of control implicit in it. We have shown that, whilst espousing the rhetoric of choice, empowerment techniques in health education/promotion extend the gaze of public health into previously private spheres of life.

The advent of HIV/AIDS as a public health issue has demanded a response both at the population level and towards specific targeted segments. Previously, medical discourse through public health has employed large-scale campaigns in its monitoring and regulation of sexual behaviour. Any less explicit regulation through techniques such as sex education has been minimal and deemed to be outside the domain of health.

Empowerment as a technique is particularly relevant in the government of sexual relations, as sex 'belongs' in the privacy of the family. As discussed earlier, knowledge of the population is located within its constituent elements (families), whilst those individuals or groups whose lives are not lived in 'normal' families are subject to more explicit regulation, and are accustomed to more visible techniques of information-gathering in their sexual lives. However techniques of 'non-control' (Bunton 1990), such as empowerment, may be particularly relevant for monitoring 'normal' sex, and form part of the new public health's techniques for extending its role in the regulation and surveillance of sexual behaviour.

This chapter has considered the idea that 'knowledge' is socially constructed, and has suggested that a Foucauldian analysis is particularly useful for understanding the discourse of health. It has argued that those regulatory techniques are problematic for public health because they raise the issue of individual free choice and thereby expose the hidden agenda of public health. This, it is suggested, is dictated by its reliance on the discourse of rationality, which privileges the healthy choice. This ultimately obscures other discourses (or forms of knowledge) and, as a consequence, may render public health messages ineffective. Nevertheless, empowerment techniques do constitute a way in which public health can extend into previously unavailable sites, such as 'normal' sexual relations.

The increasing designation of nurses as 'health educators' suggests that it is timely to raise these issues and to question their implications. Is empowerment simply a more sophisticated form of regulation, or can it facilitate social action? Can public health ever adopt such techniques on a wide scale without compromising its own goals? It should be noted here that there is more than one actor in any relationship. Those who adopt empowerment techniques to promote their work, whatever their perspective, will find their subjects simultaneously invoking or creating strategies of resistance (see Bloor and McIntosh 1989 on client resistance in health visiting: also, generally, Foucault 1979c, p. 95). Whatever conclusions are reached regarding the impact of these techniques of 'non-control', it would appear that they should not be adopted uncritically.

This chapter began by asking 'what is knowledge?' and considered the debate using 'public health knowledge' and the regulation of sex as a particular example. Whilst this is interesting in itself, it is clear that these are not just philosophical abstractions. They are also of importance in carrying out the day-to-day business of providing health care.

References

Armstrong, D. 1993: Public health spaces and the fabrication of identity. *Sociology* **27(3)**, 393–410.

Ashton, J. and Seymour, H. 1988: *The new public health*. Milton Keynes: Open University.

Bilton, T., Bonnett, K., Jones, P., Sheard, K., Stanworth, M. and Webster, A. 1987: *Introductory sociology*, 2nd edition. Basingstoke: Macmillan.

Bloor, M. and McIntosh, J. 1989: Surveillance and concealment: a comparison of techniques of client resistance in therapeutic communities and health visiting. In

Cunningham Burley, S. and McKeganey, N. P. (eds), *Readings in medical sociology*. London: Tavistock.

Bunton, R. 1990: Changes in the control of alcohol misuse. *British Journal of Addiction* **85**, 605–615.

Foucault, M. 1979a: On governmentality. *Ideology and Consciousness* **6**, 5–21.

Foucault, M. 1979b: *Discipline and punish: the birth of the prison*. Harmondsworth: Penguin.

Foucault, M. 1979c: *The history of sexuality. 1: an introduction*. London: Allen Lane.

Graham, H. 1993: Smoking among working class mothers. *Primary Health Care* **3(2)**, 15–16.

Holland, J., Ramazanoglu, C. and Scott, S. 1990a: Managing risk and experiencing danger: tensions between government AIDS education policy and young women's sexuality. *Gender and Education* **2(2)**, 193–202.

Holland, J., Ramazanoglu, C., Scott, S., Sharpe, S. and Thompson, R. 1990b: *Don't die of ignorance – I nearly died of embarrassment*. Paper presented to the Fourth 'Social Aspects of AIDS' Conference, London.

James, N. 1989: Emotional labour: skill and work in the social regulation of feelings. *The Sociological Review* **37(1)**, 15–42.

Kitzinger, C. 1987: *The social construction of lesbianism.* London: Sage.

Kuhn, T. 1970: *The structure of scientific revolutions*. Chicago: University of Chicago Press.

Mort, F. 1987: *Dangerous sexualities: medico-moral politics in England since 1830*. London: Routledge & Kegan Paul.

Mulkay, M. 1979: *Science and the sociology of knowledge*. London: Allen & Unwin.

Nettleton, S. 1992: *Power, pain and dentistry*. Buckingham: Open University Press.

Nietzsche, F. 1969: *On the genealogy of morals*, Kaufmann, W. (ed.). New York: Vintage Books.

Peter, A. 1993: Practice nursing in Glasgow after the new general practitioner contract. *British Journal of General Practice* **43(368)**, 97–100.

Popper, K. 1968: *The logic of scientific discovery*. London: Hutchinson.

Rhodes, T. and Shaughnessy, R. 1988: Compulsory screening: addressing AIDS in Britain 1986–1989. *Campaign* 23 January.

Rodmell, S. and Watt, A. (eds) 1986: *The politics of health education: raising the issues*. London: Routledge & Kegan Paul.

Ross, F., Bower, P.J. and Sibbald, B.S. 1994: Practice nurses: characteristics, workload and training needs. *British Journal of General Practice* **44(378)**, 15–18.

Smart, B. 1985: *Michel Foucault*. London: Tavistock.

Smith, P. 1992: *The emotional labour of nursing*. London: Macmillan.

Stilwell, B. 1991: The rise of the practice nurse. *Nursing Times* **87(24)**, 26–28.

Thorogood, N. and Jessopp, L. 1990: No sex please, we're British. *Critical Public Health* **2**, 10–15.

Tones, B.K. 1986: Health education and the ideology of health promotion: a review of alternative approaches. *Health Education Research* **1**, 3–12.

Weeks, J. 1989: *Sex, politics and society*. Harlow: Longman.

Wilton, T. and Aggleton, P. 1990: *Condoms, coercion and control: heterosexuality and the limits to HIV/AIDS education*. Paper presented to the Fourth 'Social Aspects of AIDS' Conference, London.

Index